VESTIBULAR MECHANISMS
IN
HEALTH AND DISEASE

VESTIBULAR MECHANISMS
IN
HEALTH AND DISEASE

VI Extraordinary meeting of the Barany Society

Edited by

J. D. HOOD

MRC Hearing and Balance Unit
Institute of Neurology
National Hospital
London, UK

1978

ACADEMIC PRESS

London . New York . San Francisco

A Subsidiary of Harcourt Brace Jovanovich, Publishers

ACADEMIC PRESS INC. (LONDON) LTD.
24-28 Oval Road,
London NW1

United States Edition published by
ACADEMIC PRESS INC.
111 Fifth Avenue
New York, New York 10003

Library of Congress Catalog Card Number 77-94303
ISBN: 0-12-354250-2

Printed in Great Britain by
Whitstable Litho Ltd.
Whitstable, Kent

Contributors

G. ASCHAN, Linköping University, Department of Otolaryngology, University Hospital, Linköping, Sweden.

M. AOYAGI, Department of Otolaryngology, Yamagata University, Yamagata, Japan.

R. BAKER, New York University, Department of Physiology and Biophysics, 11b, 14th Avenue, New York, N.Y. 10016, U.S.A.

R.W. BALOH, Department of Neurology (Reed Neurological Research Center), University of California, Los Angeles 90024, U.S.A.

G.R. BARNES, Royal Air Force, Institute of Aviation Medicine, Farnborough, Hants, U.K.

J.B. BARON, Laboratoire de Statokinesimetrie, Centre Psychiatrique, Saint-Anne, Paris, France.

J.T. BENITEZ, Division of Otoneurology, William Beaumont Hospital, Royal Oak, Michigan, U.S.A.

A.J. BENSON, Royal Air Force, Institute of Aviation Medicine, Farnborough, Hants, U.K.

A. BERTHOZ, Conservatoire National des Arts et Metiers, Department des Sciences de l'Homme au Travail, Physiologie du Travail Ergonomie, 41 Rue Gay-Lussac, 75005 Paris, France.

F.O. BLACK, Departments of Otolaryngology and Pharmacology, University of Pittsburgh, School of Medicine, Pittsburgh, Pennsylvania, U.S.A.

K.R. BOUCHARD, Division of Otoneurology, William Beaumont Hospital, Royal Oak, Michigan, U.S.A.

U. BÜTTNER, Department of Neurology and Brain Research Institute, University of Zürich, Switzerland.

J.A. BÜTTNER-ENNEVER, Department of Neurology and Brain Research Institute, University of Zurich, Switzerland.

Y. CHIKAMORI, Department of Pharmacology, Faculty of Medicine, Kyoto University, Kyoto 606, Japan.

D.L. CLARK, Department of Anatomy, Ohio State University, College of Medicine, Columbus, Ohio, U.S.A.

M.J. CORREIA, University of Texas Medical School, Galveston, Texas, U.S.A.

J. CORVERA, Department of Otolaryngology, Hospital General, Centro Medico Nacional, I.M.S.S. Mexico City, Mexico.

G.H. CRAMPTON, Wright State University, Dayton, Ohio, U.S.A.

I.S. CURTHOYS, Department of Psychology, University of Sydney,

Sydney, N.S.W. 2006, Australia.

J. DELGADO-GARCIA, New York University, Department of Physiology and Biophysics, 11b, 14th Avenue, New York, N.Y. 10016, U.S.A.

T. EGAMI, Department of Otolaryngology, University of Pittsburgh, School of Medicine, Eye and Ear Hospital, Pittsburgh, PA 15213, U.S.A.

L.C. ERWAY, Department of Biology, University of Cincinnati, Cincinnati, Ohio, U.S.A.

J.M. FREDRICKSON, Department of Otolaryngology, University of Toronto, Canada.

T. FUTAKI, Department of Otolaryngology, The Faculty of Medicine, Kyoto University, Kyoto, Japan.

S. GONZALEZ, Multiple Sclerosis Clinic, Wayne State University, Detroit, Michigan, U.S.A.

M. GRESTY, Medical Research Council, Hearing and Balance Unit, Institute of Neurology, National Hospital, Queen Square, London WC1N 3BG, U.K.

F.E. GUEDRY Jr., Naval Aerospace Medical Research Laboratory, Pensacola, Florida, U.S.A.

C.S. HALLPIKE, 44 Ashurst Road, West Moors, Dorset, U.K.

M. HALMAGYI, Medical Research Council, Hearing and Balance Unit, Institute of Neurology, National Hospital, Queen Square, London WC1N 3BG, U.K.

M.A. HAMID, Engineering in Medicine Laboratory, Imperial College, London SW7 2BT, U.K.

V. HENN, Neurological Clinic, University of Zürich, Zürich, Switzerland.

R. HINCHCLIFFE, Institute of Laryngology and Otology, London WC1X 8EE, U.K.

M. HINOKI, Department of Otolaryngology, The Faculty of Medicine, Kyoto University, Kyoto, Japan.

S. HIWATASHI, Fukui Red Cross Hospital, Japan.

S. HOLM-JENSEN, University ENT-clinic, Copenhagen City Hospital, DK1399, Copenhagen, Denmark.

S. HONJO, Department of Otolaryngology, Yamaguchi University, School of Medicine, Ube City, 755 Japan.

V. HONRUBIA, Division of Head and Neck Surgery (Otolaryngology), University of California, Los Angeles 90024, U.S.A.

H. INO, Department of Otolaryngology, Niigata University, School of Medicine, Niigata, Japan.

N.J. JOHNSEN, University ENT Department, Rigshospitalet Copenhagen, Denmark.

T. KAMEI, Department of Otolaryngology, Gunma University Medical School, Maebashi, Japan.

K. KANESADA, Department of Otolaryngology, Yamaguchi University School of Medicine, Ube City, 755 Japan.

I. KATO, Department of Otolaryngology, Yamagata University, Yamagata, Japan.

T. KAWASAKI, Department of Physiology, Toyama Medical and Pharmaceutical University, Japan.

M. KITAHARA, Department of Otolaryngology, Faculty of Medicine, Kyoto University, Japan.

T. KOBAYASHI, Department of Otolaryngology, Yamaguchi University School of Medicine, Ube City, 755 Japan.

Y. KOIKE, Department of Otolaryngology, School of Medicine, Yamagata University, Japan.

T. KUBO, Department of Otolaryngology, Osaka University Medical School, Osaka 553, Japan.

A. KUMAR, Department of Otolaryngology, University of Illinois, Abraham Lincoln School of Medicine, Chicago, Illinois, U.S.A.

B. LARSBY, Linköping University, Department of Otolaryngology, University Hospital, Linköping, Sweden.

C.G.Y. LAU, Division of Head and Neck Surgery (Otolaryngology), University of California, Los Angeles 90024, U.S.A.

S. LECHNER-STEINLEITNER, Max-Planck-Institut für Verhaltens-physiologie, Seewiesen, W. Germany.

S.R.C. LIEDGREN, Linköping University, Department of Oto-laryngology, University Hospital, Linköping, Sweden.

D.J. LIM, Department of Otolaryngology, Ohio State University, College of Medicine, Columbus, Ohio, U.S.A.

M. MACHINO, Department of Respiratory Disease, Osaka Hospital of Japanese National Railways, Abenoku, Minami 1-3-5, Osaka, Japan 545.

C.H. MARKHAM, Reed Neurological Research Center, UCLA School of Medicine, Los Angeles, California 90024, U.S.A.

H. MATSUBARA, Department of Otolaryngology, Faculty of Medicine, Kyoto University, Japan.

T. MATSUNAGA, Department of Otolaryngology, Osaka University, Medical School, Osaka 553, Japan.

I. MATSUOKA, Department of Otolaryngology, Hyogo Kenritsu Amagasaki Hospital, Hyogo 660, Japan.

A. MEYER ZUM GOTTESBERGE, ENT Clinic, University of Düsseldorf, Moorenstr. 5, D-4000, Düsseldorf 1, W. Germany.

D.L. MICHAELS, Biomedical Engineering Center for Clinical Instrumentation and Man Vehicle Laboratory, Massachusetts

Institute of Technology, Cambridge, Massachusetts 02139, U.S.A.

A.C. MILNE, Department of Otolaryngology, University of Toronto, Toronto, Ontario, Canada.

T. MIYOSHI, Fukui Red Cross Hospital, Japan.

K. MIZUKOSHI, Department of Otolaryngology, Niigata University School of Medicine, Niigata, Japan.

C.E. MORTENSEN, Emory University Atlanta, Georgia, U.S.A.

K. NAKANISHI, Department of Otolaryngology, The Faculty of Medicine, Kyoto University, Kyoto, Japan.

J.B. NELSON, Louisiana State University, Baton Rouge, Louisiana, U.S.A.

B. NOVAK, Department of O.R.L., University of Basel, Switzerland.

L.M. ÖDKVIST, Linköping University, Department of Otolaryngology, University Hospital, Linköping, Sweden.

D.P. O'LEARY, Departments of Otolaryngology and Pharmacology, University of Pittsburgh, School of Medicine, Pittsburgh, Pennsylvania, U.S.A.

C.M. OMAN, Biomedical Engineering Centre for Clinical Instrumentation and Man Vehicle Laboratory, Massachusetts Institute of Technology, Cambridge, Massachusetts 02139, U.S.A.

W. OSHIMA, Department of Otorhinolaryngology, Osaka Hospital of Japanese National Railways, Abenoku, Minami 1-3-5, Osaka, Japan 545.

E. PEITERSEN, University ENT-clinic, Copenhagen City Hospital, DK1399, Copenhagen, Denmark.

R.J. PETERKA, Biomedical Engineering Program, Carnegie-Mellon University, Pittsburgh, Pennsylvania, U.S.A.

C.R. PFALTZ, Department of O.R.L., University of Basel, Switzerland.

R. ROMERO, Department of Otolaryngology, Hospital General, Centro Medico Nacional, I.M.S.S. Mexico City, Mexico.

A.M. RUBIN, Department of Otolaryngology, University of Toronto, Toronto, Ontario, Canada.

I. SANDO, Department of Otolaryngology, University of Pittsburgh, School of Medicine, Eye and Ear Hospital, Pittsburgh PA 15213, U.S.A.

M. SASA, Department of Pharmacology, Faculty of Medicine, Kyoto University, Kyoto 606, Japan.

T. SATO, Department of Neuropathology, Brain Research Institute, Niigata University, Niigata, Japan.

Y. SATO, Department of Otolaryngology, Niigata University, Niigata, Japan.

Y. SATO, Department of Physiology, Toyama Medical and Pharmaceutical University, Japan.

B. McA. SAYERS, Engineering in Medicine Laboratory, Imperial College, London SW7 2BT, U.K.

H. SCHÖNE, Max-Planck-Institut für Verhaltensphysiologie, Seewiesen, W. Germany.

D.W.F. SCHWARZ, Department of Otolaryngology, University of Toronto, Canada.

T. SEKITANI, Department of Otolaryngology, Yamaguchi University School of Medicine, Ube City, 755 Japan.

S. SHIDA, Department of Otorhinolaryngology, Osaka Hospital of Japanese National Railways, Abenoku, Minami 1-3-5, Osaka, Japan 545.

K. SHIMAMOTO, Department of Otolaryngology, Yamaguchi University, Medical School, Ube City, Japan.

M. SHIRATO, Fukui Red Cross Hospital, Japan.

J. STAHLE, Department of Otorhinolaryngology, Akademiska sjukhuset, Uppsala, Sweden.

P. STRAUSS, ENT Clinic, University of Düsseldorf, Moorenstr. 5, D-4000, Düsseldorf 1, W. Germany.

J.-I. SUZUKI, Department of Otolaryngology, Teikyo University School of Medicine, Japan.

M. SUZUKI, Department of Otorhinolaryngology, Osaka Hospital of Japanese National Railways, Abenoku, Minami 1-3-5, Osaka, Japan 545.

S. TAKAORI, Department of Pharmacology, Faculty of Medicine, Kyoto University, Kyoto 606, Japan.

S. TAKEMORI, Department of Otolaryngology, Teikyo University School of Medicine, Japan.

M. TANAKA, Department of Otolaryngology, Yamaguchi University Medical School, Ube City, Japan.

M.J. TANGAPREGASSOM, Serv. Neuro-ophthal., CPSA 1, Rue Cabanis, Paris XIV, France.

R. THAM, Linköping University, Department of Otolaryngology, University Hospital, Linköping, Sweden.

J. THOMSEN, University ENT Department, Rigshospitalet Copenhagen, Denmark.

J.R. TOLE, Biomedical Engineering Centre for Clinical Instrumentation and Man Vehicle Laboratory, Massachusetts Institute of Technology, Cambridge, Massachusetts 02139, U.S.A.

D.L. TOMKO, Departments of Otolaryngology and Pharmacology, University of Pittsburgh, School of Medicine, Pittsburgh, Pennsylvania, U.S.A.

R.D. TOMLINSON, Department of Otolaryngology, University of

Toronto, Toronto, Ontario, Canada.

N. TOROK, Department of Otolaryngology, University of Illinois, Abraham Lincoln School of Medicine, Chicago, Illinois, U.S.A.

N. USHIO, Laboratoire de Statokinesimetrie, Centre Psychiatrique, Saint-Anne, Paris, France.

W. WAESPE, Neurological Clinic, University of Zürich, Zürich, Switzerland.

C. WALL III, Department of Otolaryngology, University of Pittsburgh, School of Medicine, Pittsburgh, Pennsylvania, U.S.A.

Y. WATANABE, Department of Otolaryngology, Niigata University School of Medicine, Niigata, Japan.

A.D. WEISS, Biomedical Engineering Centre for Clinical Instrumentation and Man Vehicle Laboratory, Massachusetts Institute of Technology, Cambridge, Massachusetts 02139, U.S.A.

T. YAGI, Reed Neurological Research Center, UCLA School of Medicine, Los Angeles, California 90024, U.S.A.

L.R. YOUNG, Biomedical Engineering Center for Clinical Instrumentation and Man Vehicle Laboratory, Massachusetts Institute of Technology, Cambridge, Massachusetts 02139, U.S.A.

K. ZILSTORFF, University ENT Department, Rigshospitalet Copenhagen, Denmark.

Preface

Robert Barany, a Nobel lauriate, pioneered clinical studies of vestibular function and is generally credited with being the founder of the specialty that has come to be known as neuro-otology.

The Barany Society was founded in 1960 to commemorate his name and to pursue his high ideals by bringing together scientists of international standing engaged in vestibular research. This field of study has expanded much since Barany's day and is still expanding due, in some measure, to the pressing problems of space travel but more particularly perhaps to the new knowledge we now possess of the extraordinarily complex and widespread connections of the vestibular system throughout the central nervous system. In consequence modern vestibular research is being increasingly directed not only at the vestibular end organs themselves and their immediate central connections but also with their complex interaction with other sensory systems. This is exemplified by the variety of topics covered by the contributions to this book which represents the Proceedings of the 6th Extraordinary meeting of the Society held at Imperial College, London, September, 11-15th, 1977, under the Presidency of Professor O. Lowenstein, F.R.S.

The main themes of the conference were Problems of Head Stability, Central Control of Vestibulo-oculomotor Function, Positional Nystagmus, and Signal Processing in the Evaluation of Vestibular Mechanisms. These are all well represented in their respective chapters. In addition, a large number of free papers were presented covering almost every aspect of vestibular function of current interest and these have fallen conveniently into a further 6 chapters. As a result, it is to be hoped that the reader will find in this book a fairly comprehensive and up to date review covering the most recent advances in all aspects of vestibular research.

A special tribute is due to the Secretary of the Steering Committee, Professor R. Hinchcliffe whose exceptional organising ability contributed much to the success of the conference.

Grateful acknowledgement is made to the following for generous financial support: Aural-aide Ltd., British Association of Otolaryngologists, Imperial College, Institute of Laryngology and Otology, Linco-Acoustics, Royal National Institute for the Deaf, Royal National Throat, Nose and Ear Hospital, Royal Society, The British Council, The Wellcome Trust.

J. D. HOOD

Contents

Anatomy

Computer Analysis

Positional Nystagmus

President's Address

O. Lowenstein, F.R.S.

Professor Engström, Ladies and Gentlemen!

The year 1977 marks the 250th anniversary of the death of Isaac Newton, whose thoughts on Gravitation emanated from this country all over the world and into every laboratory in which, a century later, vestibular function began to be studied. This year 1977 also marks the 25th anniversary of the beginning of the reign of Queen Elizabeth II. You will, therefore, find this country in a festive mood. Thus, nothing could have been more natural than to receive members of the Barany Society and guests here in London for the 6th extraordinary meeting this year.

Newton's work will be brought nearer to you at our Reception this evening in the Rooms of the Royal Society, where a copy of his Principia will be on view, and the aura of the Queen's Jubilee Year will be all around you when you walk through the streets of London.

It is my great pleasure to welcome you here for a few day's concentrated work and for the social functions which have been arranged to alleviate the labour in the Lecture Theatres at Imperial College with the pleasures of conviviality. May this London Meeting become a worthy link in the chain of memories of all previous ordinary and extraordinary gatherings of our great Society.

Personally for me this Meeting of the Barany Society is of special significance, as it falls very near the 50th anniversary of my becoming enmeshed in the labyrinth, when my teacher Karl von Frisch asked me to participate in his efforts at localizing the acoustic function within the labyrinth of the tiny Minnow *(Phoxinus laevis)*, by delineating it accurately from the purely vestibular functions residing in the pars superior of this organ.

When I set out to prepare myself for this task by a scrutiny of the literature to date, my heart sank on reading the classical papers by Flourens, Ewald, Mach, Breuer, Crum-Brown, as well as the reviews on the subject by Magnus, de Kleijn, Versteegh and Fischer and the mathematical articles by Schmaltz in the then new volumes of Bethe's Handbook. Steinhausen and Dohlman had just elevated the status of the cupula ampullaris by showing its real size and functional behaviour, and the period was also marked by the work of Lorente de No. Last and not least our Patron Barany wielded his pathfinding influence in the clinical field at Uppsala.

Here was I trying to contribute to a field in which all the important aspects were either known or being investigated by great masters. Surely, vestibular physiology was reaching a state of near completion! – I need not have worried, had the gift of precognition to see 50 years ahead allowed me a glimpse of this year's Barany Programme! We are still at it with a vengeance, and the queue of unsolved vestibular problems is as long as ever.

Four important topics viz:

I   Problems of Head Stability,
II   Central Control of Vestibulo-ocolumotor Function,
III   Positional Nystagmus,
IV   Signal Processing in the Evaluation of Vestibular Mechanisms,

have been selected as a framework for this year's scientific programme, and it was hoped that these would attract a wide range of contributions from our members and the guest speakers introduced by them. Our hopes have been amply fulfilled; so much so that our programme committee had to deal with an embarras de richesse in their tasks to allocate sufficient time for these contributions commensurate with the promise indicated by titles and abstracts.

In the programme we have arranged a solid block of four sessions on caloric and positional nystagmus and three consecutive sessions on neurophysiology, interspersed with sessions on computer analysis, anatomy, perception of head movement and on postural control. We hope the logic of this arrangement will be acceptable, and we are sure that we can look forward to reports on a weighty body of research in which will be found a fortunate blend of results of pure research and – most important – of clinical experience.

It would be futile at this moment to map out in detail the exciting "journey through the labyrinth" of vestibular problems which we are going to undertake, a journey that has been planned for us by the enthusiastic efforts of the conference Committee over which I had the good fortune to preside. Let the success of their labours be judged by the value of the experience which we shall gather this week here at Imperial College within the walls of festive London.

Primary Afferents

1. The development of function of horizontal semicircular canal primary afferents in the rat.

I.S. CURTHOYS

Department of Psychology, University of Sydney, Sydney N.S.W. 2006, Australia.

Introduction

The main aim of this study was to measure the changes which occur during development in the response of primary vestibular neurons to horizontal angular acceleration. To achieve this aim, data from the primary neurons in adult rats to long duration angular acceleration was compared to data from newborn and young rats to the same stimulus. The rat was specifically chosen because it is one of the few mammals in which the semicircular canals increase in size after birth. Clark (1973) has shown that both the radius of curvature of the horizontal canal (R) and the cross-sectional tube radius *(r)* both continue to increase for about 20 days after birth. In the light of data on other species it is highly likely that the receptor hair cells and their neural innervation are also immature in the rat at birth (Heywood, Pujol, & Hilding, 1976).

Recently a case has been made for dividing semicircular canal primary afferents into two categories according to their spontaneous activity — regularly firing and irregularly firing neurons. In the squirrel monkey Goldberg and Fernandez (1977, 1971) have shown that regular cells tend to be thinner, slower conducting neurons with a lower average sensitivity than irregular neurons. In this study, reliable differences were observed between regular and irregular primary neurons in the rat, both at adulthood and during development.

Materials and methods

Data was obtained from 83 rats (22 adults and 61 young animals) ranging in weight from 4.9g to 395g. Each had a tracheal cannula inserted under ether anaesthesia and was maintained under ether anaesthesia for the remainder of the experiment. EKG and EMG were monitored continuously to ensure depth of anaesthesia was adequate.

The animals were placed in specially designed head-holders in a Kopff stereotaxic device which was mounted on a custom-made lightweight turntable. Adult animals were held by a modified rat palate clamp. For young animals the head was fixed to a machine screw by cyanoacrylate glue and dental cement. The techniques for preparation and recording from very young rats have been described in detail elsewhere (Curthoys & Webber 1977). For animals of all ages we endeavoured to ensure the horizontal semicircular canal was in the plane of rotation of the turntable.

The lateral part of the left cerebellum was removed enabling the glass micro-electrodes to be aimed at the vestibular nerve under visual control with the assistance of an operating microscope. The electrodes were filled with 2 molar sodium chloride and had impedances of about 3 megohms.

Horizontal canal neurons were initially identified by their response to hand rotations of the turntable; and then where possible subjected to a standardized test procedure: rest, ipsilateral angular acceleration of $16.7^\circ/sec^2$ for 12 seconds; constant velocity ($200^\circ/sec$) until the neuronal response stabilized; ipsilateral angular deceleration of $16.7^\circ/sec^2$ for 12 seconds; rest. Neural firing rate from an RC integrator was recorded on one channel of a strip chart recorder, the other channel showed turntable velocity from a tachometer directly coupled to the turntable shaft.

A cell was classified as regular if the range of firing rate divided by the mean during a three second interval was less than 0.18. This criterion is approximately equivalent to the criterion of a coefficient of variation of interspike intervals of 0.0579 as used by Goldberg & Fernandez (1971). Other measures were: resting rate, peak increase in firing during the angular acceleration, the time taken to reach 63% of this peak value (the incremental time constant), and peak decrease during deceleration. From these peak firing measures incremental sensitivity (Si) was calculated, defined as the peak increase in firing during the angular acceleration, divided by the magnitude of the acceleration. Si has dimensions of extra spikes/ sec/deg/sec^2. When the cell's firing was decreased by the deceleration the same procedure yielded decremental sensitivity (Sd).

Results

Data was obtained from 983 neurons – 246 in adult animals and 737
from rats weighing between 4.9g and 35.4g. Qualitatively neurons in
newborn animals differ from those in the adult in having a lower
resting rate, a lower sensitivity, taking longer to reach peak increase
in firing during the angular acceleration and adapting quickly. They
exhibit unpredictable bursts of spikes and are more variable in
response to repeated presentations of the same stimuli.

No regular neurons could be detected in very young animals,
however the proportion of regular cells increases during growth until
in the adult about 32% of primary afferents are regular (see Fig. 1
inset). In the adult, the resting rate of regular neurons is significantly
higher than irregular neurons (Fig. 1). For both categories the resting
rate in young animals is significantly less than the adult value and it
gradually increases during growth (Fig. 1).

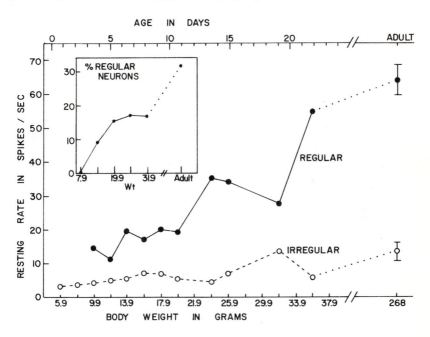

Fig. 1. Average resting rate of regular and irregular neurons during growth. The
vertical bars around the adult values in this and all following graphs are two
tailed 95% confidence intervals for the mean. The points along the bottom
abscissa are the midpoints of 2g weight intervals into which the data was
combined. The upper abscissa shows estimated age from an independent study
(Curthoys & Webber, 1977). *Inset*. Percentage of regular neurons during growth,
with 6g weight intervals.

In the adult irregular neurons are on average more sensitive than regular neurons and this difference appears consistently in the younger animals (see Fig. 2). In irregular neurons in newborn animals Si is significantly smaller than in adults, but it approximates adult values within two or three days (see Fig. 2).

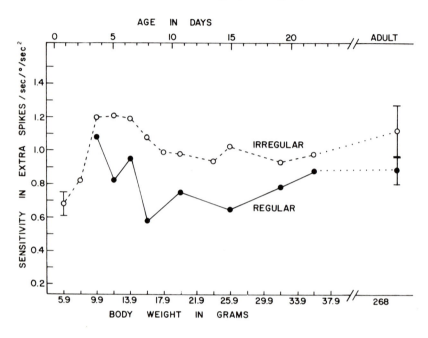

Fig. 2. Changes in incremental sensitivity during growth for regular and irregular neurons. Since the acceleration for all these points was $16.7°/sec^{-2}$, a sensitivity of 1.0 represents a peak increase of 16.7 spikes during acceleration.

In neurons in the adult, where measures of both Si and Sd can be made, the two are not significantly different. In the adult these cells are symmetrical in that they decrease their firing to a deceleration by about the same amount as they increase it to an acceleration of the same magnitude. However in primary afferents in very young animals where both Si and Sd can be measured in the one cell, Sd is significantly less than Si. This asymmetry between Si and Sd is progressively reduced during growth (See Fig. 3).

For animals up to 35g linear regression analysis shows there is a significant decrease of incremental time constant during growth (Regression coefficient = -0.03; $p < 0.05$) (Fig. 4). However the

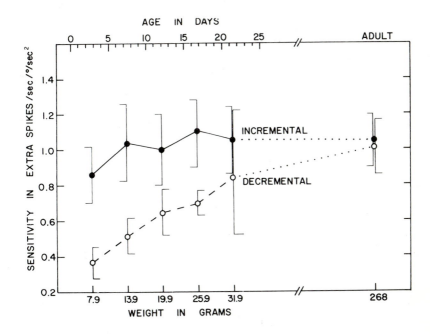

Fig. 3. Average incremental and decremental sensitivity measured in the same cells growth. The vertical bars show two-tailed 95% confidence intervals for each mean.

variability is large and the relationship is not strong: there is no significant difference between the average time constants of newborn rats weighing from 4.9–6.9g and adult rats: Newborn Mean = 3.81 ± 1.97 (standard deviation), n = 53; Adult Mean: 3.31 ± 1.25, n = 111 : t = 1.96, p > 0.05).

Discussion

It is clear that semicircular canal neurons in the rat are functioning well before the receptor system has reached its full adult size, although there are differences between newborn and adult neurons in a number of respects.

The failure to detect regular neurons in newborn rats may have been due to the microelectrode tip being too large to record from regular cells which are probably smaller on average than irregular

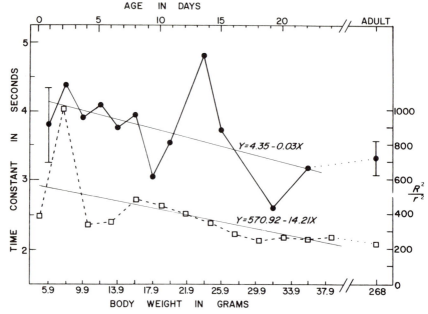

Fig. 4. Time to reach 63% of peak increase in firing at various stages during growth. (closed circles). The lower curve (open squares – use right-hand ordinate) shows how R^2/r^2 decreases during growth (data calculated from Clark (1973).

cells (Goldberg and Fernandez, 1977).

The most unexpected result was that Sd is significantly less than Si in newborn animals. The reason for this asymmetry is not clear.

In adult animals of various species the response of primary neurons has been used to assess the adequacy of the Steinhausen torsion pendulum model of semicircular canal operation. Use of developmental neurophysiological data for the same end, is much less straightforward. Not only are the physical dimensions of the canals known to be increasing, but other factors governing the physiological response such as hair-cell maturation, synaptogenesis and myelination are all changing as well. Other mechanical factors which enter into the torsion pendulum model may also be changing factors such as: endolymph viscosity, cupular stiffness, perhaps even the mode of cupular deformation (ten Kate, 1969).

In view of the potential for interaction between all these factors it is with considerable caution that neural developmental data be used in the context of the torsion pendulum model. Nevertheless it is appropriate to note here the points of agreement and disagreement between our data and the model.

During prolonged angular acceleration the time taken for the cupula to reach 63% of maximum cupular displacement — the mechanical incremental time constant — depends amongst other things on the ratio of R^2/r^2 (Jones & Spells, 1963; Blanks, Estes & Markham, 1975). In the rat this ratio decreases from birth to day 25 (Clark, 1973) and in accordance with that result our results show a decrease in the neural incremental time constant from birth to day 25 (see Fig. 4). Despite this similarity it is possible that this decrease in neural time constant may be due to other factors related to the physiology of the developing cells rather than the mechanics of the canal.

Maximum increase in firing during prolonged angular acceleration is presumably related to the magnitude of cupular displacement (Blanks *et al.*, 1975) which in turn depends upon R, endolymph viscosity and cupular stiffness. In the rat R continues to increase for 22 days following birth whereas there is no such consistent monotonic increase in Si during this time. On the other hand, Sd increases more slowly than Si and in a manner more consistent with the change in R.

Acknowledgements

This research was supported by the National Health and Medical Research Council of Australia.

I thank Susan Webber for her skilled assistance.

References

Blanks, R.H.I. Estes, M.S. and Markham, C.H. (1975). Physiologic characteristics of vestibular first-order canal neurons in the cat. II. Response to constant angular acceleration. *J. Neurophysiol.*, **38**, 1250-1268.

Clark, D.L. (1973). Correlative postnatal vestibular development. Ohio State University Research Foundation, Report 2988.

Curthoys, I.S. and Webber, S.C.A. (1977). Techniques for acute single neuron recording in newborn rats. *Physiol. and Behav.*, in press.

Goldberg, J.M. and Fernandez, C. (1977). Conduction times and background discharge of vestibular afferents. *Brain Research*, **122**, 545-550.

Goldberg, J.M. and Fernandez, C. (1971). Physiology of peripheral neurons innervating semicircular canals of the squirrel monkey. III. Variations among units in their discharge properties. *J. Neurophysiol*, **34**, 676-684.

Heywood, P., Pujol, R. and Hilding, D.A. (1976). Development of the labyrinthine receptors in the guinea pig, cat and dog. *Acta Otolaryngol.*, **82**, 359-367.

Jones, G.M. and Spells, K.E. (1963). A theoretical and comparative study of the functional dependence of the semicircular canal upon its dimensions. *Proc. Roy. Soc. London*, Series B **157**, 403-419.

ten Kate, J.J. (1969). The oculo-vestibular reflex of the growing pike. Thesis. Rijksuniversiteit te Groningen.

2. Linear system techniques for the evaluation of semicircular canal afferent responses using white noise rotational stimuli.

R.J. PETERKA*, D.P. O'LEARY, D.L. TOMKO

Departments of Otolaryngology and Pharmacology, University of Pittsburgh, School of Medicine, Pittsburgh, Pennsylvania.

* *Biomedical Engineering Program, Carnegie-Mellon University, Pittsburgh, Pennsylvania.*

Introduction

The response of semicircular canal afferents to rotational accelerations of the head are determined by the transduction mechanisms of the supporting and neural elements of the crista ampullaris. It may be assumed that the nature of those mechanisms can to some extent be inferred from responses of first-order neurons to stimuli with known properties. In addition to inferences regarding peripheral transduction mechanisms, recording from single first-order afferents reveals the information which is encoded by peripheral structures for relay to the central nervous system.

Semicircular canal afferents have been tested using constant angular acceleration pulses (velocity trapezoids) to determine a single system time constant, system asymmetries, and adaptation (Goldberg and Fernandez, 1971; Blanks, Estes and Markham, 1975) and sinusoidal rotations to estimate gain and phase at discrete points within the frequency bandwidth of the system (Fernandez and Goldberg, 1971). Recently, linear system analysis techniques using white noise stimuli have offered alternative methods for describing dynamic properties encoded by semicircular canal afferents. These techniques permit the measurement of multiple time constants and characterization of gain and phase relations over virtually the entire system bandwidth simultaneously, and in short periods of time. The objective of this paper is to explain and demonstrate the ability of a white noise rotational stimulus to provide rapid and accurate descriptions of the response properties of the semicircular canal afferents.

White Noise Rotational Stimulus

The linear system analysis we have employed takes advantage of the ability to decompose a periodic stimulus signal into a unique summation of individual sinusoidal components by Fourier analysis (Bendat and Piersol, 1971). Delivery of an appropriate complex periodic stimulus to the vestibular system is equivalent to the simultaneous presentation of a set of different sinusoids over a selectable band of frequencies. Using spectral analysis techniques, the individual components of the complex stimulus may be isolated to obtain a description of the system's response characteristics.

The pseudorandom binary sequence (PRBS) of rotational accelerations is one of a large number of possible complex stimuli which we have found convenient to implement. It consists of repeated sequences of clockwise and counterclockwise rotational accelerations of equal magnitudes and varying durations, and has been described in detail elsewhere (Davies, 1970; O'Leary and Honrubia, 1975). This stimulus is advantageous because the

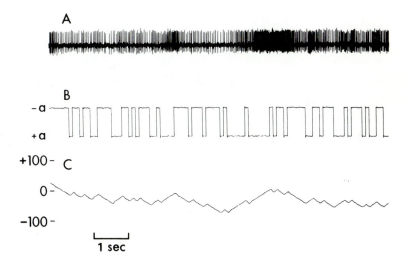

Fig. 1. A shows the neural discharges during a portion of a PRBS shown in B. In B, +a indicates a constant rotational acceleration (in this case $80°/sec^2$) in a clockwise direction, -a indicates an identical constant acceleration in the opposite direction. C shows the tachometer output of the torque motor. The tachometer shows that the table responds to state change commands in a time much less than the shortest acceleration state.

magnitude of its spectral components are approximately constant over a large bandwidth. Therefore, the delivery of a PRBS stimulus is equivalent to the simultaneous presentation of a large number of individual sinusoidal rotations of approximately equal magnitude. The determination of the gain and phase relationships between the input PRBS and the output neural response for this series of sinusoids produces the linear system transfer function which is a description of the dynamic properties of the first order afferents.

Figure 1 shows a portion of a single period of PRBS with the concommitant neural discharge evoked from a single neuron of the eighth nerve of the barbiturate anesthetized cat. We have used such data to determine the dynamic characteristics of about 100 horizontal semicircular canal afferents in the cat. For a large subset of these neurons, sufficient sinusoidal rotations and velocity trapezoids were applied as well to compare directly the results of the three techniques.

Before considering the data further, some theoretical background considerations are necessary. The system transfer function, $H(\omega)$, is estimated by determining the ratio of the cross power spectrum computed from the input PRBS stimulus and the output neuron's firing rate, $G_{xy}(\omega)$, to the PRBS stimulus power spectrum $G_x(\omega)$.

$$H(\omega) = \frac{G_{xy}(\omega)}{G_x(\omega)} \tag{1}$$

A power spectrum is a measure of the mean square value of a sinusoidal component of a signal at various frequencies, and is determined from the spectral components of the signal calculated from a discrete Fourier transform (DFT). The DFT is calculated using an efficient algorithm known as the Chirp z transform (Rabiner, Schafer and Rader, 1969). An evenly sampled estimate of the afferent neuron discharge rate is determined by filtering the series of action potential occurence times via the French-Holden algorithm (FHA) (French and Holden, 1971; Peterka, Sanderson and O'Leary, 1977). The use of the FHA is a crucial step in the data analysis procedure since the evenly spaced time samples of the cell's firing rate that the filter provides are required for the implementation of the other spectral analysis techniques. An example of the use of the FHA for the filtering of a sinusoidally modulated afferent response from a semicircular canal is shown in Figure 2.

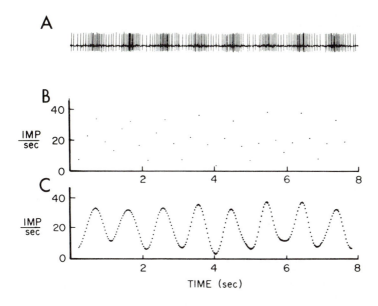

Fig. 2. A shows the neural discharges from a semicircular canal afferent modulated by a sinusoidal stimulus of 1 Hz. The French-Holden algorithm is a filter which preserves the spectral content of the original spike train below a specified cutoff frequency, in this case 2 Hz. The output of the FHA shown in B is an estimate of the neural firing rate at evenly spaced intervals of time. In C, a Fourier interpolation (Hamming, 1973) between the FHA sampled points clearly shows the sinusoidal nature of the response.

In addition to the transfer function estimate, the system coherence function, $\gamma_{xy}^2(\omega)$, can be estimated from the available power spectra:

$$\gamma_{xy}^2(\omega) = \frac{|G_{xy}(\omega)|^2}{G_x(\omega)\,G_y(\omega)} \tag{2}$$

where $G_y(\omega)$ is the power spectrum of the neuron's firing rate obtained via the FHA and the DFT. The coherence function gives an indication of how much of the response of a neuron can be accounted for by a linear transfer function between the input PRBS stimulus and the output cell firing rate. $\gamma_{xy}^2(\omega)$ varies from 0 to 1 with the high value indicating a perfect explanation of the output response to the PRBS input in terms of a linear system description. A low value of coherence indicates either that there is a nonlinearity in the system or that noise uncorrelated with the stimulus is present in the measurement of the system response. The coherence function is also used to evaluate the size of the confidence limits on the gain and phase estimates of the transfer function.

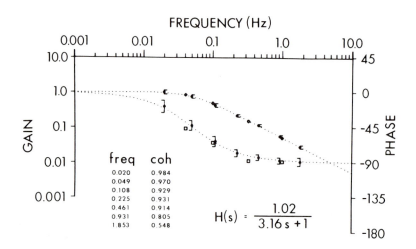

Fig. 3. Gain in (spikes/sec)/($^{\circ}$/sec^{2}) and phase estimates re acceleration are shown for cat horizontal semicircular canal afferent C17-12. The right facing brackets are 95% confidence limits surrounding the gain estimates determined from the cross spectral analysis of the responses to the PRBS stimulus. The left facing brackets are 95% confidence limits on the corresponding phase estimates. Value of coherence (coh) from the cross spectral analysis are indicated (see text for interpretation). The dotted lines are the gain (upper) and phase (lower) components of a transfer function fit H(s) to the experimental data determined using the PRBS stimulus. The diamonds and squares are gain and phase values, respectively, determined from the response of this neuron to a sinusoidal acceleration.

Figure 3 shows the gain and phase estimates of the transfer function for a typical cell, C17-12. Ninety-five percent confidence limits are included for each gain and phase value. A least squares fit to the experimentally determined transfer function reduces these data to a set of meaningful parameters (Seidel, 1975). The fit is of the form:

$$H(s) = \frac{K \prod_{i}(A_{i}s + 1)}{\prod_{j}(T_{j}s + 1)} \qquad (3)$$

where $s = j\omega$ is the Laplace operator. These fits provide a convenient description of the observed response dynamics in terms of system time constants, T_j, and sensitivity or DC gain, K.

The choice of a fit order, or the number of parameters, is arbitrary and we have adopted a criterion for the order determination. If the fit mean square error was reduced by at least 10% by choosing a more complex fit, then this fit was assumed to be a more nearly correct description of the true system properties. Typically, this resulted in fits requiring either 2 or 3 time constants for an adequate description. The example data shown in Figure 3 illustrates the rather rare case where a single time constant was adequate to describe the data, and additional parameters did not improve the fit as described above. For comparison, four discrete frequency gain and phase estimates obtained from sinusoidal rotations are included.

Figure 4 shows the gain, phase and fit to the experimentally determined transfer function for two additional sample units, one requiring two, and the other three time constants in the fit. Again the gain and phase estimates from sinusoids are in concordance with the estimates from the linear systems analysis. A statistical distribution of fit parameters of the entire population of afferents will be considered in another paper in the same proceeding (O'Leary, Tomko, Black and Peterka, 1978).

Conclusions

The use of a white noise rotational test signal and linear systems analysis provides a powerful and efficient tool for determining response dynamics in the vestibular system. It has the following characteristics:

1. Gain and phase relationships over the functional bandwidth of the system may be measured in a shorter period of time than required by sinusoidal testing over a similar bandwidth, and lead to similar conclusions.
2. The short duration pulses of angular acceleration employed by this technique resemble natural head movements more than either

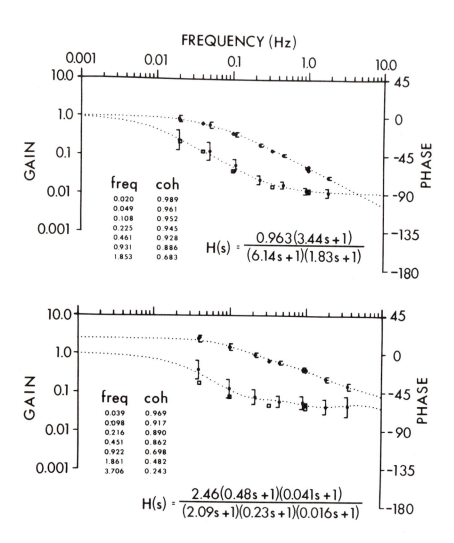

Fig. 4. The gain and phase estimates for two additional cat horizontal semicircular canal afferents (C19-3 in A and C14-1 in B) are shown. These estimates were obtained from the analysis of the response to both the PRBS and sinusoidal acceleration stimuli as described in Figure 3. The symbols and units are analogous to those in figure 3. More complex transfer functions were required (see text for fit criterion) to fit the gain and phase values determined from the response to the PRBS stimulus. The high values of the coherence function indicate approximate system linearity.

the long duration accelerations of velocity trapezoids or the pendular oscillations produced by sinusoidal stimulation.

3. Experimental determination of time constants other than the dominant one is straightforward with the linear systems analysis.
4. PRBS testing yields results over a finite bandwidth which is defined by the stimulus properties. Care must be exercised to insure that the bandwidth tested matches that of the system under test.

Acknowledgements

This work was supported in part by National Institutes of Health Grants NS12494, NS12308 and GM01455.

References

Bendat, J.S. and Piersol, A.G., 1971. *Random Data: Analysis and Measurement Procedures*, Wiley-Interscience.

Blanks, R.H.I., Estes, M.S. and Markham, C.H., 1975. The physiologic characteristics of vestibular first order canal neurons in the cat — II. Response to constant angular acceleration. *J. Neurophysiol.*, **38**, 1250-1268.

Davies, W.D.T., 1970. *System Identification for Self-Adaptive Control*, Wiley-Interscience.

Fernandez, C. and Goldberg, J.M., 1971. Physiology of peripheral neurons innervating semicircular canals of the squirrel monkey — II. Response to sinusoidal stimulation and dynamics of peripheral vestibular system. *J. Neurophysiol.*, **34**, 661-675.

French, A.S. and Holden, A.V., 1971. Alias-free sampling of neuronal spike trains. *Kybernetik,* **8**, 165-171.

Goldberg, J.M. and Fernandez, C., 1971. Physiology of peripheral neurons innervating semicircular canals of the squirrel monkey — I. Resting discharge and response to constant angular acceleration. *J. Neurophysiol.*, **34**, 635-660.

Hamming, R.W., 1973. *Numerical Methods for Scientists and Engineers*, McGraw-Hill.

O'Leary, D.P. and Honrubia, V., 1975. On-line identification of sensory systems using pseudorandom binary noise perturbations. *Biophys. J.*, **15**, (6) 505-532.

O'Leary, D.P., Tomko, D.L., Black, F.O. and Peterka, R.J., 1978. Comparative analysis of cat and isolated guitarfish horizontal canal afferent responses to rotational acceleration. *Proc. VI Extraordinary Meeting of the Barany Society.* 28-34.

Peterka, R.J., Sanderson, A.C. and O'Leary, D.P., Practical considerations in the implementation of the French-Holden algorithm for sampling of neuronal spike trains. In Press: *IEEE Trans. on Biomed. Eng.*

Rabiner, L.R., Schafer, R.W. and Rader, C.M., 1969. The chirp z-transform algorithm. *IEEE Trans. Audio Electroacoust.*, **AU-17**, 86-92.

Seidel, R.C., 1975. Transfer-function-parameter estimation from frequency response data — a FORTRAN program. NASA Technical Memorandum, NASA TM X — 3286, Sept., 1975.

3.   Influence of neck afferents on activity in the cat vestibular nuclei.

S.R.C. LIEDGREN, A.M. RUBIN, G. ASCHAN, L.M. ÖDKVIST, B. LARSBY

From the Departments of Otolaryngology, University of Toronto, Toronto, Ontario, Canada and University of Linkoping, Linkoping, Sweden

Introduction

The association of a disturbed balance with neck disease has long since been known by the clinician. The modern otoneurological examination of patients complaining of vertigo often suggests a pathology in the neck region. A neural and/or a vascular basis have been proposed as explanations for these conditions (for a review see Decher, 1969).

The former is especially supported by basic neurophysiological work; e.g. cats and monkeys deprived of neck afferents demonstrate serious disturbances in their motor control (Magnus and Storm van Leeuwen, 1914; Cohen, 1961). The close relation between the vestibular and the proprioceptive system has been documented at different levels of the central nervous system, from the spine caudally to the cerebral cortex rostrally (Fredrickson *et al.*, 1966, Lund and Pompeiano, 1968, Shapovalov, 1969, Grillner *et al.*, 1969, 1970, 1972, Schwarz and Fredrickson 1971, Bruggencate and Lundberg, 1974, Ödkvist *et al.*, 1975, Schwarz *et al.*, 1975, Liedgren *et al.*, 1976).

A co-operation between the vestibular system and the somatic proprioceptive receptors in the neck region seems logical in vertebrates where the labyrinths only give information about head position and not total body position. Fredrickson and co-workers (1966) in their studies in cats frequently observed convergence of vestibular and deep somatic afferents, mainly from the neck and the proximal joints, on neurons in the vestibular nuclear complex (VNC).

Somatosensory input to the VNC has been shown to arise primarily from joint and muscle receptors (Wilson *et al.*, 1966, 1968, Wilson, 1970) exclusive of Ia muscle afferents (Pompeiano and

Barnes, 1971) but also to some degree from skin receptors (Allen *et al.*, 1971). This somatosensory influence on the VNC appears to travel mainly via the reticular formation and the cerebellum (Wilson *et al.*, 1966, Bruggencate *et al.*, 1975).

It has been the purpose of this study to decide if neck muscle afferents to the VNC are restricted to certain vestibular nuclei or nuclear subdivisions. We have further tried to analyze the information content of the neural signals during neck manipulation to decide if it tends towards position, angular velocity or angular acceleration of the head in analogy with previous studies concerned with the vestibular apparatus (Melvill Jones and Milsum, 1971).

Material and Methods

The study is based on two different experimental series. The first one was made to collect quantitative and topographic knowledge about the distribution of neck afferents to the VNC. 16 adult cats were investigated under continuous halothane-$N_2 O$ anesthesia delivered via a trachoestomy tube. The cleidotrapezius, the splenius and the occipitoscapular muscles were dissected on both sides and their respective nerve supply mounted in plastic chambers containing bipolar stainless steel electrodes. Electrical stimulation (square waves, 0,1 msec, 1Hz) was used with an intensity twice the threshold value as determined by evoked afferent volleys. This stimulus strength should recruit most of the enclosed nerve fibers. The extracellular recording in the VNC and the subsequent histological procedure were identical with the technique employed below. In the following experiments 21 cats were used. The anesthesia was initiated as described above. The VNC was reached through a combined craniolaminectomy. Before the recording session started the animal was allowed to recover from the anesthesia and wounds and pressure points were heavily infiltrated with Xylocaine. Immobilization was achieved with repeated doses of Flaxedil. Respiration was then artifically assisted. Indications of pain were absent.

During the recording the cat was placed in a movable cast supporting the body. The head was mounted in a David Kopff stereotaxic frame in the usual reference position. A mechanical device was designed to move the body laterally to each side with the head remaining fixed, thus permitting movement of the body in the neck region. The position of the body with respect to the head was continuously recorded and will be referred to as neck-position or angle. The whole set up rested on a manually operated rotating table.

Glass microelectrodes (2 M NaC1, 3-8 megohm) were driven

obliquely into the brain stem to the VNC without penetrating the intact cerebellum. On-line poststimulus time histograms of single cell responses were generated by a PDP 8E computer and displayed on an oscilloscope. Neural responses and neck position were also stored for off-line analysis.

If a VNC unit influenced by horizontal rotatory acceleration could be identified the response to horizontal torsion around the neck joints 20 degrees to either side was investigated and an analysis of neuronal response dynamics undertaken.

During and after the recording the electrode position in the VNC was marked by producing electrolytic lesions. The animal was killed with an overdose of pentobarbital and subsequent perfusion with 10% formaldehyde. Locations of electrode tracks in the brain stem were determined in frozen serial sections (100μm) stained according to the Klüver and Barrera method. The boundaries used to separate individual vestibular nuclei were those described by Brodal and Pompeiano (1957) and Berman (1968).

Results

A. Response to electrical neck nerve stimulation. A total of 569 VNC neurons (56%, n = 1019) was observed to receive afferent information from somatosensory body receptors. Input from face, trunk and limb areas was investigated through manual stimulation of skin, fur, whiskers, deep tissues and joints. The majority of these units (63%, n = 569) responded to electrical stimuli applied to the dissected neck nerves. No nucleus was devoid of neck afferents but a high percentage of somatosensory units responded to neck input in all four major vestibular nuclei; superior vestibular nucleus (SVN), 77%, n = 43; medial vestibular nucleus (MVN), 68%, n = 178; descending vestibular nucleus (DVN), 63%, n = 176; lateral vestibular nucleus (LVN), 56%, n = 172.

Excitatory and inhibitory responses were seen with the former dominating. However, irregular spontaneous neuronal discharges may have masked some of the inhibitory influence, making this observation less valid. Response latencies varied over a wide range, the most rapid being 1,2 msec. Table 1 shows the distribution of VNC "neck" units without separating the various muscle nerves. Ipsilateral effects (108) were more prominent than contralateral (64) but many neurons could be affected by bilateral stimulation (188). No neuron was noted to have an input from all six muscles or even five of them. Usually an effective stimulus included only two or three muscles. No consistent pattern of interaction between the different muscles can be claimed. However, a reciprocal relation seems to exist at least between the cleidotrapezius and the splenius muscles as e.g. an excitation elicited by stimulating the nerve to the former frequently was followed by an inhibition when stimulating the latter.

TABLE 1
Excitation and/or inhibition of VNC neurons by electrical stimulation of ipsi- (IL) and contralateral (CL) nerves to the cleidotrapezius, occipitoscapular and splenius muscles.

Figures indicate number of units. BL = bilateral.

	SVN	MVN	DVN	LVN VLVN	DLVN	TOTAL
IL NECK	6	48	29	18	7	108
CL NECK	12	16	30	5	1	64
BL NECK	15	56	51	40	26	188
TOTAL	33	120	110	63	34	360

On comparing the ventral and dorsal parts of the LVN (Table 1) certain differences were seen. Only 36% of the "somatosensory" units in the dorsal part responded to neck nerve stimulus. The corresponding figure for the ventral part was as high as 82% (n = 91). The majority (56%, n = 97) of LVN units responded to bilateral neck nerve stimulation. Over half of these units (62%) received either exclusively excitatory or exclusively inhibitory bilateral input. More than one-third of these "bilateral neck responsive" units received a mixed input, stressing the complexity of neck input integration. For the majority of LVN units the responses had similar latencies (± 1 msec). However, for a few units, latencies varied by as much as 5 msec. Also for the other nuclei, bilateral input influenced the cells at about the same time.

Many neurons in the SVN received bilateral neck input (45%, n = 33) which was almost invariably similar, i.e. if excitatory from one side then also excitatory from the other side.

The most common pattern seen for units belonging to the MVN was that of bilateral neck input (48%, n = 56) with 40% of the neurons responding to ipsi- and 13% to contralateral input. SVN and MVN appear to have opposite patterns of neck preference with regard to body half, a factor to be remembered when considering the functional role of the two nuclei in the vestibulo-oculomotor system. DVN neurons seemed to receive neck inflow from ipsi- and contralateral regions without significant priority for any side.

B. **Response to neck torsion.** In this part only neurons with background responding to rotation were analyzed. The spontaneous neuronal discharge rate was on average higher (mean 24 spikes per sec) than in the former part of the study (mean 16 spikes per sec) depending almost certainly on the different types of anesthesia. 164 VNC neurons were collected responding to angular acceleration; 68 type I, 89 type II, 4 type III and 3 type IV units were encountered according to the classification of Duensing and Schaefer (1958). To be kept in mind is the fact that their terminology refers to angular acceleration in the plane of the horizontal canal whereas ours deals with a mixed canal response. Almost all neurons fired in a relatively regular manner. Eight neurons displayed an irregular discharge with sporadic bursts of activity. However, during rotatory acceleration their response pattern equalled that of the regularly firing units.

30% (n = 164) responded to lateral movement of the body at the neck joint. 22 units increased and decreased their spontaneous activity when the body was moved towards and away from the recording electrode respectively. 19 units displayed exactly the opposite pattern. 7 units increased their discharge rate during body movements in both directions while none was observed to be inhibited by this kind of a stimulus.

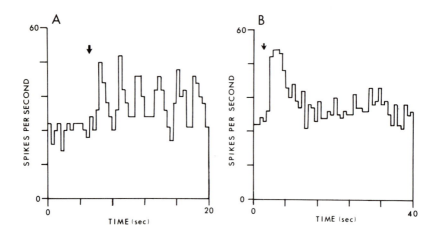

Fig. 1. LVN neuron responding to both vestibular and neck stimuli. A. Neuronal excitation resulting from alternating rotatory acceleration at around 0,5 Hz categorizing this unit as type III. B. An excitatory response was also seen when the body was moved laterally 20 degrees towards the recording side. The phasic nature of response is evident as the neck angle was kept constant throughout the recording. Spontaneous discharge level can be seen prior to onset of stimulation as indicated by the arrows.

Figure 1 shows a typical response from a single cell in the LVN with convergent labyrinthine-neck input. The response to angular acceleration of the whole animal is found in A where the discharge rate can be seen to increase during acceleration in both directions (type III). B illustrates the response of the same cell to ipsilateral torsion of the body. An increase of discharge rate above the spontaneous level was observed when the neck angle was increased to 20 degrees. This position was held for 40 sec during which time the discharge rate decreased to a spontaneous level. 94% (n = 48) of the studied units displayed this type of a phasic response with a change of firing frequency independant of neck angle.

To examine the relationship of neck velocity and acceleration to neuronal discharge rate the body was moved in a sinusoidal fashion with the head held fixed. A correlation between change in firing rate and neck velocity, not acceleration could then be observed. To quantify this relation neck position was averaged over each cycle of sinusoidal laterotorsion and cycle histograms were constructed illustrating the neuronal responses. The average neck position curves and the average post-stimulus histograms over 5 cycles were then subjected to Fourier analysis to determine the best fitting curves. Sixteen cells were analyzed in this way. The average phase shift between neck position and unitary response was $85° \pm 4°$. Figure 2 shows the relationship between neural response and neck velocity by superimposition of the two on the same time scale. The average velocity curve was obtained by differentation of the equation produced by the Fourier analysis of the average position curve for a single unit. The close fit of the velocity curve with the average cycle histogram supports the supposition that the analyzed VNC units respond to changes in position, i.e. velocity. From the data in fig. 2 the average neural gain of VNC unitary responses can be calculated. The average sensitivity factor was 0,37 spikes per sec/degrees per sec with a range of 0,28 to 0,44.

Neural responses to neck torsion and rotation were opposite for 84% of the cells. An acceleratory rotation, e.g. towards the side of the recording electrode could elicit an excitation while lateral body movement to the same side inhibited the same unit. Three units responded tonically to neck torsion. A sustained inhibition was observed when the body was kept in a lateral position away from the recording electrode. The opposite position resulted in an excitatory response for one of the units as long as the neck angle was kept constant. No change of spontaneous activity occured in the other two cases.

The majority of the neurons, 58% (n = 164), was located in the

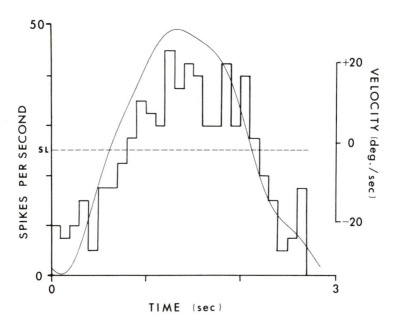

Fig. 2. The neck velocity curve superimposed on the neuronal response cycle histogram. SL = average discharge level. See text for further explanations.

MVN. Few "neck" units were, however, found in this nucleus which appeared to receive a predominantly labyrinthine input. The distribution of neurons receiving convergent vestibular and neck input (n = 48) did not differ significantly between the four main vestibular nuclei.

Discussion

The results of the present study confirm those of Fredrickson *et al.*, (1966) with regard to the importance of neck afferent input into the VNC from a quantitative point of view. This input is generally agreed to be of major importance for balance reflexes and postural body regulation but opinions diverge with regard to its contribution to the stabilization of eye movements.

Receptors for tonic neck reflexes have been demonstrated to be localized exclusively within the neck joints (McCough *et al.*, 1951, Gernandt *et al.* 1959). Electrical stimulation of group I a fibers arising from muscle spindles produced no responses in the VNC according to Pompeiano and Barnes (1971). In support of their findings is the observation that pressure to muscles in the neck region was equally ineffective (Fredrickson *et al.*, 1966). The electrical stimulus in our study to the dissected neck muscle nerves was well over threshold for group I - III activation (Silfvenius, 1972). The possible contribution of joint afferents is uncertain as they are known to travel with cutaneous and muscle nerves. Our results indicate a vast neck influence on the entire VNC since about one third of the investigated neurons modified their spontaneous activity during neck nerve stimulation. Response latencies as fast as 1,2 msec allow for a delay in one or two synapses. The attempt failed to correlate the distribution of "neck" neurons to anatomically or functionally defined territories of the VNC. Only in the dorsal and ventral parts of the LVN a significant difference in representation could be observed with a majority of responsive neurons in the latter region.

The effective semicircular canal stimulus is angular acceleration ultimately transformed into position information by way of the oculomotor output. The first step of the double integration necessary with respect to time takes place in the labyrinthine peripheral receptor. Primary vestibular afferents (Fernandez and Goldberg, 1971) and neurons in the VNC (Melvill Jones and Milsum, 1971) carry head rotation velocity information. Our data suggest a similar coding in the VNC for input from neck receptors as the units activated by neck torsion responded to velocity of neck movements and not to absolute neck position or acceleration. Only for three units neck input was coded in terms of position rather than velocity. We have, however, been dealing with a selected neuronal population responding to rotatory acceleration and thus focused our interest in canal-kinesthetic interaction. It is highly probable that if a utricular stimulus had been included then more tonically active neurons would have been found. Interaction between otolith and neck activity has been demonstrated previously (Kim and Partridge, 1969, Erhardt and Wagner, 1970).

von Holst and Mittelstaedt (1950) reported opposite information content in vestibular and neck messages during the tilting situation. More than eighty percent of our units with labyrinthine-neck convergence received antagonistic input from these two sensory systems. This so called vestibulocervical antagonism was first observed experimentally by Fredrickson *et al.* (1966) and its importance in postural motor regulation further emphasized.

Recent work by Thoden and Wirbitsky (1976) in which the influence of passive neck movements on eye position and VNC neuronal activity was investigated supports our findings since their post-stimulus frequency histograms during sinusoidal neck movement

movement were in phase with the input signal for velocity.

Acknowledgements

This study was supported by the MFR, Sweden (grant 14 X-4503) and by the MRC, Canada (grant MA 3311).

References

Allen, G.I., Sabh, N.H., Toyama, K. (1971). Effect of fore- and hindlimb nerve stimulation on Deiters' neurones. *Brain Res.* **25**, 645-650.

Berman, A.L. (1968). The brain stem of the cat. A cytoarchitectonic atlas with stereotaxic coordinates. Madison, Wisc.: Univ. of Wisconsin Press.

Brodal, A. Pompeiano, O. (1957). The vestibular nuclei in the cat. *J. Anat. (Lond.)* **91**, 438-454.

Bruggencate, G.T. Lundberg, A. (1974). Facilitatory interaction in transmission to motoneurones from vestibulospinal fibres and contralateral primary afferents. *Exp. Brain Res.* **19**, 248-270.

Bruggencate, G.T., Teichmann, R., Weller, E. (1975). Neuronal activity in the lateral vestibular nucleus of the cat. IV. Postsynaptic potentials evoked by stimulation of peripheral somatic nerves. *Pflügers Arch.* **360**, 302-320.

Cohen, L.A. (1961). Role of eye and neck proprioceptive mechanisms in body orientation and motor coordination. *J. Neurophysiol.* **24**, 1-11.

Decher, H. (1969). Die zervikalen Syndrome in der Hals-Nasen-Ohren-Heilkunde. Aktuelle Oto-Rhino-Laryngologie, Heft 2. Stuttgart; G. Thieme.

Duensing, F., Schaefer, K.P. (1958). Die Aktivität einzelner Neurone im Bereich der Vestibulariskerne bei Horizontalbeschleunigungen unter besonderer Berücksichtigung des vestibulären Nystagmus. *Arch. Psychiat. Nervenkr.* **198**, 225-252.

Ehrhardt, K.G., Wagner, A. (1970). Labyrinthine and neck reflexes recorded from spinal single motorneurons in the cat. *Brain Res.* **19**, 87-104.

Fernandez, C., Goldberg, J. (1971). Physiology of peripheral neurons innervating semicircular canals of the squirrel monkey. II. Response to sinusoidal stimulation and dynamics of peripheral vestibular system. *J. Neurophysiol.* **34**, 661-675.

Fredrickson, J.M., Schwarz, D.W.F., Kornhuber, H.H. (1966). Convergence and interaction of vestibular and deep somatic afferents upon neurons in the vestibular nuclei of the cat. *Acta Otolaryngol.* **61**, 168-188.

Gernandt, B.E., Iranyi, M., Livingston, R. (1959). Vestibular influences on spinal mechanisms. *Exp. Neurol.* **1**, 248-273.

Grillner, S., Hongo, T., Lund, S. (1969). Descending monsynaptic and reflex control of gamma-motorneurones. *Acta Physiol. Scand.* **75**, 592-613.

Grillner, S., Hongo, T., Lund, S. (1970). The vestibulospinal tract. Effects on alpha-motoneurones in the lumbosacral spinal cord in the cat. *Exp. Brain Res.* **10**, 94-120.

Grillner, S., Hongo, T. (1972). Vestibulospinal effects on motoneurones and interneurones in the lumbosacral cord. *In:* 'Basic aspects of central vestibular mechanisms'. Ed. by A. Brodal and O. Pompeiano. pp 243-262. Amsterdam: Elsevier.

von Holst, E., Mittelstaedt, H. (1950). Das Reafferenzprinzip. *Naturwissenschaften*, **37**, 464-475 (1950).
Kim, J.H., Partridge, L.D. (1969). Observations on types of response to combinations of neck, vestibular and muscle stretch signals. *J. Neurophysiol.* **32**, 239-250.
Liedgren, S.R.C., Milne, A.C., Rubin, A.M., Schwarz, D.W.F., Tomlinson, R.D. (1976). Representation of vestibular afferents in somatosensory thalamic nuclei of the squirrel monkey (Saimiri Scirueus), *J. Neurophysiol.* **39**, 601-612.
Lund, S., Pompeiano, O. (1968). Monosynaptic excitation of alphamotoneurones from supraspinal structures in the cat. *Acta Physiol. Scand.* **73**, 1-21.
Magnus, R., Storm van Leeuwen, W. (1914). Die akuten und die dauernden Folgen des Ausfalles der tonischen Hals und Labyrinthreflexe. *Pflügers Arch. ges. Physiol.* **159**, 157.
McCough, G.P., Deering, I.D., Ling, T.H. (1951). Location of receptors for tonic neck reflexes. *J. Neurophysiol.* **14**, 191-195.
Melvill Jones, G., Milsum, J.H. (1971). Frequency response analysis of central vestibular unit activity resulting from rotational stimulation of the semicircular canals. *J. Physiol. (Lond.)* **219**, 191-215.
Ödkvist, L.M., Liedgren, S.R.C., Larsby, B., Jerlwall, L. (1975). Vestibular and somatosensory inflow to the vestibular projection area in the post cruciate dimple region of the cat cerebral cortex. *Exp. Brain Res.* **22**, 185-196.
Pompeiano, O., Barnes, C.D. (1971). Effect of sinusoidal muscle stretch on neurons in medial and descending vestibular nuclei. *J. Neurophysiol.* **34**, 725-734.
Schwarz, D.W.F., Fredrickson, J.M. (1971). Rhesus monkey vestibular cortex. A bimodal primary projection field. *Science* **172**, 280-281.
Schwarz, D.W.F., Rubin A.M., Tomlinson, R.D., Milne, A.C., Fredrickson, J.M. (1975). Studies on the integrative activity of the vestibular nuclei complex. *Can. J. Otolaryng.* **4**, 378-382.
Shapovalov, A.I. (1969). Posttetanic potentiation of monosynaptic and disynaptic actions from supraspinal structures on lumbar motoneurones. *J. Neurophysiol.* **32**, 948-959.
Silfvenius, H. (1972). Projections to the cat cerebral cortex from fore- and hindlimb group I muscle afferents. Medical dissertation thesis, Umea, Sweden.
Thoden, U., Wirbitsky, J. (1976). Influence of passive neck movements on eye position and brain stem neurones. Deutsche Physiologische Gesellschaft. Suppl. vol. 362 R 37.
Wilson, V.J., Kato, M., Thomas, R.C., Peterson, B.W. (1966). Excitation of lateral vestibular neurons by peripheral afferent fibers. *J. Neurophysiol.* **29**, 508-529.
Wilson, V.J., Wylie, R.M., Marco, L.A. (1968). Organization of the medial vestibular nucleus. Synaptic inputs to cells in the medial vestibular nucleus. *J. Neurophysiol.* **31**, 166-185.
Wilson, V.J. (1970). Vestibular and somatic inputs to cells of the lateral and medial vestibular nuclei of the cat. *In:* fifth symposium on the role of the vestibular organs in space exploration. NASA **SP-187**, 145-158.

4. Comparative analysis of cat and guitarfish semicircular canal afferent responses.

D.P. O'LEARY, D.L. TOMKO, F.O. BLACK, R.J. PETERKA*

Departments of Otolaryngology and Pharmacology, University of Pittsburgh, School of Medicine, Pittsburgh, Pennsylvania.

* Biomedical Engineering Program, Carnegie-Mellon University, Pittsburgh, Pennsylvania.

Introduction

The pioneering research of Groen, Lowenstein and Vendrik (1949) provided a fundamental basis for our understanding of the input-output characteristics of the semicircular canal system, particularly as expressed quantitatively in the form of a linear differential equation. More recent studies in animals such as the squirrel monkey (Fernandez and Goldberg, 1971), frog (Precht, Llinas and Clark, 1971) and the cat (Blanks, Estes and Markham, 1976) have greatly extended this work.

Advances in communication and control theory during the past 20 years have provided the background for development of computerized techniques for the analysis of biological control systems. A major development is the concept that a functional system can be "identified" by analysis of its responses to controlled inputs, in the form of small perturbations superimposed on normal operating conditions (Davies, 1970). White noise stimuli are particularly useful because they provide "information-rich" inputs that test a system throughout its useable dynamic range.

The type of white noise stimulus used in the present study employs pseudorandom binary sequences of rotational accelerations and was developed originally to study the response of semicircular canal afferents in the guitarfish (O'Leary and Honrubia, 1975; 1976; O'Leary, Dunn and Honrubia, 1976). The analysis of neural data generated during the presentation of this type of stimulus has been recently modified and improved for better resolution over broader bandwidths as described by Peterka, O'Leary and Tomko (1978) in this symposium.

A major goal of the present study was the empirical determination of a small number of linear system parameters which correspond to major and associated minor time constants, and the gain and phase relationships over the portion of the frequency domain of physiological significance. Because of time constraints, this report briefly describes and compares the time domain properties of horizontal canal afferent responses in the barbiturate anesthetized cat and the isolated guitarfish head using white noise stimulation. Frequency domain properties will be considered in a more detailed paper later.

Methods

A computer-controlled rotating table was used to deliver pseudorandom binary sequences (PRBSs) of rotational acceleration (Davies, 1970; O'Leary and Honrubia, 1975). Extra-cellular afferent spike trains were recorded by the use of forceps electrodes for isolated guitarfish preparations (O'Leary, Dunn and Honrubia, 1976) and with glass pipette microelectrodes from barbiturate anesthetized cats after ablation of the flocculus and adjacent portions of the cerebellum. (See Loe, Tomko and Werner, 1973 for details of surgical and recording techniques).

Results

A. Guitarfish Horizontal Canal Afferent Responses. Results were displayed during experiments as unit impulse responses (UIRs) which are derived from statistical communication theory (Lee, 1960) and are the prediction of a response to a brief pulse of rotational acceleration. Although obtained indirectly by a cross-correlation technique, UIRs are similar conceptually to vestibular responses obtained by the technique of "cupulometry", i.e. a rapid acceleration resulting from the sudden braking of a subject rotating at constant velocity. Each UIR may be characterized by its amplitude and shape. Since each one represents the time course of the afferent discharge rate that would occur in response to a brief pulse of rotational acceleration, the amplitude may be interpreted as an indication of the sensitivity of the afferent to that acceleration, and the rate of decay of response following the stimulus would be determined by the time constant or constants of the system. Thus the UIR represents for each afferent a unique "signature" profile determined by its peripheral transduction mechanisms.

Results from the isolated guitarfish horizontal semicircular canal showed UIRs that varied in the shape of their response contour (or

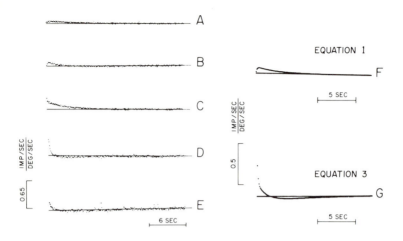

Fig. 1. Representative unit impulse responses (UIRs) from the guitarfish horizontal semicircular canal are shown in A-E. The UIRs were grouped into two general classes (or contour shapes) which are shown in F and G, as plotted from equations 1 and 3, respectively, after division by the PRBS state duration equal to 92 msec. The response classes were correlated with the receptor anatomy and innervation as described in the text. (Adapted from O'Leary, Dunn and Honrubia, 1976).

"signature") profiles. Examples are shown in Figure 1 A-E. This degree of response diversity was unexpected particularly since they were obtained under "open-loop" conditions from an isolated elasmobranch preparation, in which the efferent system was disrupted, and with only Type II hair cells. However, horizontal canal afferents of this species are divided into 5-9 individual bundles, providing an anatomical correlation with functional responses. The most sensitive afferents, (Figure 1 D & E) with fastest major time constants, were obtained from afferents located in central bundles of the nerve, whereas afferents with less sensitivity (Figure 1 A & B), and UIR response profiles resembling an overdamped second-order system were obtained from bundles located in the extreme rostral and caudal nerve bundles (O'Leary, Dunn and Honrubia, 1974; O'Leary, Dunn & Honrubia, 1976). Through the use of serial section histology, these studies have shown that central bundles project to the apex of the crista, whereas the extreme rostral and caudal bundles project to the crista slopes.

In order to obtain quantitative parameters as system descriptors, each UIR was assigned to one of four specific classes of linear systems. Each class may be described by a time domain exponential equation (O'Leary and Honrubia, 1976). The equations from the four classes of UIRs obtained from the population of guitarfish afferent responses were in units of $(imp/sec)/(deg/sec^2)$ $(x10^{-3})$:

$$h(t) = (7.34 \pm 4.28)e^{-(0.362 \pm 0.197)t} - (5.35 \pm 4.03)e^{-(7.04 \pm 5.70)t} \tag{1}$$

$$h(t) = (13.2 \pm 7.57)e^{-(0.495 \pm 0.139)t} + (41.2 \pm 40.0)e^{-(18.2 \pm 11.5)t} \tag{2}$$

$$h(t) = (24.3 \pm 9.18)e^{-(0.748 \pm 0.588)t} + (54.6 \pm 40.1)e^{-(10.9 \pm 7.16)t} - (9.08 \pm 4.94)e^{-(0.218 \pm 0.087)t} \tag{3}$$

$$h(t) = (4.78 \pm 2.33)e^{-(0.349 \pm 0.149)t} \tag{4}$$

For illustrative purposes, UIRs computed from equations 1 and 3 are shown in Figure 1F and G, respectively. Although the above equations were classified according to linear system order, an additional anatomical correlation was found. All afferents contributing to the average response described as equation 1 (Figure 1F) were found in the extreme rostral or caudal nerve bundles (i.e. crista slopes). All afferents contributing to the averaged response equations 2 and 3 (Figure 1G) were located in more central regions of the nerve (i.e. crista apex). Finally, responses contributing to equation 4 were distributed throughout all bundles of the nerve. These results were interpreted as implying that specific bundles of the nerve, innervating specific regions of the receptor, could be carrying specific classes of head movement information to centrally located vestibular pathways (O'Leary and Honrubia, 1976).

B. Cat Horizontal Canal Afferent Responses. The additional complexity provided by the existence of both Types I and II hair cells in the mammalian crista suggested that the afferent response UIRs from a mammal might be significantly different from those obtained from the isolated guitarfish. In Figure 2 are shown representative examples of UIRs obtained from individual cat afferents. Qualitatively, the general form of the cat UIRs was similar in shape to that of the guitarfish shown in Figure 1G. This general form was fitted in the guitarfish data by equation 3, with two positive exponentials with different time constants, and a negative, or overshooting, exponential term. There were quantitative differences however in the fitted parameters obtained from cat afferents, relative to those from guitarfish afferents, as described below. We did not observe UIRs from cat afferents with contours resembling the guitarfish class shown in Figure 1F. It is of course possible that this class of afferents

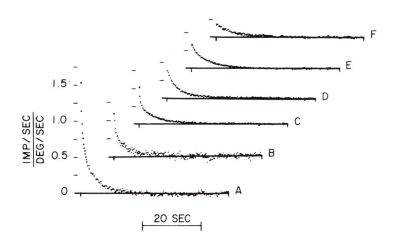

Fig. 2. Representative unit impulse responses from afferents innervating the cat horizontal semicircular canal.

does indeed exist in a localized region of the cat nerve that was not explored by our microelectrode recording procedure.

The system transfer function, $\tilde{H}(\omega)$, was estimated for each primary afferent by determining the ratio of the cross power spectrum computed from the input PRBS stimulus and the output neural discharge rate to the PRBS power spectrum as described in the previous paper (Peterka, O'Leary and Tomko, 1978). The least squares fit to this transfer function provided estimates of the system time constant or constants and DC gain. Figure 3 shows histograms of the dominant time constants of afferents from the cat as described above, and from the guitarfish UIRs.

The histograms are relatively broad, implying a continuum of time constants. The time constants from the guitarfish spanned a range from less than 1 to 6 seconds, whereas the majority of the cat time constants were in the range from 2 to 8 seconds. It is useful for comparative purposes to note that the mean and standard deviation of major time constants from each animal were: 4.95 ± 1.87 for the cat and 2.66 ± 1.22 for the guitarfish. Because of the extended range of the distributions shown in Figure 3, it is doubtful that simple biophysical interpretations can be attached to the averaged value of the time constants from either species. In fact, interpretations of averaged values may obscure the possibility that differences in localized receptor transduction mechanisms occurring in different parts of the crista could be responsible for the relatively broad range of values.

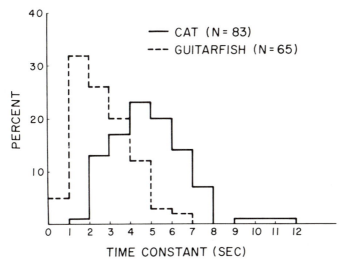

Fig. 3. Histograms of dominant time constants of horizontal canal afferent responses from the cat and guitarfish. The means and standard deviations were, cat: 4.95 ± 1.87 seconds, and guitarfish: 2.66 ± 1.22 seconds.

Conclusions

1. A comparison of the afferent response data from the guitarfish and cat showed qualitative similarities in the contours or shapes of certain of the unit impulse responses. However, a particular type of impulse response found in afferents innervating the slopes of the guitarfish crista (Figure 1F) with only Type II haircells was not observed in the cat.

2. Results from cats were in concordance with the finding from guitarfish that there exists a continuum of response parameters. The broad distribution of major time constants implies that afferent response dymanics are not dominated by the cupula-endolymph complex moving as a functional unit; in fact, the response diversity may be due to the possibility that the central-most regions of cupula may undergo more extensive deflections than those regions closer to the ampullar walls (Hillman, 1974). The observed differences in rate constants may reflect local variations in either cupula-endolymph elasticity or other trans-duction mechanisms.

3. These data support the hypothesis that specific types of head

movement are encoded by discrete sub-populations of primary afferents, i.e., that certain groups of afferents are tuned, in a matched filter sense, to certain kinds of head movements. (O'Leary, Dunn and Honrubia, 1974). In that sense, information about fast, transient head movements would be carried primarily among fibers with faster impulse responses, whereas information concerning slower head movements would be carried primarily in afferents with more gradual impulse responses.

References

Blanks, R.H.I., Estes, M.S. and Markham, C.H., 1975. Physiologic characteristics of vestibular first-order canal neurons in the cat. II. Response to constant angular acceleration. *J. Neurophysiol.,* **38**, 1250-1268.

Davies, W.D.T., 1970. *System Identification for Self-Adaptive Control,* New York: Wiley-Interscience.

Fernandez, C. and Goldberg, J.M., 1971. Physiology of peripheral neurons innervating semicircular canals of the squirrel monkey. II. Response to sinusoidal stimulation and dynamics of peripheral vestibular system. *J. Neurophysiol.,* **34**, 661-675.

Groen, J.J., Lowenstein, O. and Vendrik, A.J.H., 1952. The mechanical analysis of the responses from the end-organs of the horizontal semicircular canal in the isolated elasmobranch labyrinth. *J. Physiol.,* **117**, 329-346.

Hillman, D.E., 1974. Cupular structure and its receptor relationship. *Brain Behav. Evol.,* **10**, 52-68.

Lee, Y.W., 1960. *Statistical Theory of Communication,* New York: Wiley.

Loe, P.R., Tomko, D.L. and Werner, G., 1973. The neural signal of angular head position in primary afferent vestibular nerve axons. *J. Physiol.,* **230**, 29-50.

O'Leary, D.P., Dunn, R. and Honrubia, V., 1974. Functional and anatomical correlation of afferent responses from the isolated semicircular canal. *Nature,* **251**, 225-227.

O'Leary, D.P. and Honrubia, V., 1975. On-line identification of sensory systems using pseudorandom binary noise perturbations. *Biophys. J.,* **15**, 505-532.

O'Leary, D.P., Dunn, R.F. and Honrubia, V., 1976. Analysis of afferent responses from the isolated semicircular canal of the guitarfish using rotational acceleration white noise imputs. I. Correlation of response dynamics with receptor innervation. *J. Neurophysiol.,* **39**, 631-644.

O'Leary, D.P. and Honrubia, V., 1976. Analysis of afferent responses from the isolated semicircular canal of the guitarfish using rotational acceleration white noise inputs. II. Estimation of linear system parameters and gain and phase spectra. *J. Neurophysiol.,* **39**, 645-659.

Peterka, R., O'Leary, D.P. and Tomko, D.L., 1978. Linear system techniques for the evaluation of semicircular canal afferent responses using white noise rotational stimuli. Presented at the Sixth Extraordinary Meeting of the Barany Society, London, September, 1977. *To be published in:* Proceedings of the VI Extraordinary Meeting of the Barany Society.

Precht, W., Llinas, R. and Clarke, M., 1971. Physiological responses of frog vestibular fibers to horizontal angular rotation. *Exptl. Brain Res.* **13**, 378-407.

Neurophysiology

1. The pattern of eye movement trajectories during physiological nystagmus in humans.

C.G.Y. LAU,* V. HONRUBIA, * R.W. BALOH**

From the Division of Head and Neck Surgery (Otolaryngology)*,
and the Department of Neurology (Reed Neurological Research
Center)**, the University of California, Los Angeles 90024

Introduction

Most previous studies of the vestibulo-ocular reflex (VOR) have focused on the response characteristics of the slow component of nystagmus, (Meiry, 1971). Although several models of nystagmus have been proposed (Sugie and Jones, 1971; Barnes and Benson, 1973) the conditions under which the fast components are produced are not completely known. The present study is concerned with the way in which the threshold for the production of the fast component of nystagmus depends on eye position and eye velocity.

Methods

From ten normal human subjects, records of horizontal eye movements were obtained by means of electro-oculography, digitized at 200 samples/second and later analyzed on a PDP-11 computer system. These eye movements were induced under the following four conditions as the subject was seated in a rotatory chair within an optokinetic drum:
1. The subject was rotated sinusoidally in the light at .05 Hz and peak velocities of 30 and 60 degrees/second while maintaining gaze on the surface of the surrounding stationary optokinetic drum.
2. The subject was rotated sinusoidally in the dark at the same frequency but with peak velocities of 60 and 120 degrees/second.
3. The optokinetic drum was rotated sinusoidally about the subject at .05 Hz and peak velocities of 30 and 60 degrees/second.
4. Impulsive horizontal angular acceleration was applied to the subject in the dark, the impulse being produced by a sudden stopping

of the chair as it was rotating at a constant velocity of 128 or 256 degrees/second in the clockwise (CW) or counterclockwise (CCW) direction.

Results

1. General pattern of eye movements. Shown in Figure 1 is an example of eye movement responses obtained from one subject for each of the four types of stimulus. The nystagmus in A was

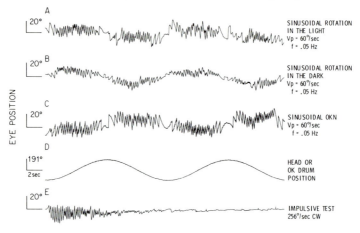

Fig. 1. Eye movement responses to sinusoidal head rotation in the light (A) and in the dark (B), to sinusoidal optokinetic stimulus (C), and impulsive angular acceleration (E). The head or optokinetic drum position as a function of time is shown in (D).

recorded during rotation in the light; in B, during rotation in the dark; and in C, during sinusoidal optokinetic stimulation. The three tests were conducted at a peak velocity of 60 degrees/second and at a frequency of .05 Hz. The fourth trace, D, shows head position or optokinetic drum position as a function of time. The bottom trace, E, is a record of eye movement responses to an impulsive angular acceleration produced by a sudden halting of the chair from constant velocity CW rotation at 256 degrees/second.

The eye movement responses in all ten subjects were not unlike those of other normal subjects tested in this laboratory, (Honrubia et al., 1977). The average gain for the slow component, which is defined as the ratio of the peak slow component velocity to the peak chair velocity, was 0.90 ± .09 for sinusoidal rotation in the light and 0.60 ± 0.14 for sinusoidal rotation in the dark. The average gain in the sinusoidal optokinetic test was 0.76 ± 0.17.

Common to all the records in Figure 1 is the deviation of the mean eye position in the direction of the fast component. The slow component moved the eye from the periphery to a more central position in the orbit and, subsequently, the fast component moved the eye from the central position to the periphery. In this group of subjects, as was found earlier in another study, (Honrubia *et al.*, 1977) the slow component amplitude was correlated with the position of the eye in the orbit at the start of the slow component (SSC).

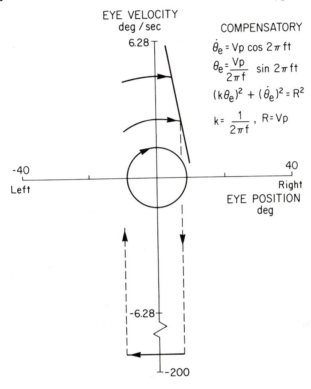

Fig. 2. Idealized eye movement trajectory on the phase-plane. The abscissa represents eye position and the ordinate represents eye velocity.

Eye position at the end of the slow component (ESC), however, seemed to be independent of the slow component amplitude, as if there were a preferred eye position, or a threshold, for the production of the fast component of nystagmus.

2. **Dependence of the threshold on eye position and velocity.** In the present study, we investigated the possibility that this threshold may be dependent on both the eye position and the instantaneous eye velocity. The complete eye movement trajectory can be re-

presented by a curve on the phase-plane, which is a plot of the eye velocity versus eye position. Figure 2 shows examples of theoretical eye movement trajectories induced by sinusoidal rotation of the head. Under subthreshold stimulus conditions, when the eye movement response is purely compensatory (or sinusoidal), the eye movement trajectory takes the form of a circle. As the magnitude of the stimulus is increased, however, the eye movement trajectory changes and the compensatory eye movement is now interrupted by the fast component of nystagmus. The slow components are represented by segments of a circle, since they are compensatory (or sinusoidal). During the subsequent fast components, the eye velocity is opposite in sign to the velocity of the slow components.

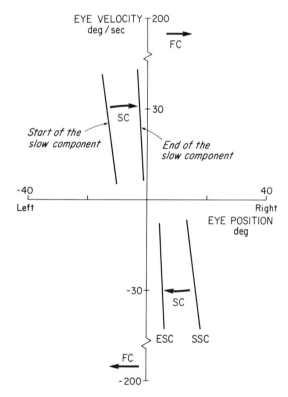

Fig. 3. Eye movement trajectory on the phase-plane and the locus of points for the start of the slow component (SSC) and end of the slow component (ESC).

On the phase-plane, one can plot the instantaneous eye position and eye velocity at the SSC and the ESC, as well as at the start and end of the fast component. The eye velocity at the SSC is obtained from the slope of the linear-regression line fit to a number of slow component data points (usually ten) at the SSC, to minimize the effect of noise on the computation of instantaneous eye velocity. Similar technique is used to obtain the instantaneous eye velocity at the ESC.

Figure 3 shows the locus of points at the SSC and at the ESC on the phase-plane. The two lines above the abscissa represent the start and end of the nystagmus slow component moving to the right, and the two lines below the abscissa represent the start and end of the slow component moving to the left. A point on the line labelled

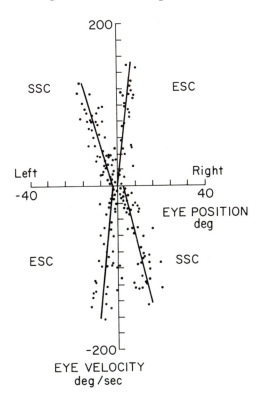

Fig. 4. Example of eye movement data on the phase-plane, taken from one subject's eye movement response to an impulsive angular acceleration. The lines drawn through the data points are the linear-regression lines for the SSC and ESC.

SSC is connected to a point on the line labelled ESC by the slow component trajectory, which is not shown in this figure. Also not shown, for the sake of simplicity, are the eye trajectories connecting the slow components with the fast components.

Shown in Figure 4 is an example, on the phase-plane, of the data taken from one subject's response to an impulsive angular acceleration in both CW and CCW directions. The lines drawn through the data points are the "x on y" linear regression lines for the SSC and the ESC, for rightward slow components (top) and leftward slow components (bottom). In this particular example, the slopes for the rightward SSC and ESC are -0.11 (with standard error 0.011) and +0.04 (with standard error 0.007), respectively. For the leftward slow component, the slopes for SSC and ESC are -0.09 (standard error 0.008) and +0.04 (standard error 0.008), respectively. This figure is representative of the responses of many subjects to the impulsive test.

TABLE 1
Mean Slope on Phase-Plane
$$\left(\frac{degrees}{degrees/second}\right)$$

	Rightward		Leftward	
	SSC	ESC	ESC	SSC
Light	-0.13	-0.09	-0.11	-0.14
(VVOR)	(± 0.15)	(± 0.15)	(± 0.14)	(± 0.16)
Dark	-0.13	-0.03	-0.01	-0.17
(VOR)	(± 0.10)	(± 0.14)	(± 0.09)	(± 0.10)
OKN	-0.12	-0.04	-0.05	-0.06
	(± 0.27)	(± 0.27)	(± 0.14)	(± 0.16)
Impulsive	-0.14	-0.04	-0.01	-0.09
(VOR)	(± 0.10)	(± 0.10)	(± 0.07)	(± 0.05)

Table 1 summarizes the data on the slopes of the regression lines for the ten subjects in each of the four tests. The magnitude of the slope is generally larger for the SSC than for the ESC, indicating the greater dependence of the SSC and lesser dependence of the ESC on the eye velocity. For the ESC on all four tests, the hypothesis that the mean slope is not different from zero cannot be rejected at the .05 significance level. These data corroborate our previous finding (Honrubia, et al., 1977) that the threshold for the production of the fast component depends primarily on eye position, and to a lesser extent on eye velocity. Table 2 shows the mean eye position at the SSC and the ESC in each of the four tests. For each test, the mean positions of the eye at the SSC and at the ESC are statistically significantly different ($p < .01$). Furthermore, the means for the ESC for right-

TABLE 2
Mean Eye Position
(degrees)

	Rightward		Leftward	
	SSC	ESC	ESC	SSC
Light	-12.94	-2.96	7.03	17.44
(VVOR)	(± 5.52)	(± 5.74)	(± 4.02)	(± 5.25)
Dark	-9.72	-1.97	3.90	12.41
(VOR)	(± 4.87)	(± 4.69)	(± 4.78)	(± 4.25)
OKN	-15.51	-6.82	2.66	12.66
	(± 7.21)	(± 5.46)	(± 3.82)	(± 3.93)
Impulsive	-9.54	0.81	2.16	12.45
(VOR)	(± 3.54)	(± 4.69)	(± 4.83)	(± 4.18)

ward and leftward slow components are also statistically significantly different (p < .01) for the visual-vestibulo-ocular reflex (VVOR) and the optokinetic nystagmus (OKN) tests.

Discussion

These data support the finding (Honrubia *et al.*, 1977; Jones 1964) that the slow component starts from the periphery and ends at a more central position, and that this pattern is valid for many types of nystagmus reaction. Furthermore, the threshold for the production of the fast component of nystagmus is largely dependent on eye position. The dependence of the threshold on eye velocity is more noticeable for individual subjects where the slopes for the ESC are statistically significant from zero. In other words, for each individual subject, the threshold depends largely on eye position and to some extent on eye velocity. When the group of subjects is taken as a whole, however, the mean slope is not statistically significant from zero because some slopes are positive and some are negative.

The eye position and eye velocity at the start and end of the fast component (SFC and EFC) can also be plotted on the phase-plane. For this group of human subjects, the fast component generally starts with a velocity of 200 degrees/second and ends at 150 degrees/second. The response characteristics of the slow component are well known, and for a given frequency of stimulus, are specified by the gain and the phase. With the conditions for the SSC, ESC, SFC and EFC specified on the phase-plane, it is possible to formulate models for the prediction of the complete eye movement trajectory, including that of the fast component, for many types of nystagmus reaction. This information can now be used to obtain a better understanding of the underlying mechanism for the production of the fast component of nystagmus, and to help in the clinical evaluation of vestibular function.

Acknowledgements

Assistance in data analysis by Ms. Sally Longmire and editorial aid by Ms. Marilyn Oreck are greatly appreciated. This study was supported by a grant from the National Institutes of Health, NS 09823.

References

Barnes, G.R., Benson, A.J. (1973): A model for the prediction of the nystagmic response to angular and linear acceleration stimuli. *In:* Guedry, F.E. (ed.), Advisory Group for Aerospace Research and Development Conference No. 128, NASA.

Honrubia, V., Baloh, R.W., Lau, C.G.Y. and Sills, A.W. (1977). The patterns of eye movements during physiologic vestibular nystagmus in man. *Trans. Amer. Acad. Ophthalmol. Otolaryngol.* **84**, ORL339-ORL347.

Jones, G.M. (1964). Predominance of anti-compensatory oculomotor responses during rapid head rotation. *Aerosp. Med.* **35**, 965-968.

Meiry, J.L. (1971). Vestibular and proprioceptive stabilization of eye movements. *In:* Bach-y-Rita, P., Collins, C.C. and Hyde, J.E. (eds.) *The Control of Eye Movements.* New York, Academic Press.

Sugie, N., Jones, G.M. (1971): A model of eye movements induced by head rotation. *IEEE Trans. Syst. Man Cyb.* **SMC-1**, 251-260.

2. Cerebellar and brainstem responses to eye muscle stretch in the cat.*

R.D. TOMLINSON, D.W.F. SCHWARZ, J.M. FREDRICKSON

Department of Otolaryngology, University of Toronto.

The medial portion of the cat's cerebellar vermis (Fig. 1) including lobule VI and VII receives afferent input from the retina, the cochlea (Snider & Stowell, 1944), the neck (Berthoz & Llinas, 1974) and eye muscle proprioceptors (Fuchs & Kornhuber, 1969; Baker *et al.,* 1972; Batini *et al.,* 1974; Schwarz & Tomlinson, 1977), and has been proposed to be involved in the generation of saccadic eye movements (Aschoff & Cohen, 1971; Ron & Robinson, 1973; Wolfe, 1971; Llinas, 1974; Kornhuber, 1974). If this part of the cerebellar cortex

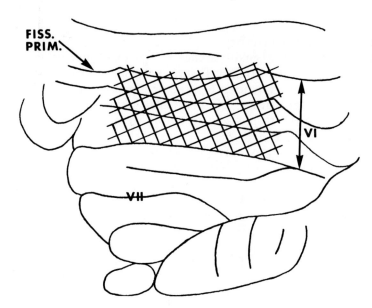

Fig. 1. See text.

* Supported by M.R.C. of Canada.

is removed surgically, a very interesting type of saccadic dysmetria results (Ritchie, 1976); there is an undershoot if the saccade is directed from primary position to an excentric target, however saccades from a lateral (or medial) position towards the midline are too long, overshooting the target. This suggests that saccadic commands, generated elsewhere in the brain, are not able to account for viscoelastic properties of orbital tissues, particularly eye muscles. It must therefore be a function of the cerebellar cortex to update the movement program according to forces which can change during life and are unnecessary for the formulation of the program itself.

One reason why the many studies of various afferent inputs to this portion of cerebellar cortex have provided no key to its role in motor control is that aspects related to movement have not generally been examined. We attempted to define parameters which might be used for cerebellar saccade adjustment, originating in extraocular muscle stretch receptors.

These receptors were stimulated by subjecting the four rectus muscles of each eye to a stretch of controlled length and tension via threads attached to the tendons at their insertions to the globe. Both optic tracts were sectioned to exclude retinal input and the cats were maintained as encephale isolé preparation under N_2O analgesia after discontinuation of surgical halothane aneasthesia. The area shown cross-hatched in Fig. 1 was systematically explored with micro-electrodes since it had been reported to receive eye muscle afferent input. However, only small patches of cortex, concentrated in the posterior bank of the primary fissure, contained cells responding to our stretch stimuli (latencies 6 msec or longer). Control recordings with stretch stimulation of periocular skin and orbital tissue ascertained that the responding receptors were indeed located in the muscles moving the eye.

Only phasic responses were seen, that is, there was no relationship between the durations of stretch plateau and response (Fig. 2). Thus eye position is not encoded in stretch afferent input. Although neurons responded only to initiation or release of a stretch, simple dynamics of the movement such as angular velocity or acceleration were not reflected in the response amplitude. The amplitude of the angular deviation of the eye was best related to the response amplitude, with thresholds ranging from 2° and 5°. The conclusion that the amplitude of an eye movement is encoded in the firing pattern would, however, be premature since the muscle stretch was in opposition to muscle tonus, which is actively decreased during normal active eye movements.

Only few cells (18 of 123) responded to stretch of only one

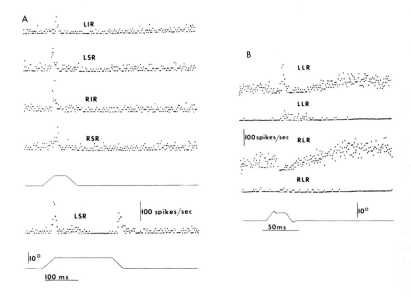

Fig. 2. See text.

muscle. The other cells, exhibiting convergence from several muscles could be divided into three groups: 1) cells with input from at least two eye muscles which would be similarly stretched during a movement of both eyes in one particular direction (37 direction-specific cells), 2) cells responding to stretch corresponding to either direction in a certain plane (22 plane-specific cells) and 3) cells with more complicated response patterns (46 complex cells).

A plane-specific cell for vertical movements is shown in Fig. 2A. This cell responded to stretch of the four vertical recti with no response to horizontal rectus muscle stretch (not illustrated). Such plane-specific cells should respond to both onset and release of the stretch, a pattern which was only seen for stretches exceeding 130 msec. The initial excitation appears to be followed by a period of response suppression which may, as in the bottom of Fig. 2A, or may not be exhibited as inhibition during prolonged stretch. Such a response suppression was usually observed when two consecutive brief stretches were used at any single muscle, regardless of the unit type tested.

A direction-specific cell for the horizontal plane is shown in Fig. 2B. This cell fired with both simple and complex spikes, simple spikes (reflecting mossy fiber input) being shown in the first and third diagram and complex spikes (climbing fiber input) in the remaining second and fourth plots. Only the lateral rectus of each eye produced responses; it will be recognized that the excitation due to left lateral rectus pull is complemented by inhibition with right lateral rectus pull. Thus excitation would occur during gaze to the right and inhibition to the left. The climbing fiber activation appears to follow this pattern, however without overt inhibition. Complex spike responses were seen relatively rarely (38 cells) in this study.

All neurons not exhibiting plane or direction specificity were classified as "complex neurons". It is, of course, possible that many of these cells also carry directional information since the oblique muscles were not adequately stimulated. A few of these complex cells responded with multiphasic excitation − inhibition patterns, which cannot be interpreted in functional terms at this time.

It can be concluded that eye muscle stretch receptors provide small patches of cerebellar cortical tissue in lobule VI with information about eye movement direction and plane. This activity pattern has also been seen in this region prior to saccades (Llinas, 1974). If this information was to be used directly to produce the program for a saccade about to occur it should be available to oculomotor output channels shortly after passing through the cerebellum. We investigated this question by applying eye muscle stretch in barbiturate anaesthetized cats and recording from identified oculomotor neurons. Both eyes were enucleated and both lateral and one medial rectus prepared for stretch stimulation whereas the nerve entering the other medial rectus was mounted on bipolar stimulation electrodes which were used for antidromic identification of medial rectus motoneurons.

The shortest latency response we have seen (range 37 − 180 msec) is shown in Fig. 3. This medial rectus motoneuron showed hardly any response to stretch of lateral rectus muscles (histograms to the left) whereas contralateral medial rectus stretch caused a clear excitation. As expected, ipsilateral vestibular nerve stimulation caused a very strong excitation with short latency. Note that the antidromic spike (inset) of this and all other units responding to muscle stretch had longer latencies than the antidromic field potential evoked by medial rectus nerve stimulation. This implies lower conduction velocities for responsive cells than for most oculomotor cells which did not respond to muscle stretch. Responsive cells seem to be a distinct group, located more ventrally in the medial rectus nucleus. We attempted to examine the possible contribution of these motoneurons to muscle contraction by attaching the medial rectus muscle to a sensitive strain gage. No

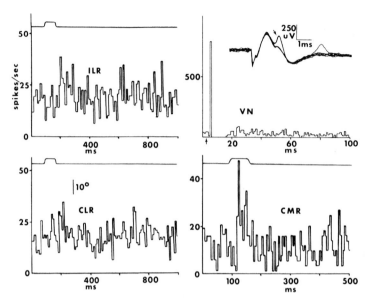

Fig. 3. See text.

change in muscle tension could be detected when any of the three muscles, that had previously been shown to cause motoneuron responses, was stretched. This tends to suggest that these responsive oculomotoneurons with low axon conduction velocities (30 − 50 msec) have a function comparable to skeletal gamma motoneurons, although encapsulated muscle spindles have not been observed in cats (Cooper & Fillenz, 1955). These results illustrate that stretch receptor information available to the cerebellar cortex is not passed on to oculomotoneurons moving the eye. It is therefore unlikely that we have observed the activity of a saccadic function generator at the cerebellar level (Kornhuber, 1974).

The short latencies of stretch responses in the cerebellum (4 − 6 msec) suggest a relatively direct input pathway. In a separate series of experiments, we have demonstrated this to be true. Cats were prepared as for recording in the cerebellar cortex, except that the microelectrodes were directed into the region of the rostral trigeminal complex (nucleus principalis and pars oralis of the nucleus of the spinal trigeminal tract). Stimulation electrodes were placed in the region of cerebellar lobule VI receiving eye muscle afferents. Responses of a trigeminal unit is shown in Fig. 4. Excitation is produced by stretch of all rectus muscles of the same side. This may suggest artifactual stimulation of extramuscular

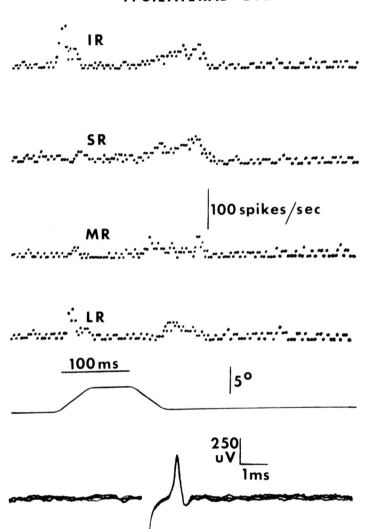

Fig. 4. See text.

receptors, which is, however unlikely in view of the fact that pull of periorbital tissues with the same stimulation parameters produced no response. Convergence patterns suggesting plane specificity were also observed at the trigeminal level. However, we cannot conclude that all the directional information seen in the cerebellum is already available at this level. The bottom trace, showing an antridromic spike in response to cerebellar stimulation proves that trigeminal cells carrying muscle stretch input project to cerebellar lobule VI. Whether these trigeminal cells are monosynaptically linked to peripheral axons is not certain.

In conclusion, our experiments have demonstrated that eye muscle stretch receptors project to the cerebellar cortex via the shortest possible route, the trigeminal complex. They converge there to supply information of great importance for control of eye movements, namely about movement plane and direction. It is, however, unlikely that this information is used to directly generate saccades, since corresponding activity cannot be demonstrated at the level of the oculomotor neurons responsible for moving the eye.

References

Aschoff, J.C. and Cohen, B.: Changes in saccadic eye movements produced by cerebellar lesions. *Exptl. Neurol.* **32**, 123-133 (1971).

Baker, R., Precht, W. and Llinas R.: Mossy and climbing fibre connection of extraocular afferents to the cerebellum. *Brain Res.* **32**, 440-445 (1972).

Batini, D., Buisseret, P. and Kado, R.T.: Extraocular proprioceptive and trigeminal projections to the Purbinje cells of the cerebellar cortex. *Arch. Ital. Biol.* **112**, 1-17 (1974).

Berthoz, A. and Llinas, R.: Afferent neck projection to the cat cerebellar cortex. *Exp. Brain Res.* **20**, 385-402 (1974).

Cooper, S. and Fillenz, M.: Afferent discharges in response to stretch of the extraocular muscles of the cat and monkey and the innervation of these muscles. *J. Physiol.* **127**, 400-413 (1955).

Fuchs, A.F. and Kornhuber, H.H.: Extraocular muscle afferents to the cerebellum of the cat. *J. Physiol.* **200**, 713-722 (1969).

Kornhuber, H.H.: Cerebral cortex, cerebellum and basal ganglia: an introduction to their motor functions. *In:* The Neurosciences Third Study Program. Ed. F.O. Schmitt and F.G. Worden. p. 267, M.I.T. Press, Cambridge (1974).

Llinas, R.: Motor aspects of cerebellar control. *Physiologist* **17**, 20-46 (1974).

Ritchie, L.: Effects of cerebellar lesions on saccadic eye movements. *J. Neurophysiol.* **36**, 1246-1256 (1976).

Ron, S. and Robinson, D.A.: Eye movements evoked by cerebellar stimulation in the alert monkey. *J. Neurophysiol.* **36**, 1004-1022 (1973).

Schwarz, D.W.F. and Tomlinson, R.D.: Convergence patterns of extraocular proprioceptive afferents to cerebellar lobule VI. *Exp. Brain Res.* **27**, 101-111 (1977).

Snider, R.S. and Stowell, A.: Receiving areas of the tactile, auditory and visual systems in the cerebellum. *J. Neurophysiol.* **7**, 331-357 (1944).

Wolfe, J.W.: Relationship of cerebellar potentials to saccadic eye movements. *Brain Res.* **30**, 204-206 (1971).

3. Influence of monoaminergic neurons on the vestibular and cochlear nuclei in cats.

I. MATSUOKA,* Y. CHIKAMORI,** M. SASA,** S. TAKAORI**

*Department of Otolaryngology, Hyogo Kenritsu Amagasaki Hospital, Hyogo 660 and ** Department of Pharmacology, Faculty of Medicine, Kyoto University, Kyoto 606, Japan*

Introduction

The locus coeruleus (LC) is composed of noradrenaline- containing neurons which project to various areas such as the cerebral and cerebellar cortices, thalamus, brainstem nuclei, etc. It has been demonstrated by Sasa *et al* (1974, 1977) that conditioning stimulation of LC produces an noradrenaline- mediated inhibition of afferent transmission of relay neurons in the spinal trigeminal nucleus (STN). An inhibitory role of LC has been also reported on the cerebellar Purkinje cells and hippocampal pyramidal cells (Hoffer *et al.*, 1973; Siggins *et al.*, 1971). In histochemical studies it has been reported that the cochlear nucleus (CN) contains a considerable number of noradrenergic nerve terminals originating in the LC, while the vestibular nucleus does not.

The present experiment was designed to determine the influence of LC on sensory input in the cochlear and vestibular nuclei.

Methods

Twenty-four adult cats of either sex weighing 2.5-3.5 kg were used. All surgical procedures were performed under diethyl ether anaesthesia. The trachea and femoral vein were cannulated. After trepanation of the inferior wall of the right tympanic bulla, the mucous membrane of the middle ear cavity was removed. A small concentric bipolar electrode for stimulating the VIIIth nerve was inserted into the lateral ampulla. After the surgical treatment was completed, the animal was anaesthetized with chloralose (30 mg/kg, i.v.) and immobilised with gallamine triethiodide (5 mg/kg/hr, i.v.). Respiration was sustained with an artificial respirator. Wound

edges and pressure points were locally anaesthetized with 8% lido-
caine spray.

A stainless-steel macroelectrode for recording field potentials and
a glass-insulated silver wire microelectrode with a resistance of
approximately 1 MΩ for recording single neuron activities were
inserted into the STN, lateral vestibular nucleus (LVN) and dorsal
CN, following the brain atlas of Snider and Niemer. Test stimuli
were given to the trigeminal nerve (the inferior alveolar nerve or
nerve trunk just distal to the Gasserian ganglion) for the STN and

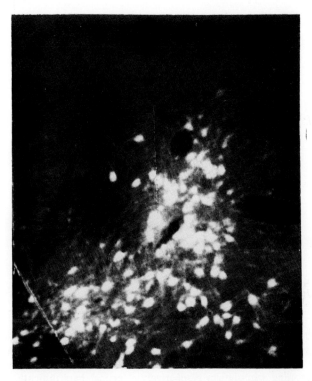

Fig. 1. Fluorescence photomicrograph of noradrenaline- containing neurons
in the locus coeruleus region of cat. There is a group of round to oval nerve
cell bodies and nerve terminals with a strong green fluorescence.

the VIIIth nerve for the VLN and CN. Conditioning stimuli of 4
train pulses (0.2 msec, 0.5-10 V, 250 Hz) were applied to the
ipsilateral LC (-2.0, 2.0, -2.0) at various intervals preceding the
test stimulus (C-T interval). The evoked field potentials and firing
spikes elicited by the test stimulus were photographed.

Statistical significance of the data was determined by Student's t-test. The location of LC was confirmed by histochemical study performed by the Falck-Hillarp method.

Results

Field potential study. Field potential in STN elicited by inferior alveolar nerve stimulation was composed of negative pre- and post-synaptic components. The postsynaptic potential was inhibited

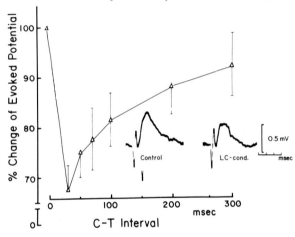

Fig. 2. Effects of conditioning stimulation of the locus coelureus on field potentials in the spinal trigeminal nucleus elicited by anterior alveolar nerve stimulation. Control and LC-cond. indicate the control potential and potentials with conditioning stimulation respectively. Vertical bars indicate the standard errors.

by conditioning stimulation of LC. The inhibitory effect of LC on STN potential was prominent during 30-100 msec of the C-T interval. Inhibitory effect of LC was also observed in the spike generation of the STN relay neurons. Therefore, when this inhibitory effect of LC stimulation was obtained, we considered that the electrode was properly situated in the LC region.

Field potential in LVN evoked by VIIIth nerve stimulation consisted of pre- (P), mono- (N_1) and polysynaptic components. LC

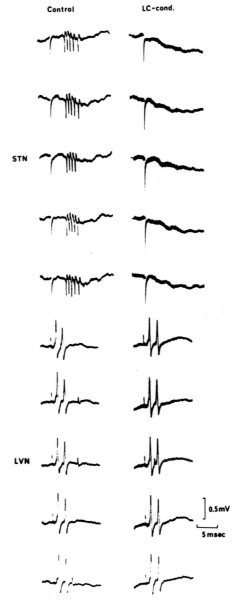

Fig. 3. Effects of conditioning stimulation of LC on neuron activities in the spinal trigeminal nucleus (STN) and lateral vestibular nucleus (LVN). Control STN and LVN show orthodromically evoked spikes without the conditioning stimulation of LC. STN indicates an inhibition of the evoked spikes by the LC conditioning stimulation. Note the evoked spikes on LVN neurons are not inhibited by the LC conditioning stimulation.

conditioning stimulation did not affect any of these components of LVN potential. In contrast to LVN potential, the field potential in CN elicited by VIIIth nerve stimulation was significantly inhibited by LC conditioning stimulation.

Single neuron study. Fig. 3 demonstrates the effects of LC conditioning stimulation on single neuron activities in the STN, LVN and CN. LC conditioning stimulation inhibited the spike generation of STN neurons elicited by trigeminal nerve stimulation. Inhibitory effect of LC conditioning stimulation was also obtained on spike generation of CN neurons elicited by VIIIth nerve stimulation.

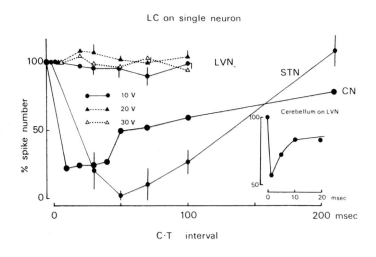

Fig. 4. Effects of conditioning of the LC on activities of the neuron in LVN, STN and cochlear nucleus dorsalis (CN). Note that the LVN neurons are not affected by the LC stimulation, however, the firing rate of LVN neuron is depressed by the cerebellar stimulation inset.

Fig. 4 shows the percent changes of orthodromic spike number in the STN, LVN and CN neurons induced by LC conditioning stimulation. There were no alterations of spike number in the LVN neurons with LC conditioning stimulation. Spike number in CN neurons, however, significantly reduced with the time course of C-T interval similar to that observed in STN neurons. An inhibition of spike generation in LVN neurons induced by conditioning stimulation of the cerebellum is shown in the inset in Fig. 4.

Discussion and Conclusion

The present study indicates that the LC, composed of noradrenaline-containing cells, produces an inhibitory effect on the CN neurons, but does not play a role in the LVN neurons. These results coincide well with the histochemical evidence that noradrenergic nerve terminals exist in the CN, but not in the LVN. Since it has been reported that the inhibition in the STN produced by LC conditioning stimulation is due to noradrenaline originating in LC, it could likewise be concluded that the inhibitory effect of LC on the CN neurons is probably mediated by noradrenaline (Sasa *et al.*, 1974; Sasa *et al.*, 1977). The inhibitory action of noradrenaline applied iontophoretically on the vestibular neurons may be due to a non-specific effect, because the observation was made only on the spontaneous firing rate of vestibular neurons (Yamamoto, 1967). It is clear that the monosynaptic spike of LVN neurons elicited by VIIIth nerve stimulation with a short latency (within 1.5 msec) was unaffected by LC conditioning stimulation. Therefore, the sensory input into the vestibular neurons may be regulated by a cholinergic and/or GABA-mediated mechanism rather than a noradrenergic one. (Matsuoka, 1972; Matsuoka *et al.*, 1973; Matsuoka *et al.*, 1975; Matsuoka *et al.*, 1975).

References

Hoffer, B.J., Siggins, G.R., Oliver, A.P. and Bloom F.E.: Activation of the pathway from locus coeruleus to rat cerebellar Purkinje neurons. *J. Pharmacol. ext. Ther.* **184**, 553-569, 1973.

Matsuoka, I.: Distribution of choline acetylase and cholinesterase and the action of cholinergic drugs on the cat vestibular system. *Equilibrium Res. Suppl.* **3**, 77-89, 1972.

Matsuoka, I., Domino, E.F. and Morimoto, M.: Adrenergic and cholinergic mechanisms of single vestibular neurons in the cat. *Adv. Oto-Rhino-Laryng.* **19**, 163-178, 1973.

Matsuoka, I., Domino, E.F. and Morimoto, M.: Effects of cholinergic agonists and antagonists on nucleus vestibularis lateralis unit discharge to vestibular nerve stimulation in the cat. *Acta Otolaryng.* **80**, 422-428, 1975.

Matsuoka, I., Chikamori, Y., Yagi, N., Domino, E.F. and Morimoto M.: Interspike interval time histogram in the single vestibular neurons in cats. Proceeding of Fifth Extraordinary Meeting of Barany Society. Ed. by Morimoto, M. p. 58-60. Kyoto, Japan, 1975.

Sasa, M., Munekiyo, K., Ikeda, H. and Takaori, S.: Noradrenaline-mediated inhibition by locus coeruleus on spinal trigeminal nucleus neurons *Brain*

Research **80**, 443-460, 1974.

Sasa, M., Igarashi, S. and Takaori, S.: Influence of the locus coeruleus on inter-neurons in the spinal trigeminal nucleus. *Brain Research* **125**, 369-375, 1977.

Siggins, G.R., Hoffer, B.J. Oliver, A.P. and Bloom F.E.: Activation of a central noradrenalinegic projection to cerebellum. *Nature (London)* **233**, 481-483, 1971.

Yamamoto, C.: Pharmacological studies of norepinephrine and related com-pounds on neurons in Deiters' nucleus and cerebellum. *H. Pharmacol. ext. Ther.* **156**, 39-47, 1967.

4. Certain single cell responses within the vestibular nuclei of cat have characteristics which may be related to secondary nystagmus.

G.H. CRAMPTON

Wright State University, Dayton, Ohio, USA

Introduction

The origins of secondary sensory phenomena such as visual after-images, kinesthetic after-effects, some visual motion illusions, vestibular after-sensations, and secondary nystagmus are of continuing interest. The generality of the effect, which includes a post-stimulus response reversal as a prominent feature, was noted as early as the mid-19th century by Plateau.

Both ocular nystagmus and subjective turning sensations show a reversal in direction following the primary or first response. Based on sensation or nystagmus data, this reversal has variously been attributed to a peripheral mechanism (Jongkees and Groen, 1946), a central acticity (Aschan and Bergstedt, 1955), or to an adaptation process (Malcolm and Melvill Jones, 1970; Young and Oman, 1969). Neurophysiological recordings have shown that a peripheral mechanism may be involved. For example (Ledoux, 1961), recording an integrated gross potential from the frog ampullar nerve, found a post-stimulus overshoot that was roughly proportional to the magnitude of the adaptation displayed during long duration stimulus applications. Lowenstein and Sand, (1940) noted an enhanced after-discharge following inhibitory accelerations and an inhibition after excitatory accelerations for some recordings from single ampullary fibres in the ray. Similar observations were reported later by Groen, Lowenstein and Vendrik (1952). And, Goldberg and Fernandez (1971) elegantly showed in peripheral nerve of the anaesthetized monkey that those units which showed adaptation were those which showed overshoot or secondary characteristics. Recordings from central

structures have also shown some overshoot or secondary characteristics, but according to Shimazu and Precht (1965) they are
relatively rare in the decerebrate cat.

The data described here are from single cells within the medulla
of anaesthetized cat. Large post-stimulus responses were found
under conditions which would have been most conducive for
secondary nystagmus in an alert, intact animal; that is, very long
duration angular accelerations separated by long periods of constant
angular velocity. It is the purpose of this paper to describe these
events and to discuss them in relation to secondary nystagmus.

Methods

Apparatus. A circular turntable, 1.25 m in diameter, was mounted
directly on the vertical shaft of a torque-motor rate table. The
single-ended signal from the microelectrode was led through a
cathode follower mounted on the stereotaxic instrument, through

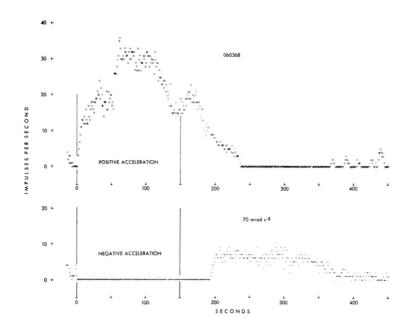

Fig. 1. Response from a Type I cell of the left superior vestibular nucleus during
and following accelerations of 150 sec duration (cat 060368). Each data point
represents the average of three values.

instrument slip rings, and thence to amplifying and recording equipment outside the lightproof and electrically shielded turntable room. Signals were filtered through a frequency band between 300 and 3000 Hz, observed on an oscilloscope, processed by an amplitude discriminator, counted in spikes per second and the data punched "on-line" on paper tape. Subsequent computer operations provided tables and graphs of data on a digital X-Y recorder, including data averages from several accelerations as required.

Electrodes and Histology. Electrodes were electroplished insect pins insulated with successive coats of baked varnish. Electrode tips were less than 6 microns in diameter and were tested by immersion in saline solution under a microscope and observing whether a small bubble was produced at the tip when a current was passed through the electrode. Following the recording, a small current was passed through the electrode by attaching the anode of a d.c. source to the electrode. Current and its time of application were adjusted to produce approximately 0.00015 coulomb. The

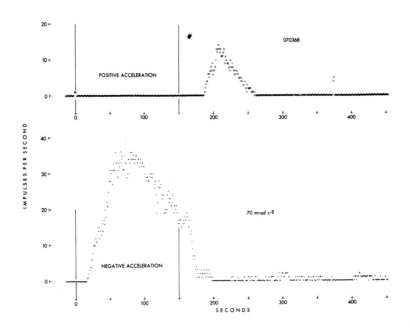

Fig. 2. Response of a Type II cell of the magnocellular portion of the medial vestibular nucleus during and following acceleration of 150 sec duration (cat 070368). Each data point represents the average of four values.

animal was then perfused with saline followed by 10% formalin to which 0.5% potassium ferrocyanide and 0.5% potassium ferricyanide had been added. The brain was removed and placed in this solution for not less than three days before subsequent processing. This procedure, adapted after the method of Green (1958), produces, by virtue of the prussian blue reaction, a small blue spot at the electrode tip site which can just be detected by the unaided eye. A series of 40-micron frozen sections in the region of the dyed spot was then cut and stained with cresylecht violet, and in some cases neutral red. Identification of electrode locations was made by reference to Brodal, Pompeiano and Walberg (1962), and Verhaart (1964).

Procedure. Cats were deeply anaesthetized with Nembutal, mounted in a stereotaxic head-holder, and a small craniotomy was made for the electrode entry. The animal was then placed on the turntable with its head centered over the axis, and the horizontal stereotaxic plane of the head parallel to the turntable surface. The electrode was tilted back 30° from the transverse plane in order to avoid the tentorium and then advanced in a sagittal plane into the medulla. The table was then gently oscillated between successive advances of the electrode until a single cell which responded to angular acceleration was engaged and clearly suitable for definitive recording. Then, in total darkness, the animal was subjected to a low acceleration of 3.8 mrad s^{-2} (1°s^{-2}) until a clockwise (CW) velocity of 5.24 rad s^{-1} (50 RPM) was reached.* The stimulus series that followed consisted of a number of constant angular accelerations of 70 mrad s^{-2} (4°s^{-2}) during which the turntable passed through zero velocity and attained a velocity equal to but opposite in direction (5.24 rad s^{-1} CCW) from that of the base velocity. A series of trials consisted of not fewer than four such maneuvers, two in each direction of acceleration, each spaced at five min intervals.

Results

Figures 1 and 2 show the important features of the central response

*Angular velocity is expressed in radians per second (rad s^{-1}); and angular acceleration, in radians per second per second (rad s^{-2}). To avoid decimal expression within the order of magnitude of greatest utility in vestibular investigations, the term milliradians per second per second (mrad s^{-2}) is employed. The "right hand rule" convention of analytical mechanics is observed. The turntable, as viewed from above, undergoes a negative angular acceleration during a period of decreasing counter clockwise (CCW) velocity or increasing CW velocity. Similarly, the turntable undergoes a positive angular acceleration during a period of decreasing CW velocity or increasing CCW velocity (see Hixson, Niven and Correia, 1966).

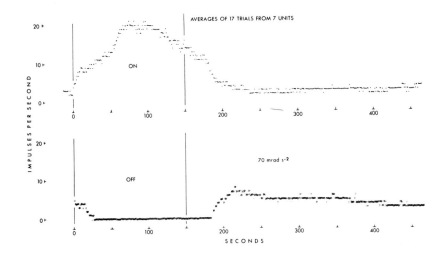

Fig. 3. Average responses derived from seven animals. Type I and II units are grouped according to the "on" or "off" character of the response, rather than by the sign of the acceleration.

to a very long stimulus duration of 150 sec. Resting discharges are usually low, if present at all, thus limiting expression of overswings to one direction, although after-discharges following the "on" response persist for 50-100 sec. Of special importance is the substantial post-stimulus rebound occuring after the "off" response. Often this rebound does not commence until after some 45-50 sec of post stimulus latency. Note that both cells were found to the left of the midline. The Type I (Fig 1) and the Type II (Fig 2) cells are classified according to the currently accepted practice (Precht, 1974). Finally in Figure 3, averages from several units are plotted for the "on" and "off" directions. This composite figure shows adaptation of the "on" response during stimulation, and also the prominent late activity to be found in the post inhibitory rebound following acceleration in the "off" direction. The general rule is that the greater the adaptation during the stimulus in the "on" direction, the greater will be the rebound following an "off" stimulation.

Discussion

Although several investigators have observed in passing that post-stimulus overshoots may be related to the secondary nystagmus, the possibility deserves greater emphasis. The overshoot of the "on" response after stimulation, as seen in peripheral nerve, is not a prominent feature of higher order units and therefore an unlikely candidate for this function. But, post-stimulus rebounds displayed following inhibitory "off"-direction stimulation are very substantial in central neurons, as shown in these data. It may be speculated that the direction of nystagmus depends upon the relative balance between the pre- and post- stimulation discharges. Consider Figs. 1 and 2 together. With a positive acceleration, the Type I unit drives the primary nystagmus whereas the Type II unit elicits the secondary. The reverse would obtain for a negative acceleration.

What of the secondary nystagmus elicited by unilateral caloric irrigation or that produced by angular acceleration in unilabyrinth-ectomized animals? The evidence does indicate that Type I responses are largely ipsilateral in origin and that Type II responses are pre-dominently served through commissural fibers from the contra-lateral labyrinth (Shimazu and Precht, 1966). If this were wholly true, a secondary nystagmus should not be seen in either of these cases. But, some Type II responses can be found following section of the contralateral vestibular nerve (Crampton, 1965, Shimazu and Precht, 1966), and even Type I responses can be found on the deafferentiated side, albeit some thirty days after the ipsilateral labyrinth is destroyed (Precht, Shimazu and Markham, 1966).

Finally, it is noteworthy that with few exceptions, the longer the stimulus duration, the more pronounced is the adaptation; and the greater a unit adapts, the more pronounced is the post-inhibitory discharge. These facts fit the general features of secondary nystagmus (Young and Oman, 1969; Malcolm and Melvill Jones, 1970; Hauty and Wendt, 1960).

References

Aschan, G. and Bergstedt, M. (1955). The genesis of secondary nystagmus induced by vestibular stimuli. *Acta Soc. Med. Upsaliensis,* **60**, 113-122.

Brodal, A., Pompeiano, O. and Walberg, F. (1962). *The vestibular nuclei and their anatomy and functional correlations,* Springfield: Thomas.

Crampton G.H. (1965). Response of single cells in cat brain stem to angular acceleration in the horizontal plane. In A. Graybiel (Chairman), *Symposium on the Role of the Vestibular Organs in the Exploration of Space,* National Aeronautics and Space Administration, NASA SP-77, 85-96.

Goldberg, J.M. and Fernandez, C. (1971). Physiology of peripheral neurons innervating semicircular canals of the squirrel monkey. I. Resting discharge and response to constant angular acceleration. *J. Neurophysiol.,* **34**, 635-660.

Green, J.D. (1958). A simple microelectrode for recording from the central nervous system. *Nature,* **182**, 962.

Groen, J.J., Lowenstein, O. and Vendrik, A.J.H. (1952). The mechanical analysis of the responses from the end-organs of the horizontal semicircular canal in the isolated elasmobranch labyrinth. *J. Physiol.,* **117**, 329-346.

Hauty, G.T. and Wendt, G.R. (1960). Secondary ocular nystagmus as a function of intensity and duration of acceleration. Report 60-29, School of Aviation Medicine, USAF Aerospace Medical Center, Brooks Air Force Base, Texas.

Hixson, W.C., Niven, J.I. and Correia, M.J. (1966). Kinematics nomenclature for physiological accelerations: with special reference to vestibular applications. U.S. Naval Aviation Medical Center, Pensacola, Florida, Monograph 14.

Jongkees, L.B.W. and Groen, J.J. (1946). Considerations regarding the secondary after-sensations caused by a stimulation of the semicircular canal system. *J. Laryngol.,* **61**, 241-244.

Ledoux, A. (1961). L'Adaptation du Systeme Vestibulaire Peripherique. *Acta Otolaryngol.,* **53**, 307-315.

Lowenstein, O. and Sand, A. (1940). The mechanism of the semicircular canal. A study of the responses of single-fibre preparations to angular accelerations and to rotation at constant speed. *Proc. Royal Soc. (B), London,* **129**, 256-275.

Malcolm, R. and Melvill Jones, G. (1970). A quantitative study of vestibular adaptation in humans. *Acta Otolaryngol.,* **70**, 126-135.

Precht, W. (1974). The physiology of the vestibular nuclei. In: Kornhuber, Ed. *Vestibular System Part I: Basic Mechanisms.* Berlin: Springer-Verlag.

Precht, W., Shimazu, H. and Markham, C.H. (1966). A mechanism of central compensation of vestibular function following hemilabyrinthectomy. *J. Neurophysiol.,* **29**, 996-1010.

Shimazu, H. and Precht, W. (1965). Tonic and kinetic responses of cat's vestibular neurons to horizontal angular acceleration. *J. Neurophysiol.,* **28**, 991-1013.

Shimazu, H. and Precht, W. (1966). Inhibition of central vestibular neurons from the contralateral labyrinth and its mediating pathway. *J. Neurophysiol.,* **29**, 467-492.

Verhaart, W.J.C. (1964). *A stereotactic atlas of the brain stem of the cat,* Philadelphia: Davis.

Young, L.R. and Oman, C.M. (1969). Model of vestibular adaptation to horizontal rotations. *Aerospace Med.,* **40**, 1076-1080.

5. Visual-vestibular interaction in motion detection and generation of nystagmus in the vestibular nuclei of alert monkeys.

W. WAESPE and V. HENN

Neurological Clinic, University of Zürich, Zürich, Switzerland

Introduction

Ever since the discovery of the vestibular system as a separate sensory system, a close interaction between the visual and vestibular system has been postulated (Mach 1875). Such an interaction is necessary to explain the continuation of nystagmus and motion sensation during rotation with constant velocity in the light, as well as the lack of post-rotatory nystagmus and the sensation of rotation after deceleration, when vision is permitted. Single neuron recordings in alert animals have shown that an interaction between visual and vestibular inputs takes place already at the level of second order neurons in the vestibular nuclei (Dichgans and Brandt, 1972; Dichgans *et al.* 1973; Henn *et al.* 1974; Allum *et al.* 1976). A summary of the results of the work with monkeys will be given below (Waespe and Henn, 1977).

Methods

Single neuron recordings were taken from the vestibular nuclei of chronically prepared alert Rhesus monkeys *(Macaca mulatta)*. Eye movements were measured by chronically implanted EOG electrodes. Monkeys were placed on a servo-controlled turntable, which could be rotated about a vertical axis and was totally enclosed by an optokinetic drum, which could be rotated about the same axis (further details: Waespe and Henn, 1977).

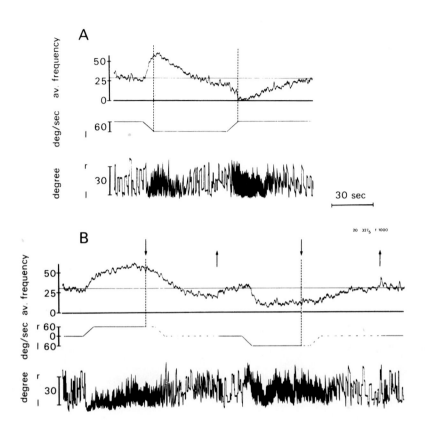

Fig. 1. Type II vestibular neuron during rotation of the animal in the dark (A), and optokinetic stimulation, while the animal is stationary (B). From above, running average (over 1 sec) of neuronal activity, turntable (A) or drum velocity (B), horizontal eye position. In A the typical response to an acceleration followed by a constant velocity of 60°/sec and deceleration. In B the same neuron during optokinetic nystagmus, followed by optokinetic afternystagmus in complete darkness. Downward arrow lights off; upward arrow lights on.

Results

More than 200 vestibular neurons, receiving their main input from the horizontal semicircular canals, have been investigated. About 2/3 of them were type I neurons (activated during acceleration to the ipsilateral side), and 1/3 were type II neurons (activated during acceleration to the contralateral side).

Fig 1A shows the typical response of a vestibular neuron, in this case a type II neuron. It has a resting discharge of 28Hz. During a step acceleration to the left there is an activation, which falls off with a time constant of 22 sec. During deceleration there is inhibition and neuronal activity returns to baseline activity with a similar time constant. Nystagmus also behaves in a similar way. During the constant rotation period before the deceleration there is a continual drop in unit activity below the level of spontaneous discharge, during which time a secondary per-rotatory nystagmus to the right can be seen. All the vestibular neurons could also be activated, when only the optokinetic drum was rotated around the stationary monkey. The turntable had to be rotated to the left to activate this neuron. Consequently, the optokinetic drum had to be rotated to the right, to elicit nystagmus in the same direction

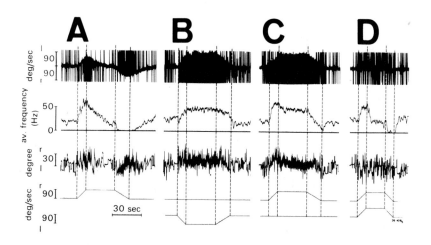

Fig. 2. Type I vestibular neuron. From above: horizontal eye velocity (fast phases were clipped off at an arbitrary level of about 100°/sec), running average (over 1 sec) of neuronal activity, horizontal eye position, turntable velocity and drum velocity. The different stimulus conditions: rotation in the dark (A), rotation of the optokinetic drum around stationary monkey (B), rotation of monkey within stationary drum in the light (C), rotation of monkey with the same velocity as drum in the light (D).

and to activate this neuron (Fig. 1B). While neuronal activity builds up, optokinetic nystagmus develops. The downward arrow marks the time when the lights were turned off. Neuronal activity falls and drops below baseline levels, to which it quickly returns when the lights are turned on again (upward arrow). Nystagmus behaves in a very similar way; after the lights are turned off, it continues as optokinetic afternystagmus (OKAN I), then reverses direction (OKAN II), and is terminated in this figure by lights on. When the drum is rotated into the opposite direction, neuronal activity is inhibited and the correlation between unit activity and nystagmus stays the same (Waespe and Henn, 1976).

Does vestibular neuronal activity always reflect the strength of nystagmus? This seems to be true only over a limited range of velocities or accelerations, although unit activity and nystagmus can always be dissociated. Fig 2 displays the behaviour of a type I neuron to illustrate this point. In A, the monkey was rotated in the dark, and the typical vestibular response to a short angular acceleration can be seen. In B, the optokinetic drum is rotated around the stationary monkey. Nystagmus now reaches 90°/sec slow phase velocity, but peak unit activity is less than in A, the pure vestibular stimulation. In C, the response to a combined vestibular-visual stimulation is shown: the monkey is rotated inside the stationary drum. The response now seems to be a combination of the responses in A and B. There is first a peak in unit activity, followed by a plateau, and very little inhibition during deceleration compared with that found with vestibular stimulation (A). Also, nystagmus shows no reversal during deceleration. In D a conflicting stimulus was given: the drum was mechanically coupled to the turntable and both were rotated together. The conflict is that the horizontal semicircular canals sense an acceleration, whereas the visual system conveys the information that no motion is taking place. There is no clear nystagmus, but the unit is activated during the acceleration and inhibited during the deceleration. However, the time constants of the return phase of unit activity are con-siderably shortened, compared to the response to pure vestibular stimulation shown in A.

The non-linear interaction between visual and vestibular inputs is further demonstrated in Fig. 3. Vestibular, optokinetic, and combined stimulation are compared. Acceleration and velocity were kept the same in each stimulus condition. During, and im-mediately after, the acceleration phase, the response is dominated by the vestibular input. During the constant velocity period the response is dominated by the visual input. During deceleration the combined stimulus leads to responses which lie between those found with the pure visual and pure vestibular stimulation.

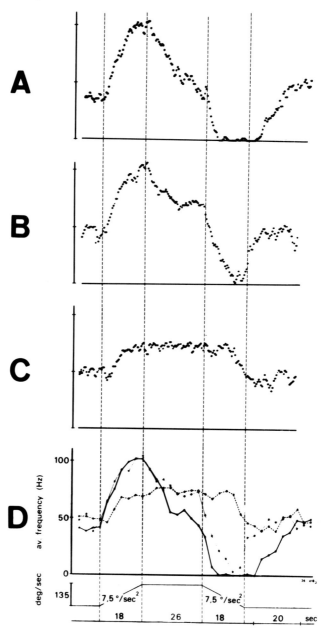

Fig. 3. Response of a type I vestibular neuron to vestibular (A), combined visual-vestibular (B) and optokinetic stimulation (C). In D individual curves (A, B, C) are superimposed for comparison. In A and B the turntable was rotated to the right, in C the drum was rotated to the left; stimulus profile below D refers to all trials.

Conclusions

In summary, it could be shown that every vestibularly driven neuron would also respond if the visual surround was moved around the stationary monkey. This means that the activity in central vestibular neurons is equivalent to relative movement between the surround and the animal. The information signalling whether activation or inhibition came through the vestibular or visual system is already lost at this stage. The vestibular end organ is specialised to sense acceleration, whereas the visual system seems to be specialised to sense velocities and low accelerations which might be below the vestibular threshold. The combination of these two responses compensates for the limited working range of either input, so that the central vestibular system receives information about velocity and acceleration in both the low and high range.

This combined visual-vestibular input is utilised in various reflex responses, one of which is nystagmus, the response we chose to analyze in some detail. There is a precise relation between the unit activity and nystagmus for vestibular and low velocity optokinetic stimulation, and for all forms of after-nystagmus. Unit responses and nystagmus dissociated for high optokinetic velocities or when conflicting stimuli are used. This means that there must be an extra optokinetic input to the oculomotor system which bypasses the vestibular nuclei. This stresses the important, although not exclusive, role of the vestibular nuclei in the generation of nystagmus.

It is tempting to speculate that this interaction might be the basis for motion sensation in general and circular-vection in particular. A further interaction of the visual and vestibular inputs has been shown to exist in the vestibular projection area of the ventroposterior thalamus (Büttner and Henn, 1976; Büttner *et al.* this vol.). This shows that visual-vestibular interaction is not confined to one level, but is repeated at different stages, so that finally the cortical signal might look very different from that present at the vestibular nuclei.

References

Allum, J.H.H., Graf, W., Dichgans, J., Schmidt, C.L. (1976): Visual-vestibular interactions in the vestibular nuclei of the goldfish. *Exp. Brain Res.* **26**, 463-485.

Büttner, U., Henn, V. (1976): Thalamic unit acitvity in the alert monkey during natural vestibular stimulation. *Brain Res.* **103**, 127-132.

Dichgans, G., Brandt, T. (1972): Visual-vestibular interaction and motion perception. *Bibl. Ophthal.* **82**, 327-338

Dichgans, J., Schmidt, C.L., Graf, W. (1973): Visual input improves the speedometer function of the vestibular nuclei in the goldfish. *Exp. Brain Res.* **18**, 319-332.

Henn, V., Young, L.R., Finley, C. (1974): Vestibular nucleus units in alert monkeys are also influenced by moving visual fields. *Brain Res.* **71**, 144-149.

Mach, E. (1875): Grundlinien der Lehre von den Bewegungsempfindungen. Leipzig: Englemann.

Waespe, W., Henn, V. (1976): Behaviour of secondary vestibular units during optokinetic nystagmus and afternystagmus in alert monkeys. *Pflüg. Arch.* **362**, Suppl. R 50.

Waespe, W., Henn, V. (1977): Neuronal activity in the vestibular nuclei of the alert monkey during vestibular and optokinetic stimulation. *Exp. Brain Res.* **27**, 523-538.

6. Responses of brainstem units to visual and vestibular stimulation in the rabbit.

T. KUBO and T. MATSUNAGA

Department of Otolaryngology, Osaka University, Medical School Osaka 553, Japan

Introduction

The interactions between the visual and vestibular systems, have been the subject of some interest and a number of studies have been devoted to these phenomena. From the observations of the optokinetic afternystagmus and sensations of self-movement during and after visual stimulation, visual and vestibular information is supposed to be integrated in certain brain areas (Collewijn, 1976; Zee *et al.* 1976). Recent neurophysiological studies in the goldfish (Allum *et al.* 1976), rabbit (Dichgans and Brandt, 1972) and primate (Waespe and Henn, 1977) prove that the vestibular nucleus is one of the visual-vestibular integrative centres. However, since visual-ocular and vestibulo-ocular pathways are presumed to lie in the pontine reticular formation (Cohen and Komatsuzaki, 1972), this area may also contribute to the integration. We have, therefore examined the visual and vestibular inputs upon the individual neurons in the vestibular nucleus, pontine reticular formation and abducens nucleus.

Methods

Experimental animals were albino rabbits, which were anaesthetized with urethane, immobilized with gallamine triethiodide and maintained on artificial respiration. Sinusoidal rotation in the horizontal plane was used for vestibular stimulation. The horizontal canals, and possibly the vertical canals, may be stimulated by this rotation, since the animal was fixed in a stereotaxic frame with the head being inclined slightly upward. For visual pathway stimulation, a bipolar steel electrode insulated except for the bared tip was vertically inserted into the optic chiasma (OX) and superior colliculus of both sides (SC). The localization of the electrode tip was assessed by observing the mass responses to a flash of light to the eye. Electrical pulses with a duration of 0.05 msec and variable intensities were applied singly or in trains of several pulses with 0.9-1.2 msec interval. Extracellular unitary activity was recorded by a glass microelectrode filled with either lithium carmine or 3 Ml KCl solutions. The recording electrode was inserted dorso-caudally at an angle of 40° from the vertical into the brain-stem with the aid of stereotaxic coordinates (Kurotsu *et al.* 1958).

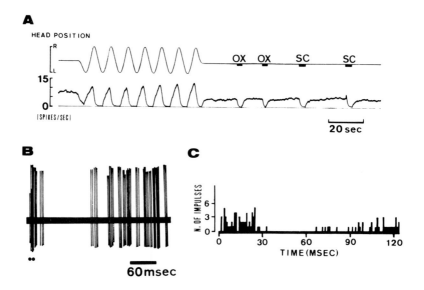

Fig. 1. Influence of sinusoidal rotation, opti chiasma (OX) and superior colliculus (SC) stimulations on left medical vestibular nucleus neuron. A. discharge rate during the rotation and repetitive stimulations applied to OX and ipsilateral SC (indicated by thick straight line). Electrical pulses with the intensity of 6V were given at 60Hz for 4-5 sec. (for details see text). B and C. Unit responses to double shock stimulation (intensity 8V, interval 1.2 msec) applied to the ipsilateral SC. Record B is composed of 20 superimposed traces, when double shock stimulation is applied at the time indicated by the dots. In C270 responses were computed to construct the post stimulus time (PST) histogram. Inhibition of the discharge is prominent during the period of 30 to more than 90 msec after the beginning of stimulation.

Unitary neural activity was amplified conventionally. The electrolytic lesions were made at the stimulating site and the recording site was marked by dye deposition. The sites of recording and stimulation were verified histologically in sections of 50 μm thickness stained with thionine.

Results

Fig. 1 illustrates the responses of a neuron in the left medial vestibular nucleus to head rotation and visual pathway stimulation. The discharge rate of this neuron increased during rotation to the right and decreased during rotation to the opposite side (type II neuron), (Duensing and Schaefer, 1958). Repetitive stimulation applied on OX and ipsilateral SC caused an immediate decrease of the discharge and almost suppressed it. When double shock stimulation was applied to the ipsilateral SC the discharge was inhibited during a period of 30-100 msec after the beginning of the stimulation (Fig. 1, B and C). However, electrical stimulation in trains of several pulses on OX provoked no positive response in this neuron. 27 vestibular nucleus neurons were examined for their responsiveness to OX and SC stimulation. 16 were susceptible to repetitive stimulation at these sites. However, none of the neurons showed a positive response from single to triple shock stimulation at the optic chiasma.

With systematic exploration in the pontine reticular formation (PRF) at the level of the nucleus reticularis pontis oralis, negative field potential could be recorded at the middle to ventral portions of the intermediate zone (1.2-2.3 mm lateral from the midline) following contralateral optic disc stimulation through silver ball electrodes or OX stimulation. Peak latencies were 6.3 and 5.6 msec, respectively. Unitary responses obtained from the cell body or axon were found at the impinging portion where the field potential appeared. In Fig. 2, a and d, it may be seen that the spikes evoked by double shock stimulation of OX are superimposed on the negative field potential with a peak latency of about 5.6 msec. The spikes were recorded from the cell body and the field potential presumably from the axon. Both units exhibited positive responses to ipsi- and contralateral SC stimulation as shown in Fig. 2, b, e and c, f, respectively. Of the PRF neurons which responded to visual pathway stimulation, some were also sensitive to head rotational stimulation. An example of a PRF neuron responding to these two classes of stimulation is illustrated in Fig. 2, g-j. The unit responded to OX and ipsilateral SC stimulations with relatively short latency (g and h). The discharge rate of this neuron increased during rotation of the head to the left and no firing was found during rotation to the opposite side, as shown in Fig. 2, i and j (type I response).

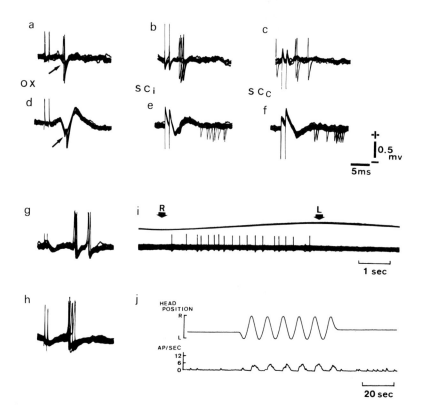

Fig. 2. Responses of 3 PRF units to visual and vestibular stimulation. Records a-c were obtained from the cell body of one unit, and d-f were presumably from the axon of the other unit. In a and d spikes and negative field potentials (indicated by the arrows) are evoked by double shock stimulation of OX. Records b, e and c, f show evoked discharge to ipsi- and contralateral SC stimulations. Traces g-j were obtained from the other neuron located in the left PRF, which responded to OX (g), ipsilateral SC (h) and rotational stimulation (i and j). Latencies of the evoked discharge to OX and SC stimulations are 7.5 and 5.9 msec, respectively. Original action potentials and the discharge rate during the rotation are shown in i and j. Unit is excited by ipsilateral rotation and inhibited by contralateral rotation (type I response). When the head is stationary the unit fires occasionally.

The type I response of this unit persisted even in the dark. Of 86 PRF neurons which responded to OX stimulation in trains of several shocks (latencies varied from 3.0 and 18.0 msec), 22 units (25.6%) exhibited a positive response to rotational stimulation, and were thus assessed as visual-vestibular convergent cells. Using rotational stimulation, 25 type I, 47 type II, two type III and one type IV neurons were encountered in the PRF. Therefore, visual-vestibular convergent cells amounted to 29.3% (22/75) of PRF neurons receiving a vestibular input. Histological examination revealed that the recording electrode sometimes hit the abducens nucleus. Most neurons recorded in the VIth nucleus or from the impinging portion (i.e. 9 out of 10 units) were susceptible to both visual and vestibular stimulation (see Fig. 3).

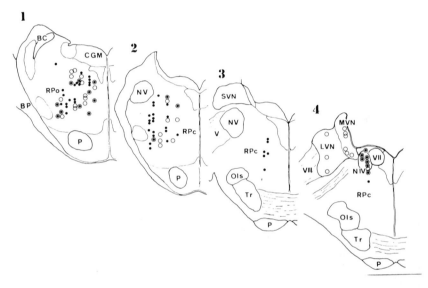

Fig. 3. Localization of brainstem neuron responding to visual and/or vestibular stimulation. Schematic drawings of 4 serial frontal sections from rostral to caudal (sections 1 to 4) are illustrated. Open circle shows the unit responded to rotational stimulation. Closed circles indicate units which exhibited a positive response to OX stimulation. Visual-vestibular convergent cells are identified by double circles. Abbreviations: BC, Brachium conjunctivum; BP, Brachium pontis; CGM, Central gray matter; N IV and V, Nucleus of IV and Vth nerve; Ols, Nucleus oliveraris superior; P, Pyramidal tract; RPo and RPc, Nucleus reticularis pontis oralis and pontis caudalis, SVN, MVN and LVN, Superior, Medial and Lateral vestibular nucleus; Tr, Nucleus trapezoideus.

The localization of brainstem neurons sensitive to visual and/or vestibular stimulation are illustrated in Fig. 3. Units receiving either visual or vestibular input are located abundantly in PRF, especially at the border between the nucleus reticularis pontis oralis and pontis caudalis (sections 1 and 2). Because of the convergence of visual and vestibular afferents in the PRF, two sorts of information frequently overlap individual neurons, as is shown by double circles in the figures. The visual-vestibular convergent cell was not found in the vestibular nucleus, though most neurons in or near the VIth nucleus received convergent impulses.

Discussion

Vestibular nucleus neurons examined in the present study did not respond to OX stimulation applied in trains of several pulses (up to 3 shocks), though repetitive stimulations of OX and SC were effective in provoking a prominent modulation of the discharge. Since it is well known that optokinetic stimulation produces a positive response in vestibular nucleus neurons of various species (Allum *et al.* 1976; Dichgans and Brandt, 1972; Waespe and Henn, 1977), the present observations may be attributed to differences in the stimuli employed. The evidence suggests that a long neural circuit, such as one via the cerebellar cortex, is intercalated between the optic nerve and the vestibular nucleus. It may be inferred that optokinetic stimulation is more effective in exciting polysynaptic neural networks than optic nerve stimulation. Similarly a PRF neuron which responded to head rotation usually was not excited until a high intensity electric current was applied to the vestibular labyrinth, so it may be presumed that the pathway is a polysynaptic neural chain. In the present experiment it was impossible to determine the stimulus intensity at which the vestibular nerve was excited without causing current spread to the auditory nerve so the vestibular input to PRF neurons was identified by using rotational stimuli.

The negative field response was recorded in a certain area of the PRF when the contralateral optic disc or OX were stimulated. Using the same experimental animal and stimulus method (Maekawa and Simpson, 1973) recorded similar field potential with a peak latency of 7-9 msec in the inferior olive. Judging from the wave form and latency characteristics it may be presumed that we have recorded the response from the visual pathway projecting onto the inferior olive. In the PRF unitary responses obtained from the axon appeared at the impinging area where the field potential could be recorded. However, responses recorded from cell bodies were diffusely located at the border between the nucleus reticularis pontis oralis and pontis caudalis; neurons receiving a vestibular input were abundant in this area. Subsequently, visual-vestibular convergent cells were frequently recorded there. Convergence of visual and vestibular information at the level of the PRF would be important in maintaining the oculomotor and postural reflexes, hence the PRF contains oculomotor related neurons (Duensing and Schaefer, 1957) and reticulospinal neurons (Torvik and Brodal, 1957; Peterson and Felpel, 1971). The visual-vestibular convergent cells found in the PRF may contributed to the generation of the optokinetic afternystagmus and sensations of self-movement both during and after visual stimulation.

Acknowledgement

We thank Mr. Koichi Yamamoto who provided skilful technical assistance through the experiments.

References

Allum, J.H.J., Graf, W., Dichgans, J. and Schmidt, C.L. (1976): Visual-vestibular interactions in the vestibular nuclei of the goldfish. *Exp. Brain Res.* **26**, 463-485.

Cohen, B. and Komatsuzaki, A. (1972): Eye movements induced by stimulation of the pontine reticular formation: Evidence for integration in oculomotor pathways. *Exp. Neurol.* **36**, 101-117.

Collewijn, H. (1976): Impairment of optokinetic after-nystagmus by labyrinthectomy in the rabbit. *Exp. Neurol.* 146-156.

Dichgans, J. and Brandt, Th. (1972): Visual-vestibular interaction and motion perception, In "Cerebral control of eye movements and motion perception," (ed. J. Dichgans and E. Bizzi), *Bibl. Ophthal.* Vol. 82, pp. 327-338.

Duensing, F. and Schaefer, K.P. (1957): Die Neuronenaktivität in der Formatio reticularis des Rhombencephalons beim vestibulären Nystagmus. *Arch. Psychiat. Nervenkr.* **196**, 265-290.

Duensing, F. and Schaefer, K.P. (1958): Die Aktivität einzelner Neurone im Bereich der Vestibulariskerne bei Horizontalbeschleunigungen unter besonderer Berucksichtigung des vestibulären Nystagmus. *Arch Psychiat. Nervenkr.* **198**, 225-252.

Kurotsu, T., Hashimoto, P.H., Matsushima, C.J. and Ban, T. (1958): Our new experimental method for stimulation in the rabbit's pons and myelencephalon. *Med. J. Osaka Univ.* **9**, 227-241.

Maekawa, K. and Simpson, J.I. (1973): Climbing fiber responses evoked in the vestibulo-cerebellum of rabbit from visual system. *J. Neurophysiol.* **36**, 649-666.

Peterson, B.W. and Felpel, L.P. (1971): Excitation and inhibition of reticulospinal neurons by vestibular, cortical and cutaneous stimulation. *Brain Research.* **27**, 373-376.

Torvik, A. and Brodal, A. (1957): The origin of reticulospinal fibers in the cat. *Anat. Record.* **128**, 113-137.

Waespe, W. and Henn, V. (1977): Neuronal activity in the vestibular nuclei of the alert monkey during vestibular and optokinetic stimulation. *Exp. Brain Res.* **27**, 523-538.

Zee, D.S. Yee, R.D. and Robinson, D.A. (1976): Optokinetic responses in labyrinthine-defective human beings. *Brain Research.* **113**, 423-428.

7. The vestibular thalamus: Neurophysiological and anatomical studies in the monkey.

U. BÜTTNER, J.A. BÜTTNER-ENNEVER, V. HENN

Dept. of Neurology and Brain Research Institute, University of Zürich, Switzerland

Introduction

For all major sensory systems anatomy and physiology provides ample evidence for pathways and the form in which information is transferred from the sensory endings to the cortical projection sites. Considering the sparse knowledge about the "presumed vestibulo-cortical pathway" the vestibular system is an exception to this rule. Evoked potential (Deecke et al. 1974) and single unit studies in the monkey (Büttner and Henn, 1976; Liedgren et al. 1976) suggest that parts of the ventroposterior nucleus (VP) complex in the thalamus might act as a relay nucleus for a vestibulo-cortical pathway.

In order to evaluate the functional significance of this vestibulo-thalamic pathway, it is important to determine what kind of vestibular information is transferred to the thalamus. Therefore in one series of experiments we recorded from single neurons in the thalamus of the alert monkey, which was exposed to natural vestibular stimulation.

Another series of anatomical experiments was undertaken with sensitive modern anterograde tracer substances to establish the existence of a vestibulo-thalamic pathway in the monkey, since classical lesion studies (Tarlov, 1969) have so far failed to demonstrate such a direct pathway.

Thalamic neuronal activity during natural vestibular stimulation

Single unit recordings were made from the ventroposterior nucleus (VP) of the alert monkey while it was rotated sinusoidally in the

*Supported by Swiss National Fund 3.044.77

dark around a vertical axis. The monkey was sitting upright with his head tilted 25° forward in order to bring the horizontal semicircular canals into the plane of rotation. Horizontal and vertical eye position was recorded by chronically implanted silver-silver chloride electrodes. The frequency of the sinusoidal turntable rotation was varied between 0.01 and 1 Hz. Peak velocities were up to 70°/sec. For quantitative analysis a fast Fourier analysis was applied to both the neuronal activity and the turntable velocity. The phase relation was determined between the first harmonic of both signals.

In general, thalamic neurons responding to natural vestibular stimulation showed a low frequency (average 10-11 impulses/sec) and irregular spontaneous activity. No modulation with eye movements was observed – a common feature of neurons in the vestibular nuclei (Fuchs and Kimm, 1975). This probably indicates that vestibular activity in the thalamus is not involved in the vestibulo-ocular reflex. The majority of vestibular thalamic neurons also responded to rotation of the visual surround (a cylinder covered with vertical black and white stripes) about the stationary monkey. Such a stimulus condition leads to optokinetic nystagmus and to motion sensation, known as circular-vection, in humans. Neurons in the vestibular nuclei also respond to rotation of the visual surround (Waespe and Henn, 1977; Waespe and Henn, this volume).

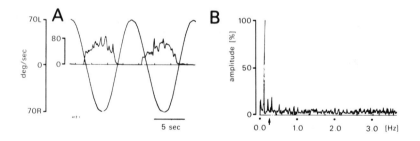

Fig. 1. Record from a vestibular-related neuron located in the thalamus on the right, which is activated during rotation to the right (type I). (A) shows neuronal activity (impulses/sec) and turntable velocity (deg./sec) at 0.1 Hz. The neuron is silent during rotation to the left side. In (B) the amplitude distribution as obtained by Fourier analysis is shown for the same neuron. Results are from 9 consecutive cycles, 2 of which are shown in (A). The amplitude spectrum is clearly dominated by the stimulus frequency (0.1 Hz). The arrow marks the 2nd and 3rd harmonic, which easily can be distinguished from neighbouring frequencies. The phase advance for the first harmonic relative to turntable velocity is 12° in this example.

When the monkey was rotated sinusoidally in the dark, neurons either responded to rotation towards the ipsilateral side (type I) or to rotation to the contralateral side (type II). About 2/3 of vestibular thalamic neurons are type I and the remaining 1/3 are type II neurons. Fig 1A shows a neuron recorded in the right thalamus during sinusoidal rotation at 0.1 Hz in the dark. The neuron is activated during rotation to the right (type I) and silenced (cut-off) during rotation in the opposite direction. The absence of all activity during rotation in the non-exitatory direction was a common feature in vestibular thalamic neurons. At frequencies between 0.1 and 1 Hz neuronal activity showed a slight phase advance relative to turntable velocity (Fig. 1A). Fig 2 shows the phase distribution of 40 neurons investigated at 0.2 Hz. It can be seen

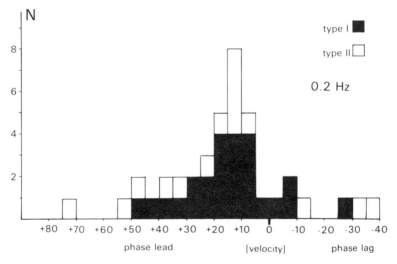

Fig. 2. Phase relation of the first harmonic relative to turntable velocity for 40 vestibular thalamic neurons (25 type I, 15 type II) at 0.2 Hz. Maximum turntable velocity was 50°/sec. Monkeys were always in complete darkness. Most neurons show a phase lead between 0-20°. In other neurons phases were grouped around this maximum with only a few neurons showing a phase lag.

that most neurons shows a phase advance between 0 and 20°. Only a few neurons showed a greater phase advance or lag on turntable velocity. Such phase characteristics for the frequency range between 0.1 and 1 Hz are very similar to the ones found in the vestibular nuclei of alert monkeys (Fuchs and Kimm, 1975).

At lower frequencies (0.01-0.05 Hz) there was only a slight increase of phase lead up to about 30° at 0.01 Hz. This small phase lead implies that the time constants of the thalamic neurons are

20-25 sec. Similar time constants are found for neurons in the vestibular nuclei when velocity steps are applied (Waespe and Henn, 1977; Waespe and Henn, this volume). Thus the vestibular thalamic neurons respond to natural vestibular stimulation in a manner similar to that of the vestibular nuclei neurons.

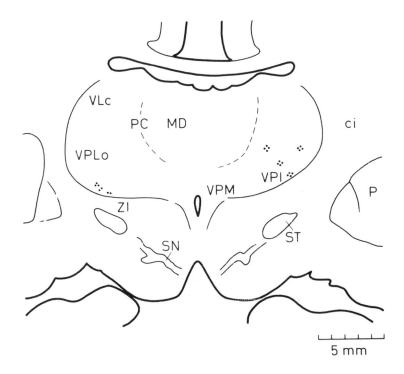

Fig. 3. Schematic transverse section through the thalamus of one monkey. Dots represent the projection sites of axons from the right vestibular nuclei complex, labelled with radioactive amino acids. Small patches are labelled in the VPL and less in the VPI on the ipsilateral and contralateral side. Abbreviations: ci = capsula interna, MD = nucleus medialis dorsalis, P = putamen, PC = nucleus paracentralis, SN = substantia nigra, ST = nucleus subthalamicus, VLc = nucleus ventrolateralis pars caudalis, VPI = nucleus ventroposterior inferior, VPM = nucleus ventroposterior medialis, VPLo = nucleus ventroposterior lateralis. pars oralis, ZI = zona incerta.

Vestibular thalamic pathways

Very careful anatomical studies (Tarlov, 1969) failed to demonstrate direct vestibular projections rostral to the oculomotor complex, whereas electrophysiological studies (Deecke *et al.* 1974) showed evidence for a direct vestibulo-thalamic pathway. New anatomical tracer methods allowed a reinvestigation of this problem. Small amounts of radioactive amino acids (a mixture of tritiated proline and leucine) were injected stereotactically into various parts of the vestibular nuclei complex in the brainstem. The radioactive amino acids, incorporated into proteins, are transported in an anterograde fashion along the axons and into the nerve endings. Their presence can be detected by standard autoradiographic techniques, which leaves a deposit of silver grains over the radioactively labelled structures (Cowan and Cuénod, 1975). Examination of the thalamus revealed that the vestibular nuclei do indeed have a direct connection to the ventro-posterior nucleus complex (VP). The projection is sparse, but definite. It is scattered in small patches as shown in Fig. 3. Both ipsilateral and contralateral projections were found.

The results show anatomically the existence of a direct vestibulo-thalamic projection in the monkey. This projection is not strong, which might easily explain why it could not be demonstrated by lesion studies (Tarlov, 1969). It also shows, that there is no cir-cumscribed, localized specific vestibular relay nucleus in the thalamus, as suggested by electrophysiological studies (Deecke *et al.* 1974). Projection sites were found scattered over the lateral and inferior part (VPL and VPI) of the ventro-posterior nucleus, which is in agreement with single unit recordings in the monkey (Liedgren *et al.* 1976). The ipsilateral as well as contralateral pro-jection might partly explain that the proportion of type I to II units is 2:1, which is the same as that in the vestibular nuclei (Waespe and Henn, 1977). A purely contralateral projection would produce the reverse relationship.

References

Büttner, U., Henn, V. (1976): Thalamic unit activity in the alert monkey during natural vestibular stimulation. *Brain Res.* **103**, 127-132.

Cowan, W.M., Cuénod, M. (1975): "The use of axonal transport for studies of neuronal connectivity.' Amsterdam, Elsevier.

Deecke, L., Schwarz, D.W.F., Fredrickson, J.M. (1974): Nucleus ventro-posterior inferior (VPI) as the vestibular thalamic relay in the rhesus monkey. I. Field potential investigation. *Exp. Brain Res.* **20**, 88-100.

Fuchs, A.F., Kimm J. (1975): Unit activity in the vestibular nucleus of the alert monkey during horizontal angular acceleration and eye movements. *J. Neurophysiol.* **38**, 1140-1161.

Liedgren, S., Milne, A., Rubin, A., Schwarz, D., Tomilson, R. (1976): Represen-tation of the vestibular afferents in somatosensory thalamic nuclei of the squirrel monkey *(Saimiri sciureus)*. *J. Neurophysiol.* **39**, 601-612

Tarlov, E. (1969): The rostral projections of the primate vestibular nuclei: An experimental study in macaque, baboon and chimpanzee. *J. comp. Neurol.* **135**, 27-56.

Waespe, W., Henn, V. (1977): Neuronal activity in the vestibular nuclei of the alert monkey during vestibular and optokinetic stimulation. *Exp. Brain Res.* **27**, 523-538.

8. The influence of the contralateral labyrinth on static and dynamic properties of brainstem vestibular neurons in the cat, guinea pig and rat.

C.H. MARKHAM,* I.S. CURTHOYS,** T. YAGI*

*Reed Neurological Research Center, UCLA School of Medicine Los Angeles, California 90024, U.S.A.

**Department of Psychology, University of Sydney, Sydney, N.S.W. 2006, Australia

Introduction

In the cat there are systematic differences between the characteristics of primary and secondary (brainstem) vestibular neurons responding to horizontal angular acceleration. The secondary cells have a lower average resting rate, but show a greater increase in firing in response to the same prolonged angular acceleration stimulus (Blanks, et al. 1975; Estes, et al. 1975; Shinoda and Yoshida, 1974). One of the aims of this study was to confirm and quantify these differences in awake animals prepared similarly for vestibular nerve and nucleus recordings and to determine whether there are comparable differences in other species – the rat and guinea pig. In addition, we sought to identify the origin of these differences. There are a number of possible causes: convergence of many primary afferents onto a secondary vestibular neuron, influences from the cerebellum or reticular formation. The most likely candidate is that the input from the contralateral labyrinth, acting via the inhibitory commissural pathway between the vestibular nuclei, enhances the response of secondary cells (Shimazu and Precht, 1965; Shimazu and Precht, 1966). This last possibility was directly tested in this study by examining the static and dynamic responses of secondary neurons before and immediately after cutting the contralateral vestibular nerve.

Materials and Methods

Data was obtained from 50 cats, 41 guinea pigs and 20 rats.

Animals of the three species were prepared similarly — each was anaesthetised with ether, received a tracheal cannula, and was placed in a stereotaxic frame. The spinal cord was transected at C_1 and the animal was maintained on artificial respiration under local anaesthesia for the remainder of the experiments. The eighth nerve was exposed by removal of the left flocculus and paraflocculus of the cerebellum. The midline cerebellum was removed in most animals to expose the floor of the fourth ventricle. These exposures enabled the glass microelectrodes to be aimed at the vestibular nerve or the vestibular nuclei under direct vision.

The microelectrodes were filled with Ringers or 2M sodium chloride and fast green FCF. Recording sites were identified by electrolytic lesions or dye spots and the majority were found in the rostral medial vestibular nucleus or the superior vestibular nucleus. Each animal's head was positoned so the horizontal semicircular canal was in the plane of rotation of the turntable and only the response of cells which were excited by ipsilateral angular accelerations (Type I cells) are reported here. Each cell was tested by a standardized velocity trapezoid (see Fig. 1), from rest; ipsilateral angular acceleration up to a constant velocity (usually $200°/sec$, or $400°/sec$ for high acceleration) which was maintained until the neuronal response stabilized; then ipsilateral angular deceleration and finally rest. The magnitudes of the accelerations ranged from $2°/sec^2$ to $33°/sec^2$, and each cell was tested at as many accelerations as possible. Not all neurons were tested at all accelerations; the results from higher accelerations were only used when the response of the cell had approached asymptote.

Neural firing rate from an RC integrator was recorded on one channel of a strip chart recorder, and another channel showed turntable velocity from a tachometer directly coupled to the turntable shaft. At each acceleration we measured the maximum firing rate and calculated incremental sensitivity (S_i) as follows:

$$S_i = \frac{\text{maximum rate} - \text{resting rate}}{\text{acceleration}}$$

S_i is thus expressed as extra spikes/sec/deg/sec². When the cells' response was decreased by the stimulus, we followed the same procedure to measure decremental sensitivity (S_d).

The contralateral vestibular nerve was cut against the temporal bone by a fine iris knife or a flattened syringe needle and the cutting was confirmed by inspection of the cut end using an operating microscope. This procedure was attempted only after sensitive secondary Type I neurons had been encountered. In a few cases

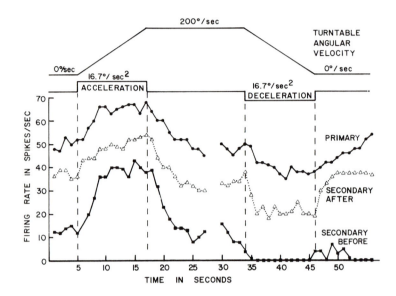

Fig. 1. Typical examples of the response of rat vestibular neurons to long duration angular accelerations (16°/sec² for 12 sec). The top rows show the angular velocity of the turntable and the duration of the angular acceleration stimulus. The graph shows the responses of a primary afferent, a secondary cell before cutting, and one after cutting the contralateral vestibular nerve.

it was possible to hold a neuron through the actual cutting, enabling direct comparison of the same neuron's response to identical accelerations with and without contralateral labyrinthine influence. The results obtained with these cells were generally confirmed by studying a number of other cells before sectioning and after sectioning the contralateral nerve.

Results

In each species the average resting rate of secondary cells was significantly less than the average resting rate of primary afferents (see Fig. 1 and Fig. 2). Immediately following section of the contralateral vestibular nerve, the average resting rate of secondary cells rose significantly (Fig. 2).

In each species the secondary neurons showed, on average, a larger increase in firing to a given angular accleration than occurred in primary afferents. The incremental sensitivity of secondary cells was very roughly between two and three times the sensitivity

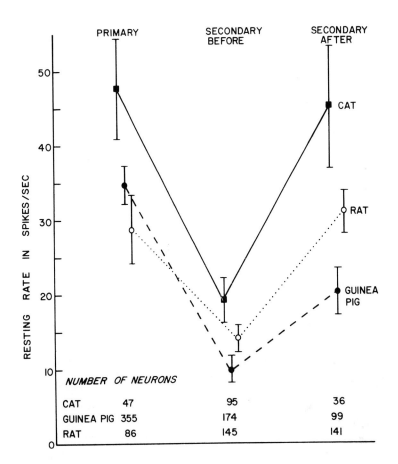

Fig. 2. Mean resting rates and two-tailed 95% confidence intervals for the three species for primary afferents, secondary cells before cutting and after cutting the contralateral vestibular nerve. The numbers of neurons for each species in each condition are given at the bottom of the graph.

of primary cells, and this enhanced sensitivity was maintained over a large range of accelerations. The average sensitivity of the secondary cells after cutting the contralateral vestibular nerve fell to about the level of primary cells (see Fig. 3).

The relation between maximum firing rate induced by acceleration and the integrity of the opposite eighth nerve is of interest, in part because of its relation to sensitivity (see Methods). In rats, 5 second order neurons were held through cutting and tested to accelerations of $16.7°/sec^2$. The peak firing rate was not significantly

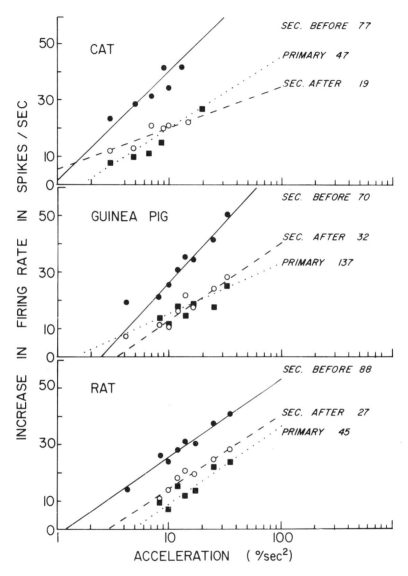

Fig. 3. Averaged increases in firing rate for different acceleration magnitudes for the three species, for primary afferents (filled squares) secondary cells before cutting the contralateral vestibular nerve (closed circles) and secondary cells after cutting the contralateral vestibular nerve (open circles). The numbers beside the categories refer to the numbers of cells studied in each condition — not all cells were measured at each acceleration. The regression lines were calculated for all the data points.

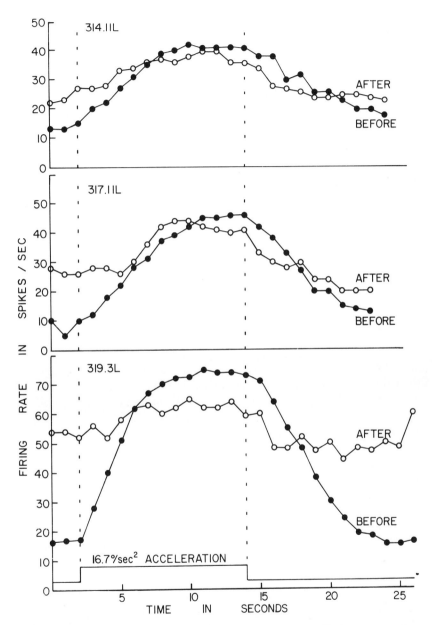

Fig. 4. Graphs of unitary firing of three rat secondary cells in response to an angular acceleration of $16°/sec^2$. Each graph shows the response of the same neuron before (solid circles) and after (open circles) cutting the contralateral vestibular nerve – these cells were held through the cutting procedure.

different before and after cutting (mean before 49.40 S.D. 15.16; mean after 53.80 S.D. 14.19; n = 5 (see Fig. 4). However the resting rate of these cells increased substantially after cutting with the result that their increase in firing to the acceleration was significantly reduced (Rat: mean before 43.57 S.D. 12.49; mean after 18.43 S.D. 4.51; n = 7). Similar results were found in 5 cat second order neurons tested in the same manner.

In the majority of secondary cells in each species the resting rate was so low that the cell's firing was suppressed to zero by even small decelerations preventing accurate measure of the decremental sensitivity (S_d). After the contralateral nerve was cut, the resting rate rose and measures of S_d so determined approximated to the S_d or primary afferents. Because of the measurement difficulties, the numbers of cells were too few to permit statistical analysis.

There seemed to be a few differences between the species but these differences (in e.g. slopes of regression lines in Fig. 3) may have been due to the variable data. The main results were consistent in cat, guinea pig and rat.

Discussion

In this study we have demonstrated differences between primary and secondary vestibular neurons in awake cats, guinea pigs and rats prepared similarly for vestibular nerve and vestibular nucleus recordings. Cutting the contralateral vestibular nerve increased the resting rate of secondary neurons and decreased their sensitivity to angular acceleration stimuli. These changes seem to be consistent with the abolition of inhibitory input stemming indirectly from the contralateral labyrinth via the contralateral vestibular nuclei (Shimazu and Precht, 1966; Precht, et al., 1966) showed that cutting the vestibular nerve virtually abolished Type I activity in the ipsilateral vestibular nucleus, with the consequence that any commissural inhibition exerted by these cells must also be abolished. The following analysis suggests how the abolition of commissural inhibition can account for our results.

In the static situation, cutting the contralateral vestibular nerve increases the resting rate of secondary neurons. This is consistent with the sudden interruption of tonic commissural inhibition.

In the dynamic situation during ipsilateral constant angular acceleration, the firing rate of normal second order neurons starts out from resting level and increases to a maximum. After the contralateral vestibular nerve is cut, the resting rate is much greater and the maximum rate produced by acceleration is either unchanged or only modestly increased. It is tempting to ascribe the reduced sensitivity found in vestibular neurons after the contralateral vestibular nerve is cut to the elevated resting rate. However, recent experiments indicated that at 4-6 weeks after contralateral nerve section, the resting rate has fallen to nearly the control value while the sensitivity remains at the level seen immediately after cutting the nerve (Markham and Yagi, unpublished data; Markham, *et al.* 1977). We would conclude that the elevated resting firing rate of second order canal neurons after cutting the contralateral vestibular nerve has an uncertain role in the reduced sensitivity.

In normal secondary cells during ipsilateral angular deceleration, the excitatory drive from the ipsilateral labyrinth decreases and inhibitory drive from the contralateral labyrinth increases. The resting rate of secondary cells is low and the decreased excitation and increased inhibition cause the cell to be suppressed to zero firing by even small values of deceleration. After cutting the contralateral vestibular nerve there is now only reduced excitatory drive from the ipsilateral labyrinth, not reinforced by the added inhibition from the contralateral labyrinth, with the result that decremental sensitivity is reduced.

This analysis does not exclude the possibility of other commissural pathways being involved in the enhancement of the response of second order neurons.

We conclude that under normal circumstances the contralateral labyrinth exerts a major influence on the static and dynamic properties of secondary neurons, causing the transformation of the predominantly bidirectional response of primary afferents into one which is predominantly unidirectional, and a more sensitive response at the level of the secondary neurons.

Acknowledgments

This study was supported by USPHS Grant NS 06658, NASA Grant NGR 05-007-418 and by the National Health and Medical Research Council of Australia.

References

Blanks, R.H.I., Estes, M.S. and Markham C.H. (1975): Physiologic characteristics of vestibular first-order canal neurons in the cat. II Response to constant angular acceleration. *J. Neurophysiol.* **38**, 1250-1268.

Estes, M.S., Blanks, R.H.I. and Markham, C.H. (1975): Physiological characteristics of vestibular first order canal neurons in the cat. I. Response plane determination and resting discharge characteristics. *J. Neurophysiol.* **38**, 1232-1249.

Mano, N., Oshima, T. and Shimazu, H. (1968): Inhibitory commissural fibers interconnecting the bilateral vestibular nuclei. *Brain Res.* **8**, 378-382.

Markham, C.H. (1968): Midbrain and contralateral labyrinth influences on brain stem vestibular neurons in the cat. *Brain Res.* **9**, 312-333.

Markham, C.H., Yagi, T. and Curthoys, I.S. (1977): The contribution of the contralateral labyrinth to second order vestibular neuronal activity in the cat. *Brain Res.* **138**, 99-109.

Precht, W., Shimazu, H. and Markham, C.H. (1966): A mechanism of central compensation of vestibular function following hemilabyrinthectomy. *J. Neurophysiol.* **29**, 996-1010.

Shimazu, H. and Precht, W. (1965): Tonic and kinetic responses of cat's vestibular neurons to horizontal angular acceleration. *J. Neurophysiol.* **28**, 991-1013.

Shimazu, H. and Precht, W. (1966): Inhibition of central vestibular neurons from the contralateral labyrinth and its mediating pathway. *J. Neurophysiol.* **29**, 467-492.

Shinoda, Y. and Yoshida, K. (1974): Dynamic characteristics of responses to horizontal head angular acceleration in the vestibulo-ocular pathway in the cat. *J. Neurophysiol.* **37**, 653-673.

9. Role of the prepositus hypoglossi nucleus in oculomotor function.

R. BAKER,* A. BERTHOZ,** J. DELGADO-GARCIA,*M. GRESTYt

*New York University, Department of Physiology and Biophysics, 11b, 14th Avenue, New York, N.Y. 10016, U.S.A.

**Conservatoire National des Arts et Metiers, Department des Sciences de l'Homme au Travail, Physiologie du Travail Ergonomie, 41 Rue Gay-Lussac, 75005 Paris, France

tMedical Research Council, Hearing and Balance Unit, Institute of Neurology, National Hospital, Queen Square, London, WC1N 3BG, England.

Introduction

The nucleus prepositus hypoglossi is one of three nuclei found in mammals which have been collectively referred to as the peri-hypoglossal nuclei because they surround the hypoglossal nucleus. The earliest function attributed to the prepositus nucleus was that of motor control of the tongue (Brodal, 1952), however, there has been anatomical evidence that the prepositus is in synaptic relation-ship with regions of the brain stem which are known to subserve oculomotor functions.

Alley, et al. (1975) have shown that the perihypoglossal nuclei project to the cerebellum and specifically to the flocculus, nodulus and lobules 6 and 7 of the posterior vermis. The reciprocal projection of the vestibulo-cerebellum to the prepositus was demonstrated by Angaut and Brodal (1967). Direct projections from the medial vestibular nucleus to the prepositus have been described by Fuse (1914) and Tagaki (1925). The culminating evidence for an oculo-motor function for the prepositus has been the demonstration of a direct projection from the prepositus to oculomotor neurones and from the paramedian pontine reticular formation (pontine centre for lateral gaze) to the vicinity of and possibly to within the prepositus nucleus (Graybiel and Hartweig, 1974; Graybiel, 1977; Ennever-Buttner, 1977).

Methods

Neurophysiological   investigations   of   prepositus   oculomotor functions have been conducted in the anaesthetised and the alert cat. In the alert preparations the animals were implanted with electro-oculographic recording electrodes, bipolar electrodes for the stimulation of individual ampullae of the semicircular canals and resealable windows which were seated into the skull to permit access to the brain for recording micro-electrodes. The cats were trained to accept restraint in an experimental situation which provided for the application of visual and vestibular stimuli.

Results and Discussion

Electrical stimulation of the labyrinth was found to provide a strong afferent input to the prepositus neurones (Baker and Berthoz, 1975), the most common events being a disynaptic EPSP evoked from the contralateral labyrinth and a disynaptic IPSP from the ipsilateral labyrinth. More infrequently the reciprocal pattern was observed. A small population of neurones showed either bilateral excitation or inhibition. In response to a natural vestibular stimulus in the form of sinusoidal oscillation in yaw, the activity of prepositus neurones was shown to be in phase lag with respect to secondary vestibular neurones and in phase lead of the abducens motorneurones (Blanks et al., 1977). In response to constant angular accelerations some prepositus neurones showed a short time constant for the increase in firing rate during the application of acceleration and a long time constant for fall off in activity following the termination of acceleration. The long time constant suggests that some prepositus cells have storage properties which, taken together with the phase data, indicates that the prepositus nucleus has performed some partial integration of the vestibular signals present in the secondary vestibular neurones. Therefore, there is the possibility that the prepositus is part of the brain stem circuit concerned with the operation of integration which has been theorised to be necessary for the central coding of eye position (Robinson, 1975).

Conclusive evidence that the prepositus neurones can effect oculomotor activity was provided by an experiment in which electrical stimulation of the prepositus evoked monosynaptic EPSPs in all third and fourth oculomotor nuclear neurones (Baker et al., 1976). The pathway mediating the projection appeared to be predominately ipsilateral.

The activities of prepositus neurones during voluntary and reflex eye movements in the alert cat conform more or less to three types (Baker et al., 1976). Burst tonic neurones were found whose activity is reminiscent of oculomotor neurones. The burst response was evident during a saccade and preceeded the E.O.G. signal by 6–10 msec. The tonic activity of such units was related to eye position in one direction and the unit was silenced during movement is the off direction. Such neurones responded to reflex and voluntary eye movements and had high position thresholds.

The activity of the second, 'tonic', type of neurone was simply related to eye position with directional selectivity and showed a similar high position threshold. Neurones of a third type, named 'bursting' cells, were found which produced high frequency firing only during saccades in the horizonatl and/or the vertical directions. Some were unidirectional and others bidirectional. Certain neurones of the burst type, located near the ventral margin of the prepositus, also exhibited clear visual receptive fields whose properties were similar to those established for superior colliculus neurones (Gresty and Baker, 1976). It is a strong likelihood that the neurones possessing visual receptive fields are relays on a descending pathway, postulated by Hyde and Elliason (1957), which runs from the colliculus through the lateral pons and posterior medulla to terminate an abducens and hence medial rectus motor neurones.

In the same vicinity as neurones with visual receptive fields, cells were found which were dynamically sensitive and directionally selective to neck movement.

In conclusion, the evidence strongly suggests that in the vicinity of and within the prepositus nucleus there are important motor mechanisms which relate vision and head movement to oculomotor command.

References

Alley, K., Baker, R. and Simpson, J.L. (1975): Afferents to the vestibulo-cerebellum and the origin of the visual climbing fibres in the rabbit. *Brain Res.* **98**, 582-589.

Angaut, P. and Brodal, A. (1967): The projection of the 'vestibulo-cerebellum' onto the vestibular nuclei in the cat. *Arch. Ital. Biol.* **105**, 441-479.

Baker, R. and Berthoz, A. (1975): Is the prepositus hypoglossi nucleus the source of another vestibular ocular pathway? *Brain Res.* **86**, 121-127.

Baker, R., Gresty, M. and Berthoz, A. (1976): Neuronal activity in the prepositus hypoglossi nucleus correlated with vertical and horizontal eye movement in the cat. *Brain Res.* **101**, 366-371.

Blanks, R.H.I., Volkind, R., Precht, W. and Baker, R. (1977): Responses of cat prepositus hypoglossi motoneurons to horizontal angular acceleration. In press, *Neuroscience*.

Baker, R. and Delgado-Garcia, J. (1977): Projection of the prepositus hypoglossi nucleus on to the oculomotor nuclei. In preparation.

Brodal, A. (1952): Experimental demonstration of cerebellar connexions from the peri-hypoglossal nuclei (nucleus intercalatus, nucleus prepositus hypoglossi and nucleus of roller) in the cat. *J. Anat. (Lond.)* **86**, 110-120.

Ennever-Büttner, J. (1977): Presentation to International Union of Physiological Sciences Satellite Symposium on 'Control of Gaze by Brain Stem Interneurones'. To be published.

Fuse, G. (1914): Beiträg zur anatomie des Bodens des IV Ventrikels. *Arb. Hiranat. Inst. Zurich* **8**, 213-231.

Graybiel, A. (1977): Presentation to International Union of Physiological Sciences Satellite Symposium on 'Control of Gaze by Brain Stem Interneurones'. To be published.

Graybiel, A.M. and Hartweig, E.A. (1974): Some afferent connections of the oculomotor complex in the cat: an experimental study with tracer techniques. *Brain Res.* **81**, 543-551.

Gresty, M. and Baker, R. (1976): Neurons with visual receptive field, eye movement and neck displacement sensitivity within and around the nucleus prepositus hypoglossi in the alert cat. *Exp. Brain Res.* **24**, 429-433.

Hyde, J.E. and Eliasson, S.G. (1957): Brain stem induced eye movements in the cat. *J. Comp. Neurol.* **108**, 139-172.

Robinson, D.A. (1975): Oculomotor control signals. *In* 'Basic Mechanisms of Ocular Motility and Their Clinical Implications'. Ed. by G. Lennerstrand and P. Bach-y-Rita, Pergamon Press, pp. 337-374.

Tagaki, J. (1925): Studien zur vergleichended Anatomie des Nucleus vestibularis triangularis. I. Der Nucleus intercalatus und der Nucleus praepositus hypoglossi. *Arb. Neurol. Inst. Univ. Wein.* **27**, 157-188.

10. Cerebellar control of the vestibulo-oculomotor reflex.

S. TAKEMORI and J.-I. SUZUKI

Department of Otolaryngology, Teikyo University School of Medicine

Introduction

The cerebellum is closely related to the vestibular system, both anatomically and physiologically, and it has an important influence on the oculomotor and vestibulo-oculomotor functions. In the clinic, it is sometimes very difficult to discern whether symptoms are caused by brain stem or by cerebellar lesions.

The purpose of this paper is to clarify the influence of the cerebellum on the vestibulo-oculomotor reflex.

Methods

Thirty-eight normal juvenile rhesus monkeys (*Macaca mulatta*) weighing from 2–4 kg were used for this study. Horizontal and vertical eye movements were electronystagmographically recorded using platinum needle electrodes. The ENG was DC-coupled and also electrically differentiated. The differentiated eye movements were clipped to display only the slow phase velocity of caloric nystagmus.

Thermal stimulation of the vestibular apparatus was undertaken to provoke the vestibulo-oculomotor reflex. Twenty ml of water at 27°C or 47°C were irrigated into the external auditory canal for 20 seconds. The maximum slow phase velocity and the duration of the induced caloric nystagmus were then measured.

Amphetamine sulfate (0.5 mg/kg) was then injected to maintain a constant state of alertness in the animals during the experiments. The monkeys sat in a primate chair with the head fixed and the arms and legs restrained.

Lesions were made electrolytically or surgically under general anaesthesia. Electrolytic lesions were made through the electrodes introduced in the vertical stereotaxic planes. Surgical lesions were made by suction-ablation through a suboccipital cranitomy using an operating microscope.

Sufficient time was allowed for the animals to recover from the surgery. Caloric stimulation was applied and the induced nystagmus was recorded before and after the lesions were made. Each animal was then sacrificed and the brains were fixed and sectioned. The extent of the lesion was determined histologically.

Results

Caloric nystagmus in normal animals

The maximum slow phase velocity of caloric nystagmus of 26 normal monkeys, induced by 20 ml of water at 27°C and at 47°C, were 144 ± 36 °/sec and 125 ± 54 °/sec, respectively, with durations of 89 ± 16 sec and 70 ± 9 sec, respectively.

Cerebellar nuclei lesions

After bilateral fastigial and interpositus nuclei lesions (two monkeys), the slow phase velocity and duration of caloric nystagmus increased markedly (Fig. 1, A and B).

In the animals with unilateral dentate nucleus lesions, (two monkeys), the slow phase velocity and the duration of caloric nystagmus, provoked by irrigation with water at 27°C and 47°C, increased duration of response until 14 days after the lesions had been made. However, peak slow phase velocity was not restored to normal until the 47th day. Additionally, there was a directional preponderance of the caloric nystagmus towards the side of the lesion (Fig. 2, A and B).

Nodulus lesion (three monkeys) (Fig. 3)

The slow phase velocity of caloric nystagmus caused by irrigation with water at 27°C was normal. When water at 47°C was used, the slow phase velocity of caloric nystagmus increased after the 31st post-operative day. The duration of the nystagmus was prolonged with irrigations at both 27°C and 47°C.

Uvula lesions (two monkeys)

The slow phase velocity of caloric nystagmus caused by hot and cold irrigations showed increased responses until six days after the lesions had been made, with recovery to normal after 37 post-operative days. The duration of the caloric nystagmus was prolonged for as much as 60 days after making the lesions.

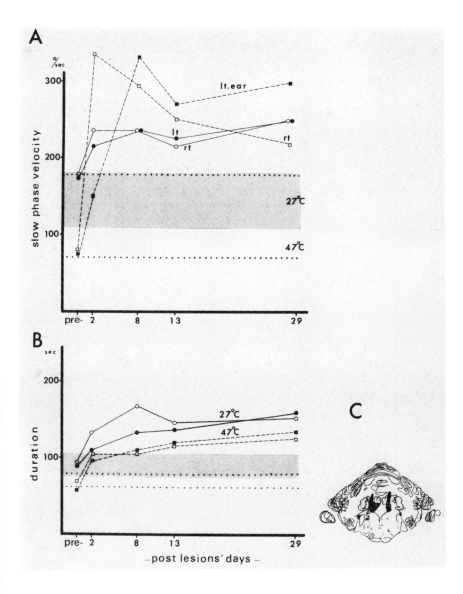

Fig. 1. Caloric responses after bilateral fastigial and interpositus nuclei lesions. The slow phase velocity (A) and the duration (B) of caloric nystagmus are shown. The shaded areas in A and B represent the mean values of slow phase velocity and of duration of caloric nystagmus caused by irrigation at 27°C in 26 normal monkeys. The areas surrounded by dotted lines represent the mean values of slow phase velocity and duration of caloric nystagmus caused by irrigation at 47°C. The open and closed circles show the caloric responses of the right and left ears, respectively. Also, the open and closed squares are the caloric responses caused by 47°C water irrigation of the right and left ears, respectively. The histology of this animal is shown in C. These are the same in Fig. 1—Fig. 4.

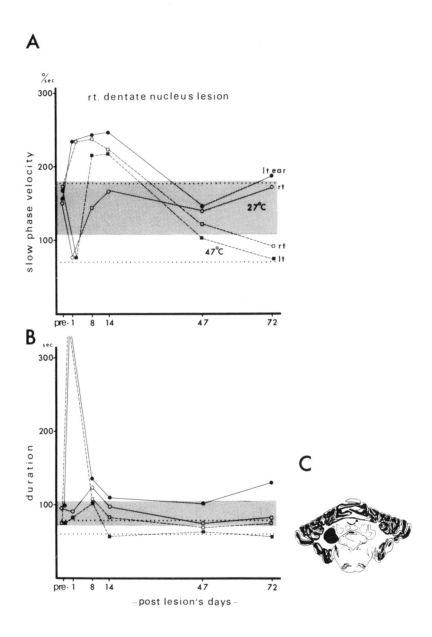

Fig. 2. Caloric responses before and after lesions were made in the right dentate nucleus. Other details as in Fig. 1.

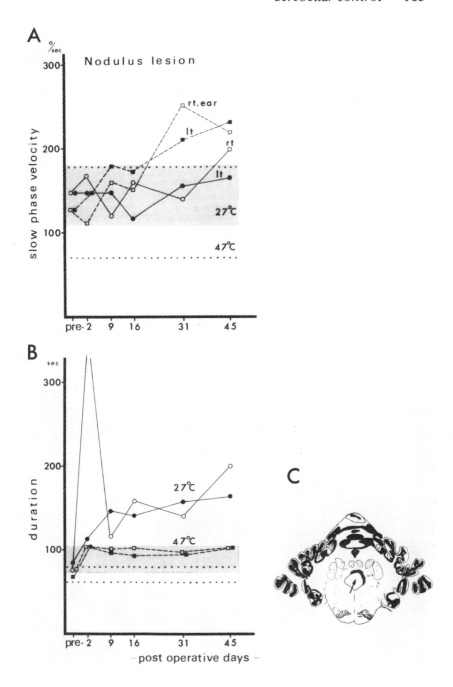

Figure 3. Nodulus lesions. Other details as Fig. 1.

Vermis lesions (seven monkeys)

In the animals in which the lesions were in lobules IV–VIII, the slow phase velocity and duration of caloric nystagmus were temporarily impaired. However, normal responses had returned by the 7th postoperative day.

Flocculus lesions (17 monkeys)

After unilateral flocculus destruction (12 monkeys), the slow phase velocity and duration of caloric nystagmus showed directional preponderance to the normal side. The responses on the intact side were within normal limits but the slow phase velocity and duration of the caloric nystagmus elicited by irrigations on the side of the lesion were smaller than normal (Fig. 4, A and B).

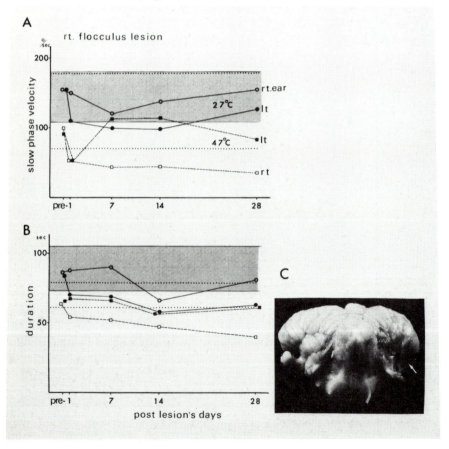

Fig. 4. Right flocculus lesions. Other details as Fig. 1.

After bilateral flocculus destruction (five monkeys), the slow phase velocity and duration of caloric nystagmus were temporarily reduced. However, they returned to normal between the 14th to the 201st post-operative day.

Paraflocculus and lateral cerebellar lesions (five monkeys)

The slow phase velocity and duration of caloric nystagmus showed reduced responses on the day after the lesions had been made, but had recovered to normal by the 7th post-operative day.

Discussion

The primary vestibular fibres terminate as mossy fibres in the flocculus, nodulus, uvula and paraflocculus in the cat. A few fibres are in the ligula and the ventral paraflocculus (Brodal and Hoivik, 1964). The secondary vestibular fibres originate from group X and the ventrolateral part of the descending vestibular nucleus (Brodal and Torvik, 1957). They terminate in the ipsi- and contra-lateral flocculus, nodulus and fastigial nuclei (Dow, 1936). Later studies by Angaut and Brodal (1967) confirm the close anatomical connection between the cerebellum, the vestibular end organs and the vestibular nuclei. The cerebellum and the vestibular nuclei also have fibre connections to the oculomotor nuclei. The vestibulo-oculomotor reflex consists of two parts, the macula-oculomotor reflex and crista-oculomotor reflex. Compensatory eye movements caused by changes of head position were preserved after cerebellectomy according to Magnus (1924). However, cerebellar influences on the otolith-oculomotor reflex is still not clear.

There have been many reports about the influence of the cerebellum on the crista-oculomotor reflex. Magnus (1924) and Dow *et al.* (1938) have reported that caloric nystagmus is not primarily affected by lesions of the cerebellum, though according to Fernandez and Fredrickson (1963), a prolongation of rotatory and caloric nystagmus was induced by lesions of the nodulus in the cat. They concluded that the nodulus acts as an inhibitor of vestibular responses.

Recently, electrophysiological studies have shown that superior vestibular nuclei are inhibited by Purkinje cell axons from the flocculus. Electrical stimulation of the flocculus caused inhibition of vestibulo-oculomotor reflex (Ito, 1972; Fukuda *et al.* 1972).

In our study, the vestibulo-oculomotor reflex, that is, the crista-oculomotor reflex caused by caloric stimulation, showed enhanced and prolonged responses after cerebellar nuclei, nodulus and uvula lesions. However, after lesions in the flocculus, vermis and other parts of the cerebellar cortex, the vestibulo-oculomotor reflex was within normal limits. Thus, it would seem that the cerebellar nuclei, nodulus and uvula have an inhibitory influence on the vestibulo-oculomotor reflex.

References

Angaut, P. and Brodal, A. (1967): The projection of the 'vestibulocerebellum' onto the vestibular nuclei in the cat. *Arch. Ital. Biol.* **105**, 441-479.

Brodal, A. and Torvik, A. (1957): Über den Ursprung der sekundären vestibulo-cerebellaren Fasern bei der Katze. Eine experimentell-anatomische Studie. *Arch. Psychiat. Nervenkr.* **195**, 550-567.

Brodal, A. and Hoivik, B. (1964): Site and mode of termination of primary vestibulocerebellar fibers in the cat. An experimental study with silver impregnation methods. *Arch. Ital. Biol.* **102**, 1-21.

Dow, R.S. (1936): The fiber connections of the posterior parts of the cerebellum in the cat and rat. *J. Comp. Neurol.* **63**, 527-548.

Dow, R.S. (1938): Effects of lesions of the vestibular part of the cerebellum in primates. *Arch. Neurol.* **40**, 500-520.

Fernández, C. and Fredrickson, J.M. (1963): Experimental cerebellar lesions and their effect on vestibular function. *Acta Otolaryng. Suppl.* **192**, 53-62.

Fukuda, J., Highstein, S.M. and Ito, M. (1972): Cerebellar inhibitory control of the vestibulo-ocular reflex investigated in rabbit IIIrd nucleus. *Exp. Brain Res.* **14**, 511-526.

Ito, M. (1972): Cerebellar control of the vestibular neurons: Physiology and pharmacology. Brodal, A. and Pompeiano, O. (Ed.), *Progress in Brain Research* vol. 37, pp. 387-390, Elsevier: Amsterdam.

Magnus, R. (1924): 'Körperstellung'. Springer-Berlin.

11. Studies on eye movement induced by electric stimulation of hippocampus in rabbits; Correlation with EEG and autonomic response during eye movement.

M. HINOKI,* K. NAKANISHI,* T. FUTAKI*, N. USHIO**

*From the Department of Otolaryngology, The Faculty of Medicine, Kyoto University (Kyoto, Japan)

**Laboratoire de Statokinésimètrie, Centre Psychiatrique Saint-Anne (Paris, France)

Introduction

Autonomic centres of a higher order are located in the hippocampus, one of the main centres in the limbic system. Thus, the function of this part of the brain has been investigated systematically from the standpoint of autonomic responses. However, there has been much discussion as to whether the hippocampus is also concerned with equilibratory reflexes, particularly with regard to nystagmus.

In our work, we found that nystagmus can be induced in rabbits when electric stimulation is repeatedly administered to the hippocampus (Hinoki *et al.*, 1975). We also found that the nystagmus of this type is closely correlated with arousal state as revealed in the EEGs from various parts of the brain, such as the hippocampus, midbrain reticular formation and neocortex, and is brought about by repeated electric stimulation of the hippocampus (Hinoki *et al.*, 1975).

Several years ago it was reported that in the hippocampus there are two types of nerve fibres involved in the production of autonomic responses, i.e., cholinergic and adrenergic (Koikegami, 1965). We found that in rabbits, the pupil tended to dilate with anisocoria when electric stimulation was repeatedly administered to the hippocampus (Nakanishi, 1976). These findings suggest that the development of nystagmus and EEG arousal may be associated with hyperexcitability of adrenergic nerve fibres in the central nervous system, particularly of those involved in the neural circuits connecting the hippocampus to the brainstem. Such was the result of a continuous, abnormal excitation of the hippocampus. The present investigation was an attempt to prove the validity of this hypothesis.

Experimental

Methods

The left side of the hippocampus of normal adult rabbits was stimulated by a train of 3V, 1 msec pulses at 30 Hz for 30 sec. The stimulus was given through chronically implanted bipolar electrodes, which had been inserted when the animals were under Pentobarbital anaesthesia. This stimulus was given once a day for 10 days.

Simultaneous recordings were made of the ENG, pulse and EEGs from the hippocampus, midbrain reticular formation and neocortex. In addition, we grossly examined pupillary reactions, particularly the size of the pupil. The animals were not anaesthetized during either stimulation or recording.

To analyse an arousal state in the EEGs, the number of *theta* waves of above 6 Hz in the hippocampus was determined every 30 sec for 20 min before stimulation and for 60 min after stimulation. The reason that we measured the occurrence of *theta* waves of above 6 Hz in the hippocampus is that the development of this type of wave is reported to be in parallel with an elevation of the activity of the brainstem reticular formation.

To analyze the activity of the autonomic nervous system, heart rate was determined from records of the pulse taken every 30 sec for 20 min before the stimulation and for 60 min after stimulation.

Results

1. **Analysis of results with reference to patterns of the EEGs**: When electric stimulation was given to the hippocampus of rabbits, a decreased arousal state in the EEG first appeared. Subsequently, this state changed into one of the following three states. (a) It returned to that noted before the stimulation (Type A, from inhibitory to normal), (b) A decreased arousal state continued during the entire period of observation, and did not return to the pre-stimulus level, (Type B, continuous inhibitory) and (c) A decreased arousal state was replaced by an increased arousal state. Thus, a rebound was noted in the EEGs (Type C, from inhibitory to excitatory).

We found that a Type A response was mostly (i.e. in 93.3% of samples) replaced by a Type C response as electric stimulation of the hippocampus was repeated daily. In contrast, there was no demonstrable change in the EEG of those animals which initially showed a Type B response in the EEG. We also found that a well defined nystagmus was present in 92.3% of those animals which showed a Type C response, and that the development of nystagmus was highly correlated with the rebound of the EEG.

2. **Analysis of results with reference to patterns of automatic responses:** When electric stimulation was given to the hippocampus in rabbits, the pulse rate decreased and the pupil constricted. In the post-stimulus phase, the response was characterised by one of three types of reactions: (a) Pulse rate and pupil size returned to that present before the stimulation (Type I, from parasympathetic to normal), (b) The bradycardia and pupillary constriction continued during the entire period of observation, and did not return readily to pre-stimulus level (Type II, continuous parasympathetic) and (c) The above mentioned reactions were replaced by a marked increase in pulse rate and dilation of the pupil with anisocoria (Type III, from parasympathetic to sympathetic).

We found that a Type I response was commonly (i.e. in 80%) replaced by a Type III response as electric stimulation of the hippocampus was repeated. In contrast, there was no demonstrable change in pulse rate or pupil diameter in animals which initially showed a Type II response. We also found that the appearance of nystagmus was marked in 84.6% of these animals which showed a Type III response, and that the development of nystagmus was highly correlated with the phase of excitation that occurred in a Type III response.

3. **Analysis of results with reference to the correlation between patterns of the EEG and of autonomic responses:** We found that the appearance of Types A, B and C responses in the EEG correlated, respectively, with that of Types I, II and III autonomic responses.

Comment

Nystagmus of central origin, particularly central nystagmus, tends to appear soon after electric stimulation of the mesodiencephalon, and to gradually disappear with cessation of the stimulation (Lachmann *et al*, 1958). This finding indicates that centrifugal impulses from this part of the brain are excitatory to the oculomotor system and influence the development of nystagmus soon after stimulation. In contrast, the nystagmus associated with hippocampal stimulation tends to appear with a considerably longer latency and to increase gradually for a certain period, despite cessation of the stimulation. Furthermore, nystagmus of this type develops only after repeated electric stimulation of the hippocampus.

With regard to the mode of action of the hippocampus upon the brainstem, there is some evidence that the hippocampus initially has an inhibitory effect on the activity of the brainstem. For example, we have found that excitation of the hippocampus inhibits the spontaneous nystagmus derived from the brainstem (Nakanishi, 1976).

From these results, it may be suggested that the nystagmus following hippocampal stimulation may be induced by a rebound in the activity of the oculomotor system, which occurs with repeated activation of the hippocampal inhibitory mechanism.

Several years ago it was demonstrated that in the hippocampus there are two types of autonomic nerve fibres, i.e., cholinergic and adrenergic (Koikegami, 1965), and we found that when electric stimulation of the hippocampus was repeated, that this was accompanied by the development of nystagmus. These findings lead to the hypothesis that the development of nystagmus may be based on over-excitation of the oculomotor system, particularly the brainstem activating system, which is due to an hyperexcitability of adrenergic fibres in the central nervous system. However, systematic investigations have not yet been carried out to validate this hypothesis.

In the present experiments, we found that in rabbits the development of nystagmus was closely correlated with the rebound excitation of the EEG (Type C response), brought about by repeated electrical stimulation of the hippocampus. This phase in the EEG was usually accompanied by autonomic responses suggestive of sympathetic hyperexcitability, i.e., the phase of excitation noted in a Type III response. In contrast, there was little evidence of nystagmus when animals showed decreased EEG arousal, such as Types A and B. Furthermore, Type A and B responses were usually correlated with Type I and II autonomic responses which are suggestive of parasympathetic hyperexcitability. These findings support the hypothesis mentioned above. In other experiments we also confirmed that nystagmus was induced, or activated, by adrenaline in animals which showed a Type III response. In contrast, neither obvious induction nor activation of nystagmus was observed when animals showed Type I and II responses, particularly the latter. A similar relationship was observed between the development of nystagmus and patterns of EEG arousal. That is, we found that nystagmus was typically induced or activated by adrenaline when animals showed a Type C response of the EEG. In contrast, no obvious change of nystagmus was observed in animals with Type A and B responses, particularly the latter. These results also support the hypothesis mentioned above.

It has previously been reported that on excitation of the hippocampus, parasympathetic and sympathetic responses alternatively appear (Akimoto, 1961, cited by Koikegami, 1965). This observation is in accord with our results, since we also found that on excitation of the hippocampus, a parasympathetic state first appeared and was followed by a sympathetic one. However, systematic investigations have not been carried out to determine how the two types of autonomic responses reported here are correlated with equilibrium reflexes, particularly with regard to nystagmus.

Conclusion

Development of nystagmus in rabbits is closely correlated with that of an arousal state in the EEG, brought about by repeated electric stimulation of the hippocampus. This arousal state is usually accompanied by autonomic responses suggestive of sympathetic hyperexcitability. From these findings and previous reports, we conclude that repeated activation of an inhibitory mechanism of the hippocampus on the brainstem eventually induces a rebound in the activity of the latter, which results in the production of nystagmus. It is suggested that this rebound is closely correlated with hyperexcitability of adrenergic nerve fibres, presumably involved in the neural circuits which connect the hippocampus to the brainstem.

Acknowledgement

Gratitude is due to M. Ohara, Kyoto University, for assistance with the manuscript.

References

Hinoki, M., Nakanishi, K., Hine, S., Ushio, N. and Imai, Y. (1975): Functional correlation between the limbic system and the oculomotor system; analysis of the mechanism of the correlation based on nystagmus induced by electric stimulation of the hippocampus in rabbits. *Proc. 5th Extraordinary Meeting of the Bárány Society (Kyoto)*, pp. 53-57.

Koikegami, S. (1965): 'The limbic system'. *Chugai-Igakusha, Tokyo*, pp. 266-271.

Lachmann, J., Bergmann, F. and Monnier, M. (1958): Central nystagmus elicited by stimulation of the meso-diencephalon in the rabbit. *Amer. J. Physiol.* **193**, 328-334.

Nakanishi, K. (1976). Functional correlation between the limbic system and the oculomotor system; observations on the correlation between changes in the ENG and EEGs caused by electric stimulation of the hippocampus in rabbits. *Pract. Otol. (Kyoto)* **69** (Suppl. 3), 1954-1982.

Anatomy

1. Scanning electron microscopic observations of the inner ear after experimental obliteration of the endolymphatic duct and sac of guinea pigs.

W. OSHIMA, M. SUZUKI, M. MACHINO*, S. SHIDA

Departments of Otorhinolaryngology and Respiratory* Disease, Osaka Hospital of Japanese National Railways, Abenoku, Minami 1-3-5, Osaka, JAPAN 545.

Introduction

Though many papers concerning the ultrastructure of the cochlear system and vestibular organs have been published, the papers treating the vestibular organs with experimental endolymphatic hydrops are few. Experimental endolymphatic hydrops seems not to damage the vestibular organ at its early stage, either physiologically or in terms of light microscopy. This study is concerned with morphological changes occurring in the vestibular organs resulting from experimental endolymphatic hydrops. Experimental endolymphatic hydrops was produced by obliteration of the endolymphatic duct and sac in guinea pigs and the vestibular organs were observed under a scanning electron microscope. The present study treats mainly with the sensory hair changes.

Materials and Methods

Ten guinea pigs with normal Preyer's reflexes and normal righting reflexes, weighing 250-350 grams were used. The left ear of each animal was operated on and the right used as a control. The endolymphatic sac was approached extradurally, the subosteal portion of the sac was drilled as far as the duct portions. A sufficient amount of bone wax was plugged into the drilled end of the endolymphatic duct to close it completely. On the 28th postoperative day each animal was sacrificed by decapitation to remove the bulla. Three were decalcified and embedded in celloidine to confirm the occurrence of hydrops under the light microscope. Two were used to examine SDH reaction in the sensory cells of the cochlea and vestibular organ obtained by a cochlear surface preparation method. Five were used for scanning electron microscopic study. Immediately after the ossicles had been removed, two percent of glutaraldehyde solution buffered with phosphate was immersed through the oval and round windows and through artificial pores at the apex of the cochlea and the three semicircular canals. The bulla was fixed for one hour at room temperature. After fixation, the saccule, utricle and cristae were taken out and the otolithic membrane and cupula were removed. The macula saculi, macula utriculi and crista ampullaris were dehydrated in a graded ethanol series and placed in iso-amyl acetate for fifteen minutes, twice. The critical point drying process using carbon dioxide was applied. The dried specimens were coated with gold by ion sputtering. For the observations a scanning electron microscope ASID attached JEM 100C was used.

Results

Following recovery from the anaesthesia during the operation no animals showed any signs of pathological symptoms. During the first week after the operation, the weight of the animals decreased. At latest at the end of the third week postoperatively, their body weights exceeded preoperative weights.

Light-microscopically no endolymphatic hydrops was observed in the right ear. In the left ear, the cochlear duct was dilated in all turns, and the saccule and utricle were also expanded. No alteration was observed in the ducts and their ampullae; the macula sacculi, macula utriculi and crista ampullaris on both sides revealed similar SDH reaction. The vestibules functioned normally: The animals showed a well balanced posture, normal righting reflexes, and normal caloric responses.

The scanning electron-microscopic study revealed various changes of sensory hairs in the vestibule of the operated ear. Sensory hairs of the right ear showed normal morphology. The macula sacculi, macula utriculi and crista ampullaris were observed.

Macula sacculi

Both in the centre and on the margin, the disappearance of the sensory hairs was remarkable. Remaining sensory hairs fused to form elongated bundles, and globular clots with wrinkled surface. Rarely, kinocilia kept their original length. At the cell-surface, projected microvilli and narrow gaps between the foot of the sensory hairs and cell surface were seen.

Macula utriculi

Sensory hairs disappeared less often in the striola portion of utricule than in saccule and in crista ampullaris. The sensory hairs fused to form a bundle or a globule with a wrinkled surface (Fig. 1). The remaining kinocilium was often bent.

Crista ampullaris

In the central portion of the lateral semicircular canal, sensory hairs frequently disappeared. At the periphery, kinocilia kept straight and stereocilia fused slightly (Fig. 2). In the intermediate zone between the centre and the periphery, sensory hairs fused to form various shapes. At the cell surface projected microvilli and minute protrusions were observed. Altered patterns of sensory hairs in the three semicircular canals were very similar.

Discussion

According to Kimura (1967, 1968) experimental endolymphatic hydrops appeared in the saccule two weeks postoperatively in the guinea pig. The saccule membrane first touched the opposite wall or foot plate of the stapes. Hydrops in the utricle was not always marked and some cases showed no hydrops. In the cochlea and in the saccule the hydrops was more prominent than in the utricle. Constant occurrence of the hydrops in the utricle was seen after one to two postoperative months. Konishi and Shea (1975) also described the following.

After one week to two months postoperatively, the hydrops was evident in the vestibular organ except in the semicircular ducts and the ampullae. During this period there were no alterations of the semicircular ducts and their ampullae. There was slight dilation of the crus commune but no obvious changes were disclosed in the sensory cells under the light microscope.

It follows that one month postoperatively is the time when the experimental endolymphatic hydrops must have had some influence upon vestibular sensory cells ultrastructurally. Scanning electron microscopy provided further information about the morphological alteration in sensory hairs.

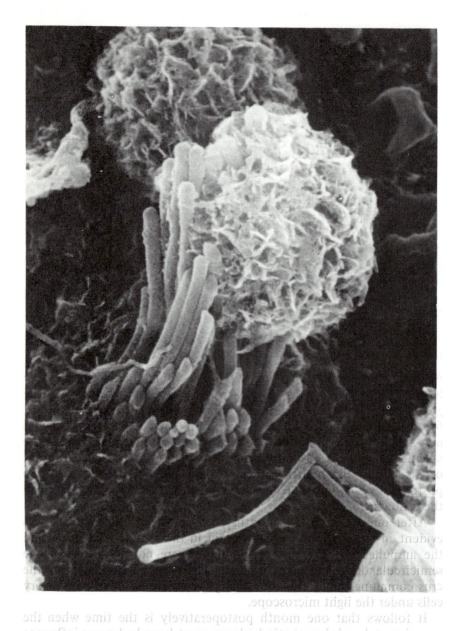

Fig. 1. Scanning electron micrograph of the peripheral part of macula utriculi. Two globule-body with wrinkled surface may be protrusions from cytoplasm. Some sensory hairs were shorter, but step-like feature of hair arrangement was preserved. A bent kinocilium was seen in the lower part. Mag X 10,000.

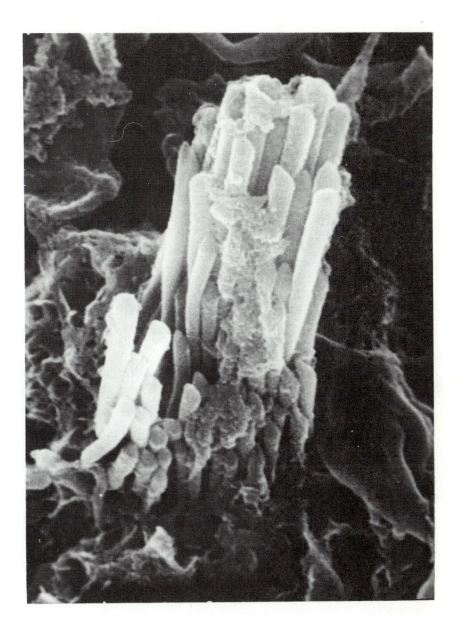

Fig. 2. Scanning electron micrograph of the intermediate part of crista ampullaris. Fusion and shortening of stereocilia was noted. The arrangement pattern of hairs was incompletely preserved. Cell surface looked uneven. Mag X 10,000.

Changes of the sensory hairs have been described in experimental animals with ototoxic agents (Durall and Wersäll, 1963: Harada, 1973; Lundquist and Wersäll, 1967: Lundquist, 1969: Wersäll et al., 1971), on genetically deaf animals (Ernston et al., 1970), and on X-ray animals (Bredberg et al., 1970). Changes such as fusion, bleb-formation, globule formation, diminuition of length, complete loss varied. In the case of Menière's disease, the sensory hairs disappeared in the central part of the crista ampullaris and short or irregularly waved hairs lost the so-called step-like pattern arrangement in the marginal part. On the surface, minute protrusions were seen, suggesting protoplasmic origin (Harada, 1973).

In otolithic organs, the lesion resulting from administration of ototoxic antibiotics was more severe in the utricle than in the saccule (Nagaba, 1968; Lindeman, 1969; Watanuki and Meyer zum Gottesberge, 1971; Wersäll et al., 1971). In our experiment, sensory hairs of the saccule were damaged most severely; sensory hairs of the central portion of crista ampularis were more severely affected in the marginal portion. This alteration in the crista was similar to the alteration observed in the human ear with Menière's disease (Harada, 1973). With respect to the pattern of sensory hair degeneration, the changes with endolymphatic hydrops are thus analogous to the degenerating process which has been reported in the above literature. The relationship between the endolymphatic hydrops and Menière's disease is still controversial (Kimura, 1967, 1968; Harada, 1973). The question to be solved in the near future is whether the mechanical or the chemical disorder influences the sensory hairs in the vestibule and can damaged sensory hairs recover?

Minute globular protrusions and unevenness of the sensory cell surface were noted. Protrusions induced by antibiotics contained cytoplasmic organelles (Wersäll et al., 1971). Unusual protrusions on the sensory cell surface may have cytoplasmic origin (Harada, 1973).

References

Bredberg G., Lindeman H., Ades H., West R. and Engström H. (1970): Scanning electron microscopy of the organ of Corti. *Science* 170, 861-863.

Duvall J.A. and Wersäll J. (1963): Site of action of streptomycin upon inner ear sensory cells. *Acta Otolaryngol* 57, 581-598.

Ernston S., Lundquist P.G., Wendenberg E. and Wersäll J. (1969): Morphological changes in vestibular hair cells in a strain of the waltzing guinea pig. *Acta Otolaryngol* 67, 521-534.

Harada Y. (1973): Observation of morphological changes in the vestibular sensory epithelia. *Equilibrium Res.* 3, 48-54.

Kimura R.S. (1967): Experimental blockage of the endolymphatic duct and sac. Its effect on the inner ear of guinea pig. A study on endolymphatic hydrops. *Ann. Otol.* **76**, 446-452.

Kimura R.S. (1968): Experimental production of endolymphatic hydrops in 'Menière disease', pp. 557-592, Saunders, New York.

Konishi S. and Shea J.J.Jr. (1975): Experimental endolymphatic hydrops and its relief by interrupting the lateral semicircular duct in guinea pig. *J. Laryngol Otol.* **89**, 577-592.

Lindeman H.H. (1969): Regional differences in sensitivity of the vestibular sensory epithelia to ototoxic antibiotics. *Acta Otolaryngol* **67**, 177-189.

Lundquist P.-G. (1969): Ototoxicity of gentamycin. *J. infect. Dis.* **119**, 410-416.

Lundquist P.-G. and Wersäll J. (1967): The ototoxic effect of gentamycin – an electron microscopical study in 'Gentamycin first international symposium', pp. 26-46, Schwabe & Co., Basel.

Nagaba M. (1968): Electron microscopic study of semicircular canal organs and otolith organs of squirrel monkeys after administration of streptomycin. *Acta Otolaryngol* **67**, 117-189.

Watanuki K. and Meyer zum Gottesberge A. (1971): Toxic effects of streptomycin and kanamycin upon the sensory epithelium of the cristae ampullaris. *Acta Otolaryngol* **72**, 59-67.

Wersäll J., Bjorkroth B., Flock A. and Lundquist P.-G. (1971): Sensory hair fusion in vestibular sensory cells after gentamycin exposure. A transmission and scanning electron microscope study. *Arch. klin. exp. Ohr-, Nas-u. Kehlk- Heilk.* **200**, 1-14.

Winther F.O. (1970): X-ray irradiation of the inner ear of the guinea pig. Thesis cited in the above literature.

2. Pathology of the vestibular aqueduct and endolymphatic sac in temporal bones with endolymphatic hydrops.

T. EGAMI and I. SANDO

Department of Otolaryngology, University of Pittsburgh, School of Medicine, Eye and Ear Hospital, Pittsburgh, PA 15213 and Department of Otolaryngology, University of Colorado Medical Center, Denver, Co 80220

Introduction

Hallpike and Cairns (1938) reported two cases of Meniere's disease which demonstrated endolymphatic hydrops and endolymphatic sac (ES) pathology, with perisaccular fibrosis replacing loose connective tissue in the temporal bones. Black *et al.* (1969) reported vestibular aqueduct (VA) pathology in a case of Meniere's disease. The purpose of this paper is to present the relationship between hydrops and VA or ES pathology as observed in 11 temporal bones.

Materials and Methods

Eleven temporal bones (10 cases) with histological endolymphatic hydrops were selected for this study. One case showed bilateral hydrops; nine others had unilateral hydrops. Symptoms, history, and clinical diagnoses of these cases are listed in Table I.

The criteria for definition of histological hydrops were as follows: (1) extension of Reissner's membrane in the cochlea, excluding cases with hydrops restricted to only the apical turn; (2) bulging of the labyrinthine membrane beyond the line of the reinforced arch in the saccule; (3) out-pouching of the labyrinthine membrane of the utricle or semicircular canals.

The temporal bones were removed from refrigerated cadavers, fixed with 10% formalin, decalcified, embedded in celloidin, sectioned horizontally at 20 microns, and every tenth section was stained with hematoxylin and eosin for light microscopic study.

The primary sites studied were the VA and ES. Measurements of the Sinus II portion of the ES as described by Anson and Nesselrod (1936), and of its neighbouring portion of VA, were made with the microprojector. In four temporal bones which had no obvious Sinus II portions of the ES, the mid-portions of the ES and VA were arbitrarily selected as the measuring points. The condition of the epithelial cells and perisaccular tissue of each ES was also investigated.

In addition to these observations, a medial view of each VA and posterior semicircular canal (Egami, Sando, and Black, 1977) was reconstructed by modifying Schuknecht's cochlear reconstruction method (Schuknecht, 1953), so that the funnel-shaped dilatation and course of the VA in the vertical plane could be evaluated. The medial-view reconstruction was essential to correct erroneous impressions of VA configuration created by various horizontal sectioning angles.

Findings

The locations of hydrops and other major pathological findings in each ear are shown in Table I. The tracings of the VA and ES at the Sinus II portion, and pathological findings in the VA and ES, are shown in Figure 1. This Figure facilitates the comparison of VA and ES configurations from the two sides in each case.

Case 1 showed small, short, straight, simple, tube-like VA and ES bilaterally. The distal VA was small and oval-shaped, rather than spindle-shaped and elongated, as shown in the horizontal section. Medial-view reconstruction of these ears revealed absence of the funnel-shaped dilatation of the distal VA and an abnormally antero-superiorly-located distal VA and operculum. There was no inferior bending of the VA at the isthmus portion. No rugose portion was seen in the ES, and epithelial cells were flattened. The bony wall between the posterior cranial fossa and the posterior semicircular canal was very thin, and no peri-aqueductal air cells were present. In addition, this case showed bilateral multifocal otosclerotic foci, but no invasion was seen around the VA of either ear.

Case 2 (Lt) and case 3 (Rt) also showed small, oval-shaped VA, rather than spindle-shaped, elongated VA, in the horizontal sections. The medial-view reconstructions of these cases showed hypoplastic, funnel-shaped VA dilatations, and steep inferior bending of the VA at the isthmus portions.

The location of the operculum in the hydropic ears was more infero-anterior than in the opposite, normal ears. The rugose portion of the ES of the affected ears was seen only in the distal end of the VA, which demonstrated a small lumen and flat epithelial cells.

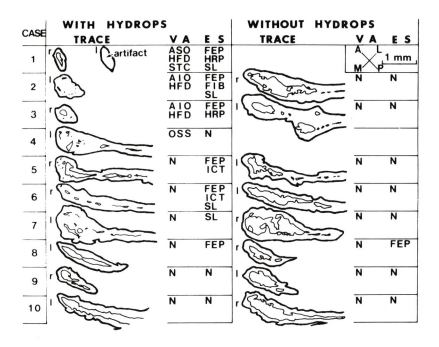

Fig. 1. *Tracings and Pathological Findings of the Vestibular Aqueduct (VA) and Endolymphatic Sac (ES) in Hydrops.* The thick line of the tracing outlines the VA and the thin line outlines the ES. The left-ear tracings are mirror images to facilitate comparison with the right ears. Note that case 1 had bilateral hydrops; therefore, both traces were placed on the 'hydrops' side. The existence of hydrops in case 4 could not be evaluated due to processing artifacts. Abbreviations: AIO = antero-inferiorly located cranial orifice; ASO = antero-superiorly located cranial orifice; FEP = flattened epithelial cells; FIB = fibrosis; HFD = hypoplastic funnel-shaped dilatation; HRP = hypoplastic rugose portion; ICT = increased connective tissue; N = normal; OSS = ossification; SL = small lumen; STC = straight course; A = anterior; P = posterior; L = lateral; M = medial.

Peri-aqueductal air cells were less marked than those on the opposite, normal sides.

Case 4 (Lt) showed bony obliteration of the VA in the isthmus portion. However, the part of the VA and ES distal to that bony lesion was well developed and contained normal epithelial cells. Extensive ossification and fibrosis, presumably due to bacterial labyrinthitis, were seen throughout the inner ear.

TABLE I

Clinical History, Location of Hydrops, and other Major Pathological Findings in 11 Temporal Bones

Case No.	Age Sex	Ear	Clinical Diagnosis	Vestibular Symptom	Average Hearing Loss	Duration of Hearing Loss	Hydrops Location*	Other ear Pathology Present
1	62 yrs M	R&L	Ménière's disease Otosclerosis	several attacks	fluctuated R 102dB L 95dB	37 yrs	R: C U P L: C U Sa P	Otosclerosis (bilateral)
2	55 yrs M	L	Hered. hemorrhagic telangiectasia	unsteadiness	progressive 70 dB	4 yrs	C Sa P	
3	78 yrs F	L	Chronic lymphocytic leukemia	an attack with deafness	sudden 82 dB	4 mos	C Sa	Hemorrhage Fibrosis/Ossification
4	84 yrs M	L	Spinal meningitis	none	sudden, total deafness	75 yrs	C U Sa P	Labyrinthitis ossification
5	69 yrs F	R	Ménière's disease	several attacks	fluctuated 41 dB	5 yrs	C	Circumscribed ossification
6	72 yrs M	R	Sensorineural deafness	none	since age 8 yrs 76 dB	64 yrs	C Sa	
7	63 yrs M	L	Sudden deafness	none	sudden, total deafness	37 yrs	C (hook portion)	Viral (?), Circumscribed ossification
8	51 yrs M	L	Peri-arteritis nodosa	dizziness prior to deafness	sudden, total deafness	6 yrs	C	Fibrosis/Ossification
9	33 yrs M	R	Renal insufficiency	an attack with deafness	sudden, total deafness	4 mos	C	Hemorrhage Fibrosis/Ossification
10	3 wks M	L	Trisomy 13	unknown	unknown	3 wks	C	Mondini-type anomaly

* C = cochlea; U = utricle; P = posterior semicircular canal; Sa = saccule.

Cases 5 (Rt), 6 (Rt), and 7 (Lt) showed only ES pathology with normal VA. The pathological findings included: small endolymphatic sac lumina (cases 6 and 7), flattened epithelial cells (cases 5 and 6), and increased amounts of perisaccular connective tissue (cases 5 and 6).

Cases 8 (Lt), 9 (Rt), and 10 (Lt) failed to show significant pathology in the VA or ES via light microscopy. The flattened epithelial cells of the ES in case 8, however, were seen not only in the left ear with hydrops, but also in the right ear without hydrops.

Quantitative comparisons of the VA and ES in ears with and without hydrops were made. The values (mean ± standard deviation) of the width of the VA were 0.45 ± 0.17 mm in the ears with hydrops and 0.56 ± 0.20 mm in the ears without hydrops. The lengths of the VA in ears with and without hydrops were 2.30 ± 1.56 mm and 3.10 ± 1.61 mm, respectively. The difference in these values for the ears with and without hydrops was not statistically significant by t-test (P > 0.05). The values for the width of the ES were 0.14 ± 0.05 mm in the ear with hydrops and 0.29 ± 0.11 mm in the ear without hydrops. These values were significantly different (P < 0.05).

Discussion

The pathological findings in the VA and ES in endolymphatic hydrops are summarized in Figure 2.

Case 1 (Rt and Lt), case 2 (Lt), and case 3 (Rt) appeared to be the result of congenital hypoplasia of the VA and ES. All of these bones demonstrated absence of funnel-shaped VA dilatation, small width of the aqueduct without any evidence of acquired bony pathology, and dislocation of the VA and ES anteriorly.

These anomalies represent decreased anatomical capacity of the VA and ES lumina. This finding may then be related to the endolymphatic hydrops present in these ears by assuming that the hydrops was the result of insufficient function of the ES or difficulty in control of the volume of endolymph fluid (Kimura, 1967). Thus, from an anatomical point of view, ears with hypoplastic VA and ES would appear to be more susceptible to endolymphatic hydrops than ears with well-developed VA and ES.

Other observations of this study that are important from a clinical viewpoint include: the difficulty of radiological visualization of the VA due to its displacement and hypoplasia; the difficulty of surgical exposure of the ES due to anterior displacement of the VA; and the implications of poorly developed peri-aqueductal air cells. These observations are all important considerations in the diagnosis and treatment in some cases of Meniere's disease.

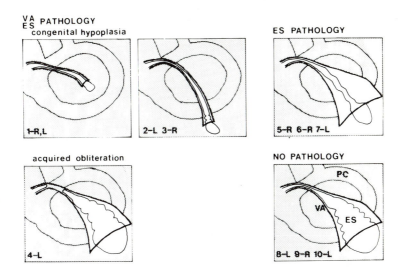

Fig. 2. *Schematic Drawings of the Vestibular Aqueduct (VA) and Endolymphatic Sac (ES) Pathology (Right Ear) in Hydrops.* The shape, course, and relationship with the posterior semicircular canal of the VA are based on the medial-view reconstruction. The numbers (1–10) and letters (R or L) indicate the case number and the side of the ear.

Congenital or acquired ES pathology with a well-developed VA, as in cases 5 (Rt), 6 (Rt), and 7 (Lt), is difficult to detect radiologically; however, flattened epithelial cells, increased connective tissue, and a small lumen seemed to be related to insufficient function of the sac and may have some bearing on the etiology of hydrops.

The bony obliteration of the VA observed in case 4 (Lt) seemed to have been acquired secondary to bacterial labyrinthitis. The significance of bony obstruction in the development of hydrops is unknown, because hydrops is usually seen in bacterial labyrinthitis without any significant primary pathology of the VA and ES.

Cases 8 (Lt), 9 (Rt), and 10 (Lt) had no detectable pathology in the VA or ES. However, pathology not visible by light microscopy may exist in the ES or other structures which relate to the control of the volume of the endolymph.

References

Anson, B.J. and Nesselrod, J.P. (1936): Endolymphatic and associated duct in man. *Arch. Otolaryng.* **24**, 127-140.

Black, F.O., Sando, I., Hildyard, V.H., *et al.* (1969): Bilateral multifocal otosclerotic foci and endolymphatic hydrops. *Ann. Otol. Rhinol. Laryngol.* **78**, 1062-1074.

Egami, T., Sando, I. and Black, F.O. (In preparation): Hypoplasia of the vestibular aqueduct in endolymphatic hydrops.

Hallpike, C.S. and Cairns, H. (1938): Observation on the pathology of Ménière's disease. *Proc. R. Soc. Med.* **31**, 1317-1336.

Kimura, R. (1967): Experimental blockage of the endolymphatic duct and sac and its effect on the inner ear of the guinea pig. A study on endolymphatic hydrops. *Ann. Otol. Rhinol. Laryngol.* **76**, 664-668.

Schuknecht, H.F. (1953): Techniques for study of cochlear function and pathology in experimental animals. *Arch. Otolaryng.* **58**, 377-397.

Computer Analysis

1. Computer analysis of electronystagmography.

Y. WATANABE, K. MIZUKOSHI, H. INO

Department of Otolaryngology, Niigata University School of Medicine, Niigata, Japan

Electro-nystagmography has become the routine method for clinical diagnosis of nystagmus responses in equilibrium examination. So far, ENG recordings have been interpreted solely on the basis of a visual and manual evaluation of the pattern of the waves. In order to facilitate an objective diagnosis of nystagmus responses, the authors have developed a method of computer analysis of the ENG recordings.

In the present studies, a procedure has been developed for the identification of nystagmus and for the evaluation of nystagmus parameters in clinical examination. The block diagram for recording eye movements is shown in Fig. 1. In the present study, the influence of the time constant and the noise filter was ignored.

The sampling rate for the analog-to-digital conversion was set to 100 times/sec. For calibration purposes, $10°$ of eye movement was made to correspond to 10mm of pen deflection.

The program for computer analysis of ENG recordings is written in FORTRAN IV and is composed of four parts.

In the first step of the procedure, the quick phase of nystagmus was identified.

In the second step, the points which marked the start and the end of each beat of nystagmus were identified, based on the detected quick phases. Fig. 2-A shows the sampled waveform of eye movements (caloric induced responses) and the vertical lines indicate the delimiting points of the slow and quick phase identified previously. In Fig. 2-A, wave 1 and wave 2 are not true nystagmus beats. In the procedure described so far, it is often the case that the detected waves include these irregular waves which should be eliminated in the analysis of nystagmus. We have selected typical waves of nystagmus by the methods of linear discriminant function and the formula is as follows.

Fig. 1. Block Diagram for recording of eye movements.

Recording and Processing Equipment for Nystagmus Test.

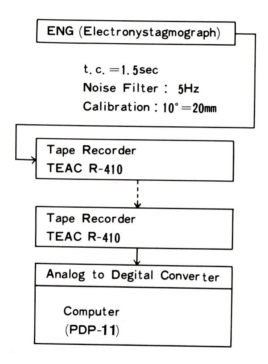

Fig. 1. Block Diagram for recording of eye movements.

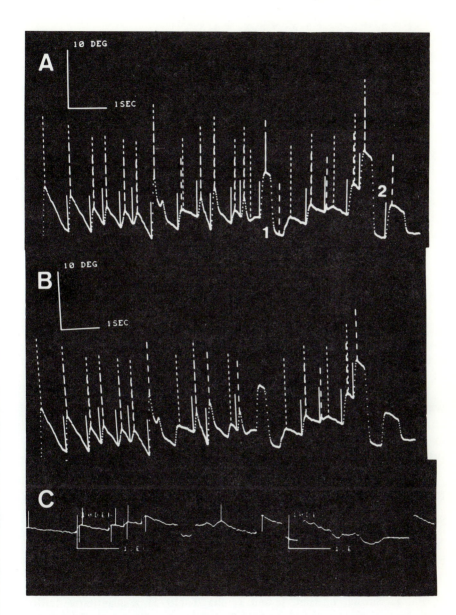

Fig. 2.
A: The sampled wave (caloric induced nystagmus) and the delimiting points of the slow and the quick phase.
B: The same picture after selection of typical waves on nystagmus.
C: The sampled wave (spontaneous nystagmus) and the delimiting points after selection of typical waves of nystagmus.

$$F = a_0 + a_1 x_1 + a_2 x_2 + a_3 x_3 + a_4 x_4,$$

where

x_i (i = 1, ---, 4): Factors which represent the degree of irregularity of a given wave, and were computed for each beat of nystagmus.

a_i (i = 0, ---, 4): Coefficients computed with 75 typical waves of nystagmus and 70 irregular waves.

Applying the discriminant function, the authors have been able to assign an appropriate value to each detected waveform. In these studies, we selected those waves as waves of nystagmus which were assigned positive values.

In Fig. 2-B, vertical lines are displayed only on the waves of nystagmus selected by the procedure described.

Fig. 2-C is the sampled waveforms of spontaneous nystagmus and fine nystagmus are identified correctly, being distinguished from irregular waves.

For evaluation of nystagmus responses such as optokinetic nystagmus, caloric induced nystagmus and so on, the amplitude and the eye velocity of nystagmus were computed for each selected wave and of the nystagmus responses.

In clinical application, it has been possible to identify nystagmus waves, even fine nystagmus such as spontaneous nystagmus. The computer analysis of ENG recordings has demonstrated its usefulness in the diagnosis of nystagmus responses and can be expected to provide more detailed information than conventional methods.

References

Sills, A.W., Honrubia and Kumley, W.E. (1975): Algorithm for the multiparameter analysis of nystagmus using a digital computer. *Aviation, Space, and environmental Medicine.* July, 934-942.

Herberts, G., Abrahamsson, S., Einarsson, S., Hofmann, H. and Linder, P. (1968): Computer analysis of electronystagmographic data. *Ata Oto-laryngolica,* **65**, 200-208.

Tokita, T., Suzuki, T., Hibi, T. and Tomita, T. (1975): A quantitative test of optokinetic nystagmus and ito data processing by computer. *Acta Otolaryngol. Suppl.* **330**, 159-168.

2. A microprocessor based vestibular test battery.

L.R. YOUNG, J.R. TOLE, C.M. OMAN, A.D. WEISS

Biomedical Engineering Center for Clinical Instrumentation and Man Vehicle Laboratory, Massachusetts Institute of Technology, Cambridge, Massachusetts 02139, U.S.A.

The advent of microprocessor technology has permitted us to develop a convenient and quantitative test battery for application to diagnostic testing of patients complaining of dizziness and disorientation. One portion of the system analyzes nystagmus eye movements and prepares a data summary of nystagmus intensity and directional preponderance. A digital filtering scheme detects saccadic eye movements, and permits the nearly immediate computation of nystagmus cumulative eye position, slow phase velocity, time of maximal velocity, nystagmus duration and frequency. Details are provided in an accompanying paper. The other portion of the system is a set of microprocessor controlled vestibular stimuli. These include an air caloric system, a two degree of freedom moving chair for testing semicircular canal and otolith function, optokinetic and galvanic stimuli, as well as devices for testing positioning and positional nystagmus. Preliminary results with a prototype version of the system as well as the anticipated clinical version, will be described.

In recent years, several research groups, including our own, have developed computer programs for analysis of the nystagmus data (Tole and Young, 1971; Honrubia *et al.*, 1971; Gentles, 1975; Allum *et al.*, 1975). These programs usually separate and process slow and fast phases of nystagmus, provide data storage in digital form, automate filtering and calibration of EOG signals and print out major parameters extracted from the data. Computers also make possible semi-automatic sequencing and error checking of a vestibular test battery although this capability has been seldom utilized by programs written to date. Unfortunately, the cost to operate such systems makes them available only to large institutions. Such systems also

Research Supported by NIH Grant 1-POIGM22392-01. The authors gratefully acknowledge the excellent technical support of R. Renshaw, W. Morrison, E. Wassmouth, D. Michaels, J. Yorker, and C. Burch in the development of this system.

often require the user to be versed in computer technology and thus may not lend themselves to use by the average clinician. This paper describes a modular microprocessor based instrumentation system for conducting a clinical vestibular test battery which performs multiple functions, yet is simple to operate.

The instrument has been designed by our group in the Biomedical Engineering Center for Clinical Instrumentation at MIT and utilizes a modular microprocessing instrumentation system based on the 8080 microprocessor. Much of the control software for the instrument is written in STOIC, a language developed at the Center for use on such instruments. (Sachs, 1976). The hardware is common to a number of the Center's instrument development projects (Michaels and Tole, 1977).

System function may be separated into several parts: collection and processing of eye movement data, semiautomatic sequencing of tests, and control of a number of stimulation devices.

The eye movement system incorporates the following features: two channels of EOG may be accepted via optically isolated pre-amplifiers. These channels are ordinarily used for one horizontal and one vertical channel, but may be used for separate analysis of the vertical or horizontal movement of either eye. The input module also contains logic and a current injection scheme for estimating imped-ance and offset of the EOG electrodes, and indicating to the user the electrode at fault and a description of the failure.

Raw nystagmus is processed to obtain slow phase velocity, cumu-lative slow phase position, fast phase frequency, and response duration. As byproducts of the analysis, a saccade interval indicator and eye acceleration are also available.

The programs for nystagmus analysis employed in the system are described elsewhere (Michaels and Tole, 1977) and in the accompany-ing paper (Tole *et al.*, 1977).

The hardware for the instrument is housed in two half rack modules; the first, which performs nystagmus analysis, also contains the operator front panel, and the second handles stimulus control. The first module together with a CRT display and chart recorder are shown in Fig. 1.

Control of the instrument is via a lighted pushbutton front panel. A flow chart of the major operations is shown in Fig. 2. When the device is turned on, the operator is asked to enter the data and then a patient identification number for use later in automatic marking of output records. Subsequently, the option is given of choosing a non-standard input/output configuration. If this option is not exercised, the instrument will assume both horizontal and vertical eye positions

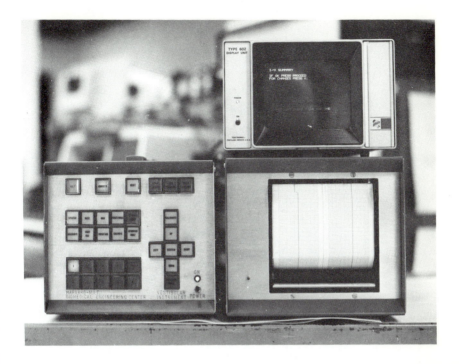

Fig. 1. Front panel of the vestibular instrument together with peripheral devices.

are to be recorded, and will display sampled horizontal position and average slow phase velocity on both the CRT display and the strip chart recorder. In addition, the event marker on the strip chart indicates those sections of the eye movement identified as fast phases.

Alternatively, the operator may choose to accept only one of the eye movement channels and to output other parameters from among position, velocity, cumulative slow phase position, fast phase frequency, and acceleration as well as the fast phase indicator flag.

Following these choices, the operator presses the calibration button. This initiates a check of electrode status. The offset potential, and then the impedance for each electrode are calculated. If the offset potential is greater than 10 millivolts or the impedance is greater than 10K ohms, the fault is signalled by operator panel lights and an error message is displayed on the CRT. When the faulty electrode has been reapplied, the procedure is repeated.

If all electrodes check acceptably or if the test is overridden, the instrument then indicates the next procedure ordinarily performed

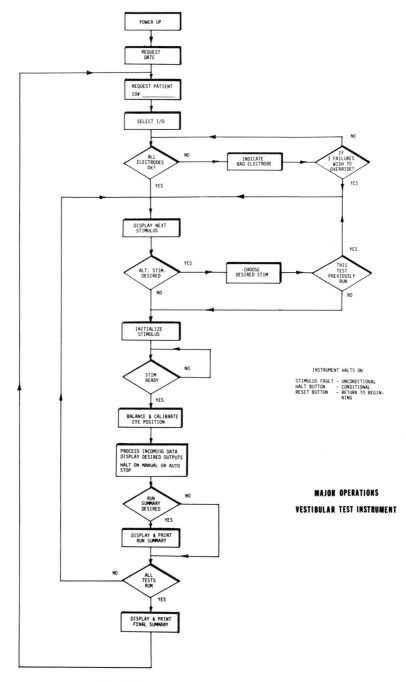

Fig. 2. Major operations of vestibular instrument

in the test battery. The operator may choose an alternate test (e.g. to repeat a previous run judged unacceptable) or may accept the current test by pressing the proceed button. The stimulus ready light will be lit when the proper initial conditions for the chosen test are met (e.g. caloric stimulator temp correct, or seat belts fastened for rotation test.)

A matrix of 5 calibration lights located behind a translucent screen is controlled by a corresponding series of pushbuttons on the front panel. During the calibration sequence, the patient is asked to direct his gaze toward the currently illuminated light. When the operator determines the subject is looking in the prescribed direction, the corresponding button on the front panel is pushed causing a 1 sec. sample of eye position to be taken.

When the subject is viewing the centre light (the first lamp to be lit) the instrument automatically balances the EOG amplifiers to bring their outputs to zero thus compensating for electrode offset potentials. Gain is automatically corrected by the program to a level acceptable for use by the analysis programs. The horizontal and vertical calibrations are plotted on the chart recorder while the patient number, date, and run number are printed on the lower margin of the record.

Once the calibration is successfully completed, and provided stimulus initial conditions are met, a message to begin the test is given. Pressing the proceed button initiates the test which continues until concluded by either program or operator control.

During the run, drift is compensated via the automatic balancing system so that the displayed eye position signal is always "on scale". This feature allows calculation of the total amount of drift with time and hence an error may be indicated if the rate of drift approaches the estimated slow phase velocity. This feature also retains the advantage of A.C. recording while allowing true D.C. position measurement for those who use it.

While the eye movement processor will work in connection with any stimulator, we have attempted to design an integrated series of test devices allowing a wide range of possible stimuli while utilizing the processing and control power of the microprocessor. The main stimulus elements of our system are shown in Fig. 3. These are a multi-degree of freedom chair which is used for rotational, positional, and vertical oscillation, as well as a patient seat for other tests; air caloric and galvanic stimulators, and an optokinetic projection system which may be operated either horizontally or vertically. Provision will be made for a fixation light which rotates with the chair for the study of visual suppression of vestibular nystagmus. The

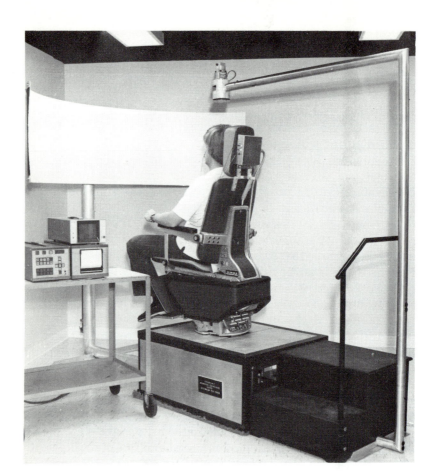

Fig. 3. Overall configuration of the vestibular test battery.

instrument is also programmed to accept and analyze spontaneous and gaze nystagmus.

Brief description of some of the novel features of the stimulators follow:

Rotation Chair

Rotation is achieved via a gear belt driven, ½ h.p. d.c. motor controlled by a digital servo system which accepts commands from the microprocessor controller. This device is a modification of a commercially available examination chair (SMR MAX II). The base of the chair houses the rotation servo as well as an air pump for the caloric stimulator and some miscellaneous controls. The servo has a resolution of 1 deg/sec from 1–250 deg/sec with peak acceleration exceeding 100 deg/sec^2.

We are also interested in the use of a vertical oscillation as a possible test of otolith function. A preliminary study (Vidic *et al.*, 1976; Vidic, 1976) suggests that labyrinthine defective patients show degraded performance in a visual tracking task during vertical body motion. We have incorporated a vertical oscillation mode into our test battery to study this response further. The chair moves vertically over a 20 in. range at a constant speed of 5 ips.

The chair is also motorized in pitch and has a motorized head rest which will be used for positional testing. The pitch mode is convenient in subject positioning and allows us to study the tilt caloric test, in which the thermal gradient across the canal is allowed to stabilize before the stimulus is made effective by tilting to the usual canal vertical position. (Viets, 1938; Oman, 1972).

A number of safety features are incorporated in the chair including interlocks for seat, shoulder, and foot harnesses, and overspeed and over acceleration detection. In addition, electrical interlocks prevent operation of more than one mode simultaneously and only allow rotation when the chair is fully down and upright. Electrically sensitive foot mats further prevent chair movement if the operator is within a 30 in. radius of the vertical axis.

Air Caloric Stimulator

The air caloric stimulator is of our own design (Tole and Weiss, 1975). A study by our group, (Tole, 1976) has found that air and water stimuli produce approximately equivalent responses in normal subjects when temperatures of 30° and 44°C and stimulus durations of 90 sec. are used. A disposable ear speculum is placed into each ear under visual control. A thermistor mounted in the speculum allows closed loop control of the temperature to within ± 0.2°C in the range from ambient to 55°C. The stimulus flow is delivered by timed control of the air pump. In order to overcome thermal lag in the heat exchanger, a separate closed loop, controlled preheating, is employed when the system is in the standby mode. Testing is not allowed to proceed until the proper preheating condition occurs for each stimulus temperature. This arrangement allows the stimulus to reach the desired temperature within 5 seconds after the flow is initiated, well below the thermal time constant of the temporal bone.

Galvanic Stimulator

For galvanic stimulation, 1 inch diameter wet electrodes impregnated with electrode jelly held within a plastic ring are applied anterior to the tragus of each ear. A large common electrode is placed over one forearm. A d.c. current is delivered under processor control, either monaurally or binaurally, with choice of polarity. The room is darkened. For the galvanic test only, eye movements are currently measured by means of a photoelectric monitor, set to measure horizontal movement of the right eye. When the run begins, the patient is instructed to look at the fixation light straight ahead of him, which flashes on momentarily every 4 seconds to avoid wandering of gaze (Tole, 1976). The patient is instructed to continue to look at the light bulb directly in order to discern its flashes throughout each run. After 8 seconds of baseline recording, a galvanic current is initiated and rises from zero at a steady rate to the maximum 2 milliamperes over a 4 second interval. The current remains at that intensity for 16 seconds, at which time it returns linearly to zero with the light flashing at 4 second intervals throughout. This procedure is repeated for each of the six possible combinations of electrodes. The nystagmus processor program produces the same derived values as were discussed under the caloric stimulation mode. The program, in this case, also looks at the baseline spontaneous nystagmus prior to the onset of galvanic stimulation.

Optokinetic Nystagmus Stimulation

For optokinetic nystagmus we have constructed a projection type stimulator, with a striped housing which rotates at commanded velocity around a fixed light source. It is also possible to stimulate both the foveal and peripheral fields separately or together by appropriate masking of the display. The screen shown in Fig. 3 can be rotated to a vertical position as can the projector to allow vertical OKN testing.

We plan to begin in-service clinical trials of these instruments and the tentative protocols in the near future, and to collect both normative data and user feedback.

References

Allum, J.H.J., Tole, J.R. and Weiss, A.D. (1975):' 'MITYNS II – A digital program for on-line analysis of nystagmus'. *IEEE Trans. Biomed. Eng.,* **BME-22**, 196-202.

Gentles, W. (1974): *Application of automated techniques to the study of vestibular function in man.* PhD Thesis, Dept. Elect. Eng., Univ. of Toronto.

Honrubia, V., Jenkins, H., Ward, P., Katz, R. and Strelioff, D. (1971): 'Computer analysis of induced vestibular and optokinetic nystagmus'. *Ann. Otol., Suppl.* **3**, CXXX.

Michaels, D.L. and Tole, J.R. (1977): 'A microprocessor-based instrument for nystagmus analysis'.*Proc. IEEE,* **CXV**, 730-735.

Oman, C.M. (1972): *Dynamic response of the semicircular canal and lateral line organs.* PhD Thesis, Dept. Aero/Astro., M.I.T., Cambridge, MA.

Sachs, J. (1976): 'An introduction to STOIC'. Biomed. Eng. Cent. for Clinical Instrum., M.I.T., Cambridge, MA, Tech. Rep. BMEC TR 001.

Tole, J.R. (1976): *A quantitative study of diagnostic techniques for peripheral vestibular disorders.* ScD Thesis, Dept. Aero/Astro., M.I.T., Cambridge, MA.

Tole, J.R., Weiss, A.D. (1975): 'A new air caloric stimulator for vestibular testing'. An abstract presented at the 3rd New England Bioeng. Conf. held at Tufts Univ., Boston, MA.

Tole, J.R. and Young, L.R. (1971): 'MITNYS, a hybrid program for on-line analysis of nystagmus'. *Aerosp. Med.* XCII, *508-511,*

Tole, J.R., Oman, C.M. Michaels, D.L., Weiss, A.D. and Young, L.R. (1977): 'Nystagmus analysis using a microprocessor based instrument'. VI Extraordinary Meeting of the Barany Society, London.

Veits, C.: Zur Technik der kalorischen Schwachreizung. *Ztsch.F. Hals-, Nasen- u. Ohrenh.* **19**, 542, 1928. As described by Joseph J. Fischer, M.D. *The Labyrinth: Physiology and Functional Tests* Grune & Stratton, New York 1956.

Vidic, T.R. (1976): *Clinical test for abnormal human response to vertical acceleration.* Dept. Elec. Eng., M.I.T. SB Thesis.

Vidic, T.R., Barlow, J.S., Oman, C.M., Tole, J.R. and Weiss, A.D. (1976): 'Human eye tracking during vertical and horizontal motion'. An abstract presented at the Sixth Annual Society for Neuroscience Meeting, Toronto, Canada.

3. Nystagmus analysis using a microprocessor based instrument.

J.R. TOLE, C.M. OMAN, D.L. MICHAELS, A.D. WEISS, L.R. YOUNG

Biomedical Engineering Center for Clinical Instrumentation and Man Vehicle Laboratory, Massachusetts Institute of Technology, Cambridge, Massachusetts 02139, U.S.A.

Introduction

Using the microprocessor based instrumentation system described in the accompanying paper, we have implemented a novel algorithm for the analysis of nystagmus. The algorithm permits calibration of eye position, and near on line, continuous estimates of cumulative slow phase eye position, slow phase velocity, and saccadic frequency. Saccades are recognized via a finite impulse response digital filter which is sensitive to acceleration. Data is available in both analog form and as a numerical summary following a run. Estimates of total electrode drift and noise and other quality control features are included.

Experience to date with the algorithm and a comparison of its performance with the manual reading of nystagmus by an experienced clinician will be presented.

Background

Although conventional nystagmography is quite laborious, otologists and neurologists routinely record and analyze patient eye movements because such records are of unquestioned diagnostic utility. The usual procedure today involves the measurement of patient eye position by electrooculography, and not uncommonly, subsequent differentiation to obtain eye velocity. This is often accomplished using an analog method (Henriksson, 1955), although more recently digital devices (e.g., L.T. Instruments, Model 3100) have become available to assist the physician in extracting slow phase velocity information. With the manual methods usually employed, lengthy chart records of eye position and eye velocity plotted versus time

Supported by NIH Grant 1-POIGM22392. The authors gratefully acknowledge the assistance of J.M. Sachs.

must be calibrated, read and analyzed usually by an experienced physician. Such methods are time consuming, and prone to human error, and therefore limit the scope of information which can practically be obtained from the nystagmogram. In recent years, a number of methods for computer analysis of nystagmus have been developed (Tole and Young, 1971; Honrubia *et al.*, 1971; Allum *et al.*, 1975; Herberts, 1973; Gentles, 1975). However, these algorithms have been implemented on either laboratory minicomputers or large scale systems, and to date have had little impact on routine clinical testing due to the expense of purchasing and expertise required to operate such computers.

Processing Algorithm

A fundamental consideration in the design of our prototype instrument was the choice of an appropriate sampling frequency for analog to digital conversion. Although nystagmus may contain frequencies as high as several hundred Hertz in the fast phase component (Melvill Jones, 1973), most of the information required to analyze slow phase nystagmus lies at frequencies below 20 Hz. It therefore appeared feasible to design the instrument to sample eye position at relatively low rates, and to work with a highly filtered nystagmus waveform without losing information of clinical interest. Operating at a low sampling rate increases the amount of time available for each eye movement processing algorithm cycle, so that real time program operation can be achieved using the relatively slow 8080 microprocessor.

In our prototype instrument, a three pole analog low pass filter with a breakpoint of 30 Hz is applied to the eye position signal from the EOG preamplifiers prior to sampling. An interrupt driven routine in the microprocessor, synchronized by a crystal stabilized clock, then samples the filtered signal at 120 Hz, and averages successive samples. Low frequency aliasing error is usually much less than EOG electrode drift. Aliasing and filtering effects do result in some rounding of the transitions between slow and fast phase components in the sampled record, but the resulting signal is almost completely free of 60 Hz noise, a common artifact in the clinical environment. Prior to the start of eye movement processing, software in the microprocessor initiates electrode impedance, offset, and noise checking. These aspects are discussed in the accompanying paper (Young *et al.*, 1977).

When a test run begins, detection of fast phase events is performed in software by convolving the averaged eye position signal with a 9

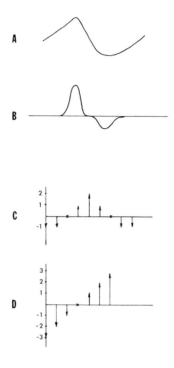

Fig. 1. Nystagmus filter considerations. A. Idealized nystagmus. B. Acceleration of waveform in A. C. Nine point finite impulse response filter (FIR) sensitive to acceleration below 7 Hz. D. Seven point FIR used in calculating velocity.

point finite impulse response digital filter sensitive to acceleration. The choice of this filter can be motivated in the following way: an idealized section of a nystagmus waveform and its second derivative (eye acceleration) are shown in Fig. 1A and B. The onset and termination of the fast phase interval may be characterized by the occurrence of two acceleration peaks of opposite sign. Computational constraints dictated that we employ a filter whose unit sample response values are powers of 2, thus permitting convolution multiplication via binary shifts. The filter chosen, whose unit sample response is shown in Fig. 1C, is sensitive to accelerations below 7 Hz, and passes little of the input signal above this frequency, thus rendering it noise insensitive. Using this filter, the following algorithm is employed:

(1) Locate the start of a saccade when the magnitude of the filter output is greater than a predetermined threshold, typically 1200 deg/sec^2.

(2) Find the end of the saccade by locating the next peak of opposite sign in the filter output. The search for this braking deceleration of the eyes is constrained to 10 points. If no end point is detected, a duration of 0.167 sec. is assumed.

Instantaneous velocity of the eye is calculated using a seven point digital filter whose unit sample response is shown in Fig. 1D. Once a saccade has been detected, the program interpolates slow phase eye position across the saccadic interval using a linear fit based on an average of the instantaneous velocities just before and just after the saccade. Slow phase eye velocity is extrapolated across the saccadic interval based on this value. A one second running average of slow phase velocity is also calculated. Eye position and average slow phase velocity are normally displayed during a test on a device such as a chart recorder. Use of information from both sides of the saccadic interval during extrapolation necessitates that the algorithm output be delayed with respect to the sampling process. Therefore, the sampled eye position as plotted on the display device is also delayed so as to appear in correct register with the algorithm output waveforms as shown in Fig. 2.

For later numerical summary of the analysis, the algorithm determines maximum slow phase velocity and frequency and their times of occurrence, cumulative slow phase position, and response duration for the caloric test. The latter is estimated as the point at least 30 seconds from the beginning of the test at which the slow phase velocity is less than 1 deg/sec for 5 seconds. This method is probably not optimal but it has been shown (Tole, 1976) to give reasonably good comparisons with manual estimates of nystagmus duration.

Fig. 2 presents examples of some of the parameters available from the algorithm. The raw eye position (sampled and smoothed) is shown individually with (a) the output of the finite impulse response filter, (b) the saccade indicator flag, (c) cumulative slow phase position, and (d) average slow phase velocity.

It is important to compare any algorithm of this type with a manual reading of the same nystagmus record by an experienced person. This has been done by a physician in our group (A.D.W.) who has been conducting ENG tests for many years. Several criteria were imposed upon the data segments used in the verification. Segments were only used if the noise level on the signal was less than 3 degrees, regardless of frequency, and if the physician judged any response to be present. Regions in which the physician indicated 25 or more fast phases were compared to the same region analyzed by the algorithm. A separate record of raw data was used by the physician.

Comparisons were done on typical clinical records of caloric and galvanic nystagmus. These were chosen since they represent large and small responses and it was felt unfair to group them under

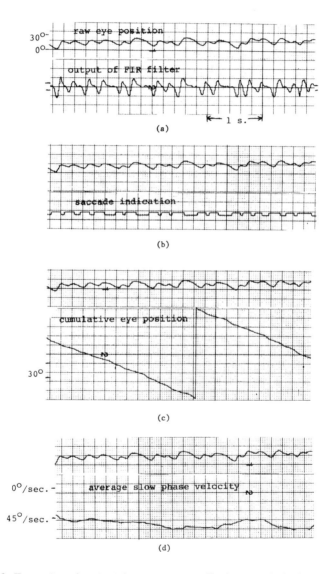

Fig. 2. Examples of output from processor. Each example is shown for the same segment of sampled eye movement.

a single comparison. Of a total of 312 comparisons for the caloric responses, 46 or 15% were identified as fast phases by the program but not by the physician. 6% of the fast phases scored by the physician were ignored by the program. The error rate was comparable for 140 comparisons on galvanic nystagmus beats. It is interesting to note that re-evaluation by the physician of the program's performance resulted in rescoring of approximately half of the events in favour of the program.

Slow phase velocity (SPV) estimates of the physician were correlated with the program estimate of the 1 second running average of slow phase velocity, yielding a correlation coefficient of 0.94. To obtain this figure, 48 data points with different magnitudes of SPV were chosen at random from caloric and positional test responses.

In its current form, the processing algorithm requires about 60% of the 8080 processor time for a single channel of EOG input. We are currently considering timing optimization methods to allow simultaneous processing of two channels, which at present must be done in sequential passes. Decoupling of horizontal and vertical channels and calculation of derived parameters such as clinical directional preponderance may be added. We plan to begin in-service clinical tests of this instrument at several sites in the coming year and to collect both normative data and user feedback.

References

Allum, J.H.J., Tole, J.R. and Weiss, A.D. (1975): 'MITNYS-II — A digital program for on-line nystagmus'. *IEEE Trans. BME,* **BME-XXII**, 196-202.

Gentles, W. (1974): *Application of automated techniques to the study of vestibular function in man.* PhD Thesis, Dept. Elect. Eng., Univ. of Toronto.

Herberts, G., Abrahansson, S., Einarsson, S., Hofmann, H. and Linder, P. (1968): 'Computer analysis of electronystagmographic data'. *Acta Otolaryng,* **LXV**, 200-208.

Henriksson, N.G. (1955): 'An electrical method for registration and analysis of the movement of the eyes in nystagmus'. *Acta. Otol.* **XCV**, 25.

Honrubia, V., Jenkins, H., Ward, P., Katz, R. and Strelioff, D. (1971): 'Computer analysis of induced vestibualr and optokinetic nystagmus'. *Ann. Otol. Suppl.* 3, CXXX.

Melville Jones, G. (1973): 'Nystagmography — A useful tool in basic and applied research'. Preprint AGARD Conf. on Use of Nystagmography in Aviation Medicine, # 128.

Michaels, D.L., Tole, J.R. (1977): 'A microprocessor-based instrument for nystagmus analysis'. *Proc. IEEE,* **CXV**, 730-735.

Tole, J.R. (1976): *A quantitative study of diagnostic techniques for peripheral vestibular disorders.* ScD Thesis, Dept. Aero/Astro, M.I.T., Cambridge, MA.

Young, L.R., Tole, J.R., Oman, C.M. and Weiss, A.D. (1977): 'A microprocessor based vestibular test battery'. VI Extraordinary Meeting of the Barany Society London.

4. Parameter variability of the post-caloric EOG response.

B. McA. SAYERS*, R. HINCHCLIFFE**, M.A. HAMID*

*Engineering in Medicine Laboratory, Imperial College, London, SW7 2BT.

**Institute of Laryngology and Otology, London, WC1X 8EE.

Introduction

The purpose of this work is to re-examine the caloric-induced nystagmus response from first principles, with a view to efficient clinical measures and instruments. In particular, we consider the spontaneous variability of the response, as demonstrated in some of the various parameter-derived variables — that are used clinically to distinguish abnormal from normal records.

At any given moment in time, each parameter of the nystagmus response to a thermal stimulus of the vestibular labyrinth is influenced by a number of factors (Table 1). But as reported previously (Sayers

TABLE 1
Factors Affecting Caloric-Induced Nystagmus

Physical	Psychological	Physiological	Pharmacological
Stimulus temperature	Alertness	Age	Alcohol
Heat transfer	Neuroticism	Gaze deviation	Smoking
Head position	Psychoticism	Optic fixation	Psychotropics
Post-stimulus time	Anxiety level	Eye closure	Vestibular
		Habituation	suppressives
		Vascular reactivity	
			Pathological

and Hinchcliffe, 1976), there is appreciable intra-response (interbeat) variability which can only with difficulty, or not at all, be accounted for by the factors listed in Table 1; so, almost certainly additional factors exist. Thus we examine the record of fluctuating EOG potential that results from a caloric stimulus, treating the record as a biological signal.

Several questions need to be asked about this signal — for example:

What are the appropriate parameters — that is, the best derived variables — that will quantify it?

How much spontaneous variability does it exhibit, and what is its origin?

How much consistent behaviour underlies the variations?

How can the sensitivity of this signal to abnormality be optimised in the light of its spontaneous variability, by specific choices of parameters?

Some of these questions can be answered.

Strategy of Analysis

The EOG signal resulting from the application of a 30-second unilateral caloric stimulus (30° or 44°, Left or Right side) can be described by the sequence of the quick-phase slopes, (speeds), slow-phase slopes, magnitudes, and intervals between successive nystagmus beats. The particular measurements illustrated in Fig. 1, like the others reported, were obtained from a normal adult subject (eyes open in the dark) supine with head tilted 30° to the horizontal but the methods discussed are quite general.

There is no typical beat in this record, because of the substantial fluctuation; it is not specifically known if the fluctuation conveys any part of the response, if it can be circumvented by the usual statistical measures, or if other measures are appropriate. It is also questioned whether one of the parameters (slopes, magnitude, interbeat interval) is more useful than the others. Thus we report here an empirical study of the two parameters (slow-phase slope and interbeat interval) that appear sensitive to abnormality; this study draws upon statistical measures and on measures of the inter-record variability to compare the stability, and so utility, of the two parameters. In this study we repeated measurements (up to 5 times spread by at least a week) on 4 different subjects. Inter-subject variability was studied in some 20 different subjects. For the purposes of this study it will suffice to use results from the first set of experiments in which the stimuli were always presented in the same order. Caloric temperatures ranging from 19° to 33°C, in addition to the usual 30° and 44°, were used to investigate the effect of stimulus intensity, and the mean slow phase speed and interbeat interval values are shown in Fig. 2.

The display technique employed here (Sayers and Hinchcliffe, 1976) disregards order-dependent effects and shows the sequence of values of the parameter in the various beats, rank-ordered according

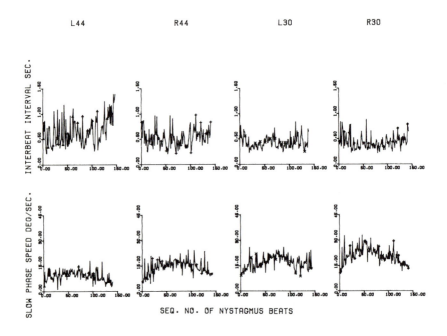

Fig. 1. Sequence of interbeat intervals and slow-phase slopes for 4 stimulus conditions (left-ear, right-ear, 30°C, 44°C).

to magnitude. This type of display is visually informative, and lends itself to formal description by the coefficients of a best-fit mathematical curve (say a third-order polynomial). Measures like the mean size of the quantal step between neighbouring magnitudes in the ranked sequence may also be useful descriptors. In practice different numbers of beats are produced in different experiments and the comparison of different records is not then directly possible. However, different sequence lengths can be considered as different-size samples and these are presumed to be drawn in each case representatively from the underlying population of values appropriate to each case. So the effect of doubling the sequence size would typically add an identical set of numbers to those values already collected. Thus expanding to a standard length the horizontal axis of the plot showing the rank-ordered sequence will suffice. Fig. 3 shows (left) the original ranked-sequences of slopes and intervals from one set of responses, and (right) the resulting expanded sequences.

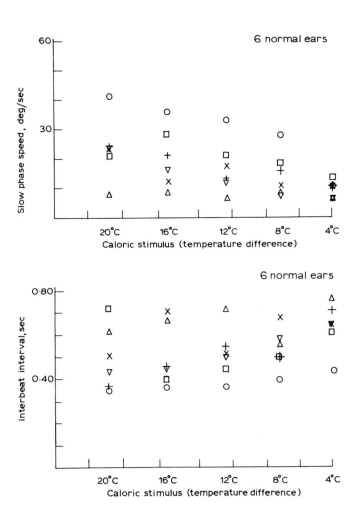

Fig. 2. The effect on mean interbeat interval and mean slow phase speed of changing the stimulus intensity (caloric temperature difference from 37°C).

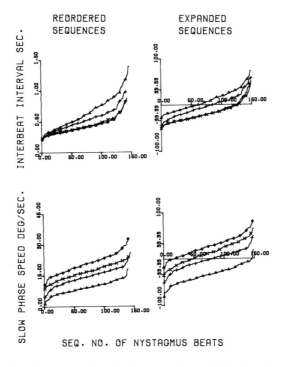

Fig. 3. Original and expanded ranked sequences of interbeat intervals (upper) and of slow phase slopes (lower); the expanded curves were normalised.

Stability of EOG Interval and Slope Measures

To decide between interbeat interval and (slow-phase) slope as parameters of the EOG caloric response their spontaneous variability must be compared; it must also be confirmed that they depict similar system properties or are at least both sensitive to significant abnormalities. The latter point will be discussed elsewhere; results so far indicate that the interval parameter is at least as sensitive as the slope measure and probably more so.

The comparative intra-subject variability of interval and of slope can be assessed only after normalisation. Again the rank-ordered sequence curves have been used, but the results with mean interval or slope or with mean quantal step confirm the visual evidence. Using the conclusions of earlier studies the L and R 30° and 44° results have been treated as equivalent; the inter-record variability between the 4 expanded sequences shown in Fig. 3 (greater for slow-phase slopes, than for intervals) is typical. Repeating the experimental measurements 5 times on this subject in the space of some 8 weeks thus produces 24 separate sequences from which the spontaneous variability can be judged. The grand mean value of all 24 interval sequences was subtracted from every individual interval value and the result divided by the grand mean, and correspondingly for the slow-phase slope (the analysis was also carried out for beat magnitude, with results broadly as for slope). Fig. 4 shows the result; on the left, with the actual ranked values and, on the right, with the sequences subsequently expanded to a standard extent.

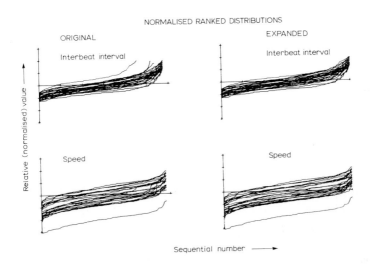

Fig. 4. Original (left) and normalised-expanded (right) ranked sequences of slopes and of intervals for 24 trials on one subject.

Thus normalised, the relative inter-record variability of the slope and interval sequences can be assessed visually, or by their mean values. The result is unequivocal. The appreciably smaller relative intra-subject scatter of the interval parameter in these records is established. Similar results have been obtained with all other subjects studied repeatedly. In our subjects the stability of the interval parameter over repeated trials was always appreciably better, by a factor of some 2–3, than the slope parameter. In our normal subjects the inter-subject variability is comparable with the intra-subject variability.

The normal values found for the interbeat interval are: mean interval 0.52 second (standard deviation 0.08); mean slow phase slope 12.48 deg. per second (SD 2.28).

Conclusions

It is concluded from these results on EOG caloric responses that:

(1)   Spontaneous variability exhibited by any descriptive parameter is very important in the assessment of its utility, especially in the EOG case. The interbeat interval is a substantially more stable parameter than speed or magnitude of the nystagmus beats. It is also at least as sensitive to apparent vestibular abnormality in the cases we have seen.

(2)   In view of previous methods of measurement of the EOG more systematic analysis has been desirable, and by the methods used here the results appear to be rewarding.

Two methods of description are useful: the mean interval and the mathematical coefficients of the best-fit curve of the ranked sequence of intervals.

We note also that dispersion can be usefully measured by quantal step size in the raw ranked sequence. Mean value and dispersion are not independent.

(3)   The methods of quantification used here lend themselves to simple implementation in a special-purpose instrument, since the intervals can be derived directly from the raw EOG and the analysis can be carried out by microprocessor. The special-purpose apparatus for this approach is operational in our laboratory and will be described elsewhere.

The methods also allow the very detailed exploration of the entire set of derived variables and their properties.

Acknowledgement

This work was supported by the Medical Research Council.

Reference

Sayers, B.McA. and Hinchcliffe, R. (1976): 'Signal analysis of neuro-otological measurements' in *Disorders of Auditory Mechanisms II.* (S.D.G. Stephens, Ed). Academic Press, 219-30.

5. Systems analysis of vestibulo-ocular system response using white noise rotational stimuli.

C. WALL III, D.P. O'LEARY, F. OWEN BLACK

Department of Otolaryngology, University of Pittsburgh, School of Medicine, Pittsburgh, Pennsylvania

Introduction

The first well-known human rotational test began with Barany's important observation that one could infer vestibular performance by looking at a patient's eye movements (nystagmus) during and after rotation in a chair. Since Barany's time, basic and clinical scientists have applied advances in electronics, computers, control theory and signal processing in attempts to gather more information from rotational testing. The torsion pendulum test at one frequency, Greiner *et al.* (1963) and sinusoidal driven tests for several consecutive frequencies, Benson (1970), Hixson (1974) and Wolfe (1977) are examples of these advances.

This report presents a technique that quickly tests the vestibulo-ocular reflex (VOR) over a wide range of rotational frequencies. It has been used to describe the VOR of 30 normal human subjects by a set of key parameters that characterize the linear systems response.

White noise rotational testing using a pseudorandom binary sequence (PRBS) acceleration stimulus with cross spectral analysis and parameter estimation has several potential advantages. First, this test signal is equivalent to testing a system with many simultaneous sine waves. Second, factors which effect the response over a medium time scale (such as changes in electrode sensitivity or in the corneal retinal potential) can be minimized since the data for all frequencies is taken at once and for the same conditions. Cross spectral calculations, Bendat and Piersol (1971) can give linear system descriptors based upon these many frequency points. These descriptors can then be validated since the technique also computes confidence intervals for the transfer function data. The cross spectral technique as applied to vestibular testing is described by Peterka *et al.* (1978).

During the period over which this test was being developed, Professor A.J. Benson (1976) provided many valuable suggestions. We would like to acknowledge his help and thank him for his encouragement.

Stimulus Delivery and Response Recording System

The test equipment consists of a steel frame chair mounted on an 80 foot-pound torque motor. The chair is equipped with the first stage of an eye movement amplification system and a head holder and bite bar to assure adequate stimulation to the semicircular canals. A Digital Equipment Corporation (DEC) LSI-11 microprocessor controls the device and digitizes the eye movement data after it has been suitably amplified and filtered. The data is then transmitted to a DEC PDP11/40 computer for storage and analysis.

A pseudorandom binary sequence (PRBS) Davies (1970) of rotational acceleration stimulus having 255 states was used (Fig. 1A). The data presented here were obtained using an acceleration of 40 deg sec^{-2} with a state duration, ΔT, of 200 milliseconds to give a test bandwidth of 0.02 to 1.67 Hz. The response of the torque motor over this frequency range was flat within .5 dB. In all cases, stimulus parameters were selected to keep the maximum test velocity below 100 deg sec^{-1} which was considered to be the maximum comfortable velocity for most normal subjects. The resulting angular velocity profile of the test device is shown in Fig. 1B.

Conjugate horizontal eye movements from subjects having normal caloric responses and no known vestibular disorders were recorded by electro-oculography using bitemporal electrodes for 5–10 consecutive presentations of the 50.5 sec PRBS. Examples are shown in Fig. 1C through E. The saccadic eye movements were more active when the table velocity was greater; and the direction of the slow phase movement changed according to the direction of the stimulus velocity.

Slow Phase Velocity (SPV) Reconstruction

An interactive computer program was used to obtain slow phase eye velocity from the raw nystagmus data. First, the fast phase movements were detected and flagged by means of minimum slope and minimum time duration criteria. Eye position was reconstructed by substituting an extrapolation of the previous slow phase movement for each detected fast phase. The next slow phase data was then concatinated onto the other end of the extrapolation. The process

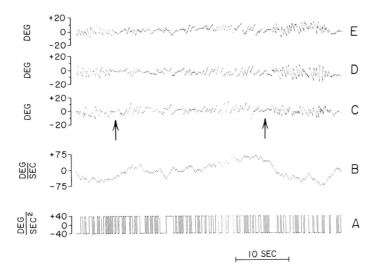

Fig. 1. Rotational stimulus and VOR eye movement response. A shows the PRBS acceleration stimulus for a single 50.5 second period. The stimulus switches between +40 and −40 deg sec^{-2}. B shows the tachometer output of the torque motor. Each constant acceleration command results in a linearly increasing velocity. C through E shows three consecutive periods of VOR response from the same subject while performing mental arithmetic recorded using bitemporal electro-ocular electrodes. Arrows mark parts of the records where direction of the nystagmus reverses in all three records. This reversal occurs approximately when the stimulus velocity, B, goes through zero degrees per second.

was repeated for each fast phase over the entire test. This signal was then differentiated to give the slow phase eye velocity which is the system output to be analyzed by cross spectral techniques.

The fast phase detection parameters of the program could be varied by the operator to optimize the results. Occasional inclusions of small undetected fast phases are less serious than in sine wave SPV reconstruction since one error in a deterministic signal reconstruction has a continued effect on the phase calculations. The problem is reduced by this method because of the statistical nature of the gain and phase calculations and also by the use of averaging which reduces the effect of random undetected fast phases. An example of the average reconstructed SPV is shown in Fig. 2A.

The SPV is actually compensatory in direction but has been reversed in sign to aid in comparison with the stimulus velocity Fig. 2B. Although the overall amplitude of the reconstructed SPV is less than that of the stimulus velocity profile, visual inspection shows a gross correlation between the two signals. Fig. 2C shows an estimate

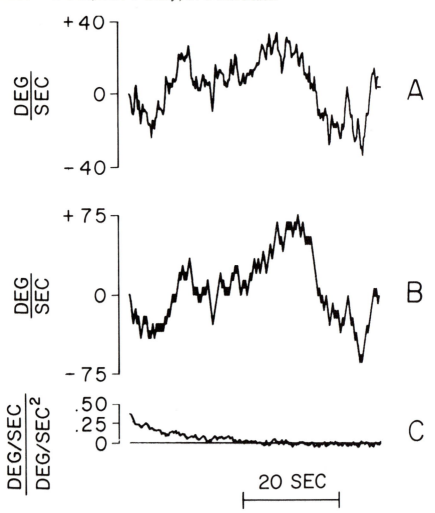

Fig. 2. A is the slow phase eye velocity (SPV) which has been reconstructed from five consecutive VOR responses similar to the ones shown in Fig. 1C – E. The SPV is compensatory in direction, however the sign has been reversed for comparison with the rotational stimulus velocity trace shown in B. The unit impulse response (UIR) shown in C is derived from correlating the data in A with the PRBS acceleration stimulus. The UIR reaches the base line at approximately two-thirds of the way through the stimulus period thus demonstrating that the stimulus parameters which test the low frequency characteristics of the system have been properly selected.

of the linear systems unit impulse response (UIR) calculated as described by O'Leary *et al.* (1978).

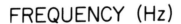

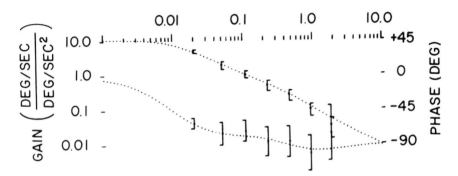

$$H(S) = \frac{10.9\,(1.03\,S+1)(.13\,S+1)}{(17.24\,S+1)(.76\,S+1)(.20\,S+1)}$$

Fig. 3. Corresponding gain and phase for data shown in Fig. 2A using cross-spectral calculations. The right-facing brackets correspond to 95% confidence intervals from the gain estimates; The left-facing brackets correspond to 95% confidence intervals for the phase estimates. The dotted lines represent a third order linear systems fit to the data. The fit parameters are written beneath in the form of the system transfer function. 'S' is the Laplace operator.

Gain and Phase Calculations

A sample gain and phase calculation using the cross spectrum is shown in Fig. 3. The response input is the reconstructed SPV that has been reversed in sign and all results are related to an acceleration stimulus. The seven frequency points shown have been obtained from averages of several adjacent frequency points to obtain a smooth spectral estimate. The brackets on the gain and phase points mark the 95% confidence intervals of the cross spectral estimate.

The dotted line which runs through or near the gain and phase points in Fig. 3A and B are least squares fits which best estimate the linear systems parameters of the response. In this case, the fit is best for a third order linear system. The 10% improvement criterion mentioned by Peterka *et al.*, (1978) was used as a basis for selecting the degree of fit.

The parameters estimated are the system steady state gain and the linear system time constants. They are written in the form of a linear systems transfer function at the bottom of Fig. 3. The time constants so obtained for the vestibulo-ocular reflex can also be compared with those obtained theoretically or experimentally from the peripheral semicircular canal responses. These parameters for the first order vestibular afferent responses in fish and cat are presented elsewhere in these proceedings (O'Leary *et al.*, 1978).

Results

The results for the group of 30 normal human subjects were obtained by ensemble averaging at each gain and phase point for all subjects. This data is presented in Table I and shown in Fig. 4. The gain

TABLE I
The Gain and Phase of the VOR Response in 30 Normal Subjects
During PRBS Rotational Testing

Frequency (Hz)	Gain $\frac{Deg/Sec}{Deg/Sec^2}$		Phase (Deg)	
	Mean	SD	Mean	SD
.02	3.77	1.32	−55.01	7.35
.05	1.54	0.49	−67.39	5.10
.11	0.79	0.27	−86.78	8.89
.23	0.38	0.16	−92.47	14.59
.46	0.17	0.07	−103.09	16.93
.93	0.08	0.03	−102.95	20.78
1.67	0.03	0.01	−89.34	54.13

points and fit of the normal data appear to decrease by a factor of 10 for each frequency decade starting at a frequency which occurs at between 0.10 and 0.20 Hz. These gain results can also be related to stimulus velocity. The VOR gain that relates slow phase eye velocity to stimulus velocity averages 0.52. This value is slightly below that of .65 reported by Barr *et al.* (1976) for subjects doing mental arithmetic under sinusoidal stimulus. When referenced to an acceleration stimulus, our data are in general agreement with the sine wave data of Benson (1970), Hixson (1974), and Wolfe (1977).

Conclusions

(1) White noise testing has provided a short, well-tolerated, information rich VOR test by the use of computer controlled rotation stimulus.

FREQUENCY (Hz)

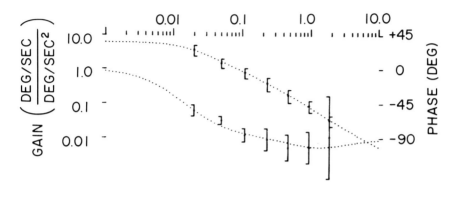

$$H(S) = \frac{6.26\,(1.95S + 1)(.15\,S + 1)}{(12.05\,S + 1)(1.72\,S + 1)(.25S + 1)}$$

Fig. 4. Mean gain and phase calculations for the group of 30 normal subjects. Data for each of the seven frequency points were ensemble averaged for all subjects. Brackets around the data represent ± one standard deviation. Dotted lines are linear systems fits for a third order system, which are also written below as the system transfer function.

(2) The resulting VOR output (slow phase eye velocity) was successfully extracted using a computer algorithm provided that extraction parameters were carefully chosen for each subject. Averaging the extracted response reduces 'noise' created by small undetected fast phase movements.

(3) The linear fits were appropriate for the averaged normal responses and a 3rd order fit was necessary to describe the data.

(4) Linear systems fit techniques yielded a set of parameters for normal subjects which provide a basis for comparison studies in patients with known vestibular disorders.

Acknowledgement

This project supported by grants from the Martha Edwards Lazear Foundation and the Richard King Mellon Foundation.

References

Barr, C.C., Schultheis, L.W. and Robinson, D.A. (1976): Voluntary, non visual control of the human vestibulo-ocular reflex. *Acta. Otolaryngol.* 81, 365-375.

Bendat, J.S. and Piersol, A.G. (1971): *Random Data: Analysis and Measurement Procedures.* Wiley-Interscience.

Benson, A.J. (1970): Interactions between semicircular canals and gravireceptors. *In: Recent Advances in Aero Space Medicine.* Busby, D.E. (Ed.), Dordrecht: D. Reidel Publishing Co., 1970, 249-261.

Benson, A.J. (1976): Personal Communication.

Davies, W.D.T. (1970): *System Identification for Self-Adaptive Control.* Wiley-Interscience.

Greiner, G.F., Conraux, C. and Picart, P. (1963): Principes physiques, experimentaux et cliniques des stimulations pendulaires l'examen vestibulaire. *Acta. Otolaryng.* 56, 388-352.

Hixson, W.C. (1974): Frequency response of the oculovestibular system during yaw oscillation. NAMRL-1212, Naval Aerospace Medical Research laboratory, Pensocola, Florida.

O'Leary, D.P., Tomko, D.L., Black, F.O. and Peterka, R.J. (1978): Comparative analysis of cat and isolated guitarfish horizontal canal afferent responses to rotational acceleration. *Proc. VI Extraordinary Meeting of the Barany Society,* 28-37.

Peterka, R., O'Leary, D.P. and Tomko, D.L. (1978): Linear system techniques for the evaluation of semicircular canal afferent responses using white noise rotational stimuli. *Ibid.* 11-17.

Wolfe, J.W. (1977): Personal Communication.

Positional Nystagmus

1. Positional nystagmus. Some introductory remarks

C.S. HALLPIKE

44 Ashurst Road, West Moors, Dorset, England

Introduction

As the subject for these introductory remarks I have chosen the condition usually known as the benign paroxysmal type of positional nystagmus. Reasons for choosing it are not hard to find. For instance, there are its clinical features, unusual and indeed spectacular, which tell, of themselves, a good deal about the pathological mechanisms that are likely to be involved. They also refresh and illuminate our ideas on a number of related and difficult problems of vestibular physiology. These clinical features have been described and are familiar enough. However, certain matters of detail are important and of these something needs to be said.

For the most part, the patients are adults of middle age or rather beyond it. They include a number in whom the condition is known to have followed a head injury. The critical head position for the elicitation of the nystagmus is shown in Fig. 1 — with one ear undermost (Hallpike, 1955). When there is evidence of damage to one

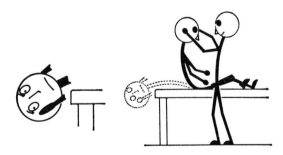

Fig. 1. Positional nystagmus of the benign paroxysmal type. The 'Lagerungs' manoeuvre.

labyrinth, resulting from head injury or otherwise, the critical position is usually found to be with the affected ear undermost. Once established in the critical position, there usually follows a latent period, lasting several seconds, sometimes longer, followed by the characteristic paroxysm of nystagmus and vertigo. If the head position is maintained the paroxysm increases rapidly and then dies away after some 5–20 seconds. The nystagmus has a very marked rotational component but with this a horizontal element can usually be discerned. It is also noted that the nystagmus is markedly exaggerated by the absence of visual fixation, a characteristic feature of caloric or rotational nystagmus known to result from excitation of the semi-circular canals. If, when the paroxysm has subsided, the subject sits upright, there often occurs another brief episode of nystagmus, this time with its direction reversed.

Nystagmographic records of the reaction are not easy to obtain. However, that shown in Fig. 2 (Hallpike, 1967) illustrates the essential findings. It was obtained with the recording electrodes at the outer canthuses, an arrangement which favours the display of horizontal nystagmus.

The subject has his right ear undermost. Visual fixation is at first eliminated by darkness and there is seen a brisk episode of nystagmus. At the point indicated, visual fixation is restored and the amplitude

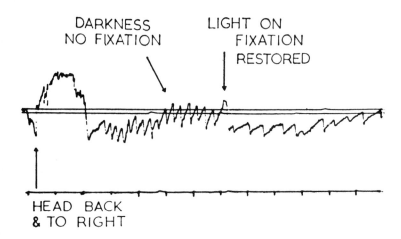

Fig. 2. Electronystagmographic recording of positional nystagmus of the benign paroxysmal type, showing inhibiting effect of visual fixation. Also, horizontal component of nystagmus to subject's left.

and frequency of the nystagmus are at once reduced. The subject's eyes can now be viewed directly and the rotational element of the nystagmus is at once apparent. Clearly shown on the record, too, there is a horizontal component directed towards the subject's left.

On rare occasions only do the patients exhibit evidence of neurological disease outside the VIII Nerve system. And it is usually appropriate to say to them what they are happy to hear – that theirs is a benign disorder; disagreeable certainly, but amenable to simple measures and *not* one that will end or shorten life.

Barany insisted that since the reaction was dependent upon a certain position of the head in relation to gravitational lines of force then it was likely to be due to a lesion of the utricle. The author and his colleagues (Dix and Hallpike, 1952; Cawthorne and Hallpike, 1957) were able in two typical cases, to carry out histological examination of the temporal bones and in both found clear evidence of lesions of the utricle in the ear placed undermost in the critical test position.

In Fig. 3 are shown the findings in one of these subjects. In A, B for comparison is seen a normal human utricle, with normal macular epithelium and sub-epithelial connective tissue traversed by fibres of the utricular nerve.In C, D is shown the affected utricle in one of the two subjects. There is much fibrosis of the sub-epithelial connective tissue with aggregations of inflammatory cells. In places, too, there are areas of new bone formation. The changes are emphatically not of a kind that could result from fixation or other type of artefact. They must, accordingly, be accorded considerable significance when it comes to explaining the pathophysiology of the condition.

The first thing to be said is that much is left to explain, not forgetting the latent period of the nystagmus reaction and its direction reversal with change of head position. Certainly, striking as they are, the finding of utricular lesions in two of these subjects can hardly be said to tell the whole story. For instance, the character of the nystagmus with its inhibition by visual fixation strongly suggests that it arises from canal excitation, and weighty arguments derived from the work of Ledoux (1953), of Schuknecht (1969) and of Gacek (1974), have done much to direct thought along these lines. It is, moreover, a view which accords with Lorenté de No's dictum: i.e. that while the utricle can modify nystagmus, the canals alone can initiate it.

Fig. 3. (Opposite and over the page). Histological Structure of human utricular macula. A, B: Normal. C, D: From a subject with positional nystagmus of the benign paroxysmal type.

Mention will first be made of the work of Ledoux who in 1953 published a well-known monograph which included a description of experiments in the course of which, while recording the 'resting' potentials in the horizontal canal nerves of the frog, he found evidence that their frequency altered with alterations of head position, so suggesting that under certain conditions the canal sense organs could themselves become gravity sensitive. Subsequently, in 1969 Schuknecht published an account of his histological findings in the temporal bone of a characteristic case of this condition, showing the presence of cellular and other debris upon the surface of the cupula of the posterior canal of the ear placed undermost in the critical test position. This, he argued, would increase its specific gravity and so render it particularly sensitive to positional changes of the head. He concluded, accordingly, that the condition should be regarded in essence as a disorder of the posterior canal. Finally, Gacek (1974) has followed this up by carrying out surgical section of the nerve from the posterior canal in a number of characteristic cases and found that in all of them the symptons were abolished. This certainly makes a very presentable picture and goes far to engage our agreement with Schuknecht's conclusions. Nevertheless, certain difficulties remain.

First of all it seems likely from the nystagmographic and other

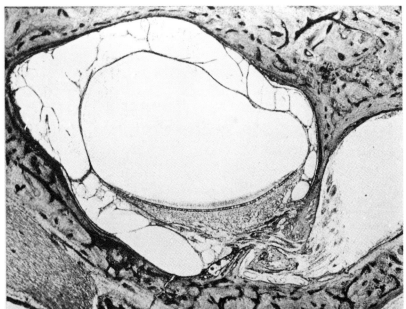

FIG. A
(magnification × 16)

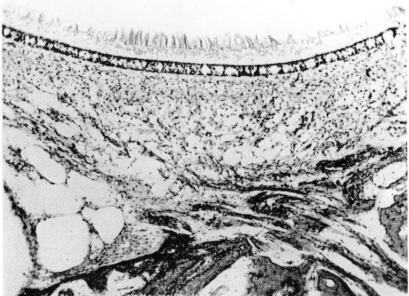

FIG. B
(magnification × 100)

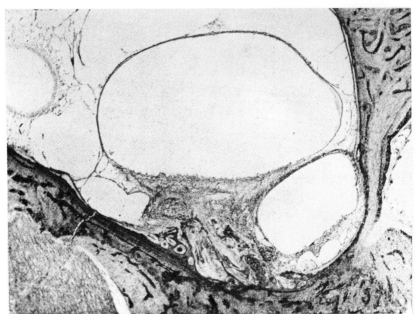

FIG. C   (magnification × 16)

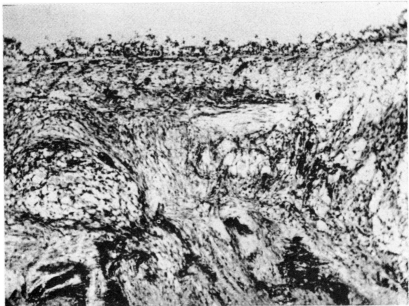

FIG. D   (magnification × 100)

characteristics of the nystagmus that it must arise from the activation of *several* canals. Schuknecht's findings, however, have been limited to the posterior canal alone.

In addition, Dix and Hallpike (1952) in the course of their clinical observations, in particular of the Caloric Test findings, derived a firm impression of a canal apparatus which was active and often normal. Its bad working as in this type of positional nystagmus, would, therefore, be best attributed to some other associated agency; and here the most obvious possibility was the utricle, itself disordered by injury or disease.

When all this has been said against Schuknecht's canal hypothesis, the position, nevertheless, remains strong. It is, after all, in clear accordance with Lorenté de No's dictum that nystagmus of this kind can arise only from a canal, and here Schunknecht has actually identified the canal.

The crux of the matter, or so it would seem, is really the status of the dictum itself. Could it be that its validity is less than complete? Could it be that, after all, nystagmus *could* be initiated by the utricle? If this were the case, then a different situation would arise. It is, however, a situation towards which a substantial move has already resulted from the work of two different groups of investigators. The first of these have used the human centrifuge. The second have employed microelectrodes in the vestibular nuclear zones of the brain-stem. The questions, vis-a-vis the dictum, which have awaited attention, are these: Firstly, what *is* the evidence that the utricle can indeed modify canal nystagmus? Secondly, if it can, then what are the electro-physiological events which underlie this transformation. Thirdly, can nystagmus be initiated by the utricle?

Question 1. Direct evidence of the modification of canal nystagmus by the utricle has been derived from certain simple applications of the human centrifuge. Bergstedt's monograph (1961) was an outstanding contribution and his studies have been continued and extended by Benson (1966), Benson *et al.* (9170) and by Crampton (1966). Crampton's findings are clearly described and will be referred to in a little detail.

In Fig. 4 is shown the turntable of a centrifuge viewed from above. The subject is seated at its periphery with his head vertical. Angular acceleration to the subject's right will excite his horizontal canals and cause nystagmus with its rapid component to the right. Now whatever the subject's location on the turntable, whether at its centre or the periphery, the magnitude of the stimulus applied to the canals remains constant. In addition, rotation of the turntable will generate a linearly acting centrifugal force which will act upon the utricles. Now

CENTRIFUGE

The subject, with head fixed in the vertical position,
is shown seated at the periphery of the turntable.

Combination of Stimuli:

I. Angular acceleration to the right. This acts upon
the horizontal canals and causes Nystagmus with
its rapid component to the right.

II. Centrifugal force. This acts linearly upon the
Otolith organs aligned in the horizontal and coronal
planes.

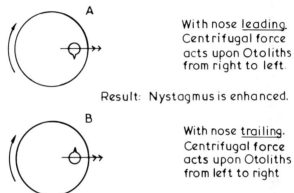

A

With nose <u>leading</u>.
Centrifugal force
acts upon Otoliths
from right to left.

Result: Nystagmus is enhanced.

B

With nose <u>trailing</u>.
Centrifugal force
acts upon Otoliths
from left to right

Result: Nystagmus is inhibited.

Fig. 4. Modifying effect in the human subject of otolith activation upon
nystagmus evoked by impulsive rotational stimulation of horizontal canals.

the magnitude of *this* force *can* be varied, increasing with displacement
of the subject towards the periphery of the turntable. Furthermore,
it is possible, by varying the position of the subject himself upon his
own vertical axis, to vary the direction of action of the centrifugal
force upon his utricles.

It is possible, therefore, with this equipment, to apply a known
nystagmogenic stimulus to the horizontal canals, and at the same
time observe how this nystagmus is modified by the simultaneous
application to the utricles of centrifugal forces of known magnitude
and direction.

The findings were quite clear. When, as shown at A, the head is
exposed to a centrifugal force acting in the line joining the utricles
with the force vector arrow emerging as shown from the left ear, then
nystagmus to the right is enhanced. When, as at B, the arrow emerges
from the right ear, the nystagmus to the right is inhibited.

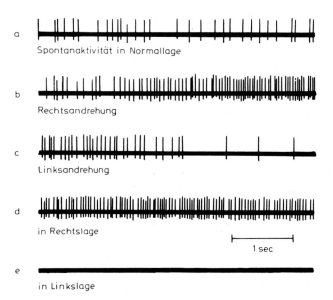

a
Spontanaktivität in Normallage

b
Rechtsandrehung

c
Linksandrehung

d
in Rechtslage

├─────────┤
1 sec

e
in Linkslage

Fig. 5. Convergence of canal and otolith afferents upon a single cell of a vestibular nucleus (Nucleus triangularis). The normal resting action potentials (Record a) are increased in frequency by angular acceleration to the right (Record b): decreased by angular acceleration to the left (Record c). Similar frequency changes result from otolith activation by positioning of the animal on its right (Record d) or left (Record e) sides.

This finding, therefore gives a clear answer to the first question. It exemplifies and confirms Lorenté de No's dictum that the utricle can modify canal nystagmus.

The other two questions concern the electrophysiological background of this modifying action. What, for instance, when it takes place, is happening to the pattern of action potential activity in the utricular and canal nerves?

Here, information of great value has been provided by Duensing and Schaefer (1959) who used micro-electrodes and recorded from single cells of the vestibular nuclei of cats and rabbits. In Fig. 5 are shown some of their published records. The electrode tip is located in a cell of the right vestibular nucleus of a rabbit. (Nucleus triangularis). The uppermost tracing is taken with the head at rest in its normal upright posture. Record (a) shows the normal resting action potentials. Angular accelerations to the right and left are applied as shown, with resultant increase and decrease of the action potential frequency, a finding which identifies the nerve cell as being connected with the cupular mechanism of the right horizontal canal. In addition, the animal's head can also be turned into one or other of the positional nystagmus positions, with either the left or right ear undermost. The utricles will now react to a linearly directed force, this time gravity, acting along the line connecting them. The resulting utricular response now reacts with and modifies the pattern of action potential activity emanating from the canal.

The first inference that may be drawn from these findings is that the vestibular nuclei are not merely relay stations but perform important integrative functions. This arrangement would seem likely to have considerable functional significance. In fact, it would appear to confer upon the utricle a certain responsibility for the maintenance of order in the system. This is all the more important since its zone of influence covers all three canals. It is clear that in this situation derangement of the utricular mechanism would derange the system. The outcome could well be the transmission of a confused mixture of nystagmogenic action potential combinations, emanating from all three canals, not unlike the result that can be seen in a typical paroxysm of positional nystagmus.

This brings us to Lorenté de No's conclusions about the utricle and canal nystagmus. It cannot cause it directly but it can do so indirectly. For showing how this could happen, much credit is due to the work of Duensing and Schaefer. All in all, it would seem right to conclude that the utricle should be brought more to the centre of this complex picture. This is where Lorenté de No left it.

Central Mechanisms

The tendency is to think of this benign paroxysmal type of positional nystagmus as an entity dependent upon peripheral mechanisms and to expend much effort in explaining how these work. All the same, it cannot be denied that certain of its features give the impression that central mechanisms are at work. There is the strangely variable latent period of the reaction. Also, a certain uncertainty about its appearance at all. On some occasions it is readily elicited. At others, not. When it comes to asking about the central mechanisms that might be involved, it is natural to turn to the contents of Nyléns famous monograph (1931). Nylén examined a substantial number of subjects; for the most part with lesions of the brain stem within the posterior fossa. In six of the subjects the temporal bones were subjected to histological examination and nothing abnormal was reported. The nystagmus, though different in some ways from that of the benign paroxysmal type, is in other ways not so different. To

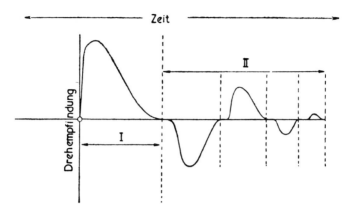

Fig. 6. Time course of turning sensations which follow an impulsive rotational stimulation (Stop stimulus) of horizontal canals. The primary episode of turning sensation (1) is followed by others, progressively smaller and of alternating direction.

be noted in particular is its dependence upon the same critical head position. It must therefore be that the nystagmus in Nylén's subjects arose from central mechanisms, and hence it is known as the central type of positional nystagmus. The question that arises is this: Could one or other of these mechanisms also have played a part in the genisis of the peripheral type of positional nystagmus?

Some of these mechanisms are familiar ones, and an example is shown in Fig. 6 — the after nystagmus phenomenon of Wodak and Fischer (1924). A rotational stimulus has been applied and there ensues an episode of turning sensation and nystagmus. This is followed by other episodes, progressively smaller and of alternating direction.

It will be apparent that this transfers the subject under discussion to that difficult area of nystagmology that goes by the name of nystagmus alternans. (Kornhuber, 1959). It is appropriate to ascribe the phenomenon in question to the alternating activities of nystagmogenic mechanisms upon the two sides of the brain stem. The mechanisms have not been identified but could be part of the vestibular nuclear complex. Discussion of the problem involved is difficult and here certain inadequacies of terminology play a part. The term 'Right-left Tonus See-Saw,' applied to the whole mechanism would be helpful and this is proposed.

Patients exhibiting the phenomenon of nystagmus alternans, and they constitute a well known neurological entity, nearly always show clear evidence of brain-stem damage — neoplastic or post-encephalitic. When such a patient lies quietly upon his back a succession of episodes of nystagmus can be observed, directed alternatively to right and left. This is the See-Saw in action.

The question that arises is: could its mechanism, in the absence of evidence of any brain stem malignancy be subject to other non-malign agents which would render it abnormally sensitive to strong otolithic stimulation; resulting, e.g. from the head positioning movement — the so called 'lagerungs' manoeuvre and so bring it into the pathophysiological picture of the paroxysmal type of positional nystagmus. If this were the case, then the alternating character of the See-Saw mechanism could help to explain the direction reversal of the nystagmus which is often evident when the patient assumes the vertical position. It might also be argued that this same alternating character might help to explain the characteristic uncertainty which goes with the elicitation of an episode of nystagmus of the paroxysmal type. Let it be assumed, for instance, that the See-Saw is set into action by impulses from the utricle triggered by the 'lagerungs' manoeuvre. Now this could quite possibly involve some synchronisation of the manoeuvre with a certain phase of the See-Saw cycle. If, however, it coincided with the opposite phase of the cycle, then the paroxysm of nystagmus could be inhibited or even suppressed. The clinical observer would then be left to ask 'what has happened to it?

Acknowledgements

The author's thanks are due to the Editors and Publishers of the following publications for kind permission to Reproduce the Figures which appear in this paper as follows:
Fig. 1. Postgraduate Medical Journal.
Fig. 2. Proceedings, Royal Society of Medicine.
Fig. 3. Annals of Otology Rhinology and Laryngology.
Fig. 5. a. Archiv fur Psychiatrie u. Nervenkrankheiten.
    b. Hals-Nasen – Ohrenheilk. George Thieme Verlag, Stuttgart.
Fig. 6. Fortschritte der Hals-Nasen und Ohrenheilkunde. S. Karger. A.G. Basel.

References

Benson, A.J. (1966): NASA. SP-115, 119.
Benson, A.J., Guldry, F.E. and Melvill Jones, G. (1970): *J. Physiol.* **210**, 475.
Bergstedt, M. (1961): *Acta. Otolaryng. (Stockh).* Supplement **165**.
Cawthorne, T.E. and Hallpike, C.S. (1957): *Acta. Otolaryng. (Stockh).* **48**, 89.
Crampton, G.H. (1966): NASA. SP-115, 169.

Dix, M.R. and Hallpike, C.S. (1952): *Ann. Otol. Rhinol. and Laryngol.* **61**, 987.
Duensing, F. and Schaefer, K.P. (1959): *Arch. Psychiat. Nervenkr.* **199**, 345.
Gacek, R.R. (1974): *Ann. Otol. Rhinol. and Laryng.* **83**, 596.
Hallpike, C.S. (1955): *Postgrad. Med. J.* **31**, 330.
Hallpike, C.S. (1967): *Proc. Roy. Soc. Med.* **60**, 1043.
Jongkees, L.B.W. (1953): *Fortschritte der Hals-Nasen und Ohrenheilk.* **1**, 124.
Karger, S. and Basel, A.G.
Kornhuber, H.K. (1959): *Archiv Ohren-usw., Heilk., Bd.* **174**, 182.
Kornhuber, H.K. (1966): *Hals-Nasen – Ohren-Heilk.* **III/3**, 2311. George Thieme
    Verlag. Stuttgart.
Ledoux, A. (1953): *Acta. Oto.-Rhino-laryng. Belg.* **12**, 109.
Lorenté de No., R. (1931): *Ergebn. Physiol.* **32**, 99.
Nylén, C.O. (1931): *Acta. Otolaryng. Stockh.* Supplement **15**.
Schuknecht, H. (1969): *Arch. Otolaryng.* **90**, 765.
Wodak, E. and Fischer, M.H. (1924): *Monatschr. f. Ohrenheilk.* **58**, 70 and 527.

2. Experimental evidence of etiology in postural vertigo

N. TOROK and A. KUMAR

Department of Otolaryngology, University of Illinois, Abraham Lincoln School of Medicine, Chicago, Illinois

Introduction

Head movements may elicit mild to severe equilibratory disturbances in a very large number of patients complaining of dizziness. The variety of movements creating the symptoms and the length and character of the resulting turning, spinning or other forms of disequilibrium are numerous. A nystagmus may also be produced which may or may not be correlated with the sensation of motion and finally it can be the positioning or the posture per se which is the triggering factor creating the symptoms. Still another variable factor is the fatiguability of the posture elicited vertigo and nystagmus.

One of the most frequently encountered forms of the postural vertigo is that seen in patients predominantly between the ages of 45 to 65, in which there is a brief but sometimes violent feeling of turning. While this symptom is unpredictable as to the frequency with which it is reproducible, it is always precipitated by certain head movements. The recurrences may last for days or weeks with gradual improvement and a final recovery. There is no spontaneous nystagmus, the vestibular sensitivity is not affected and there are no related auditory symptoms or findings. This clinical entity was first observed and described by Dix and Hallpike and has since been termed the 'Benign Paroxysmal Postural Vertigo' syndrome (B.P.P.V.).

The searching clinician without more objective aids has tried to correlate observable details of the evoked postural nystagmus with the assumed location of the disease. The direction of the nystagmus in relation to the head position became the key to differentiating dizziness of labyrinthine origin from that of the central nervous system. The concept of Nylen (1950) became widely accepted as a differential diagnostic clue. Experience has shown that these criteria are generally not valid.

The subject of this study is not the postural vertigo and nystagmus as a symptom caused by diagnosed pathological conditions of the inner ear, the central nervous system or skeletal and muscular disorders of the neck. More specifically, an answer is sought about the origin and pathology of the frequently encountered clinical entity, the 'benign paroxysmal postural vertigo' syndrome.

Obviously, a wide spectrum of pathological conditions could cause various forms of positioning or postural vertigo and nystagmus. From a clinical standpoint however, two major groups can be differentiated. Patients with established or suspected diagnosis of inner ear, central nervous system or other neural pathology may exhibit postural nystagmus and vertigo along with symptoms generated by the basic disease condition. Here B.P.P.V. is just another symptom. In contrast, if the patient is complaining of the positioning vertigo without evidence of vestibular abnormality or central nervous system pathology, the symptoms are representing the disease.

(1) Barany (1921) observed a fatiguing postural vertigo and nystagmus and suspected some otolithic disorder. Dix and Hallpike (1952) described the syndrome both in patients with no evidence of ear disease and a larger group where a variety of middle or inner ear pathology was known. In a single case, in this later group histopathologic examination of the temporal bones could be performed and in one ear the otolithic membrane was absent and the sensory epithelium disorganized. This finding lead to a widespread belief that disease of the otoliths is responsible for the symptoms of Benign Paroxysmal Postural Vertigo (B.P.P.V.). Otolithic abnormality can hardly explain the symptoms. The damaged macula could cause a lifting or sinking type sensation but not an outright spinning as it occurs in B.P.P.V. The resulting vestibulo-ocular sign would be perhaps some counter rolling but not a nystagmus. An acute endorgan lesion would rather create somewhat prolonged symptoms of B.P.P.C.

(2) Circulatory involvement has often been implicated. However, pathological evidence − except for a few angiographic studies − is lacking. It is questionable that a temporary complete or partial obstruction in the vertebro-basilar system should affect the vestibular receptors whereas the equally sensitive cochlear function is spared as is the entire content of the posterior fossa. It is difficult to explain both the fatiguability of the symptoms and the self limiting nature of the disease on the basis of a circulatory disorder. Barber and Dionne (1971) examining 100 patients with a definite diagnosis of vertebro-basilar ischemia or insufficiency, could not detect vestibular abnormalities or B.P.P.V.

(3) Somatic sensors of the neck are capable of eliciting postural nystagmus and perhaps dizziness as well. (Magnus, 1914; de Kleijn, 1921; Grahe, 1926; Frenzel, 1928). Their involvement in B.P.P.V. disease is unlikely, particularly without evidence of neck muscle pathology or symptoms of the spinal column and their ligaments. The same is the case concerning the brachial plexus. (Biemond, 1969). Reversible lesions without other neural manifestations are difficult to imagine as being responsible for the single symptom of B.P.P.V.

(4) The term 'cupulolithiasis' is indeed an attractive speculation (Schuknecht, 1962), but the concept is more speculative than factual. Loose otoconia in histologic specimens could just as well be artifacts rather than pathological evidence. It is true that in some patients, there is a few seconds latency before dizziness and nystagmus occurs following the respective positioning of the head but more commonly the postural reactions are seen instantly, without delay. Another speculative counterproposal would be that if in vivo, some otoconia were detached from the macular surfaces, noticeable symptoms must be expected. Some annoying disequilibrium — similar for instance to that initially experienced by astronauts for 2–3 days in the weightless environment — was never experienced by any patient prior to their first attack of dizziness associated with postural change. Finally, if the loose otoconia caused posterior canal cupular deflection as suggested, then a vertical nystagmus would appear, which is however seldom observed.

(5) None of the space occupying or other brain lesions with postural symptoms fulfill the criteria of B.P.P.V. disease since such a diagnosis is restricted to cases with no detectable organic disease.

(6) The sympathetic vertebral plexus and the cervical sympathetic ganglia were suspected in the pathogenesis of the postural symptoms (Barre *et al.,* 1926) fifty years ago. The assumption that irritation or interruption of the cervical sympathetics could elicit vestibular symptoms or elicit postural signs was not sufficiently proven in spite of numerous surgical attempts in experimental animals and man.

Previous anatomical studies of the extreme flexibility of the neural and vascular elements of the neck by head movement, turning, bending or twisting were as impressive as they were surprising. Observations made on cadavers showed that a 90° turn of the head in one direction combined with tilting toward the shoulder shrinks and twists the ipsilateral vertebral artery by 5–6 cm and the contralateral vessel is elongated to the same extent as it runs through the foramina of the lateral processes of the cervical vertebrae (Pfaltz and Richter, 1961). If this anatomical situation is involved in the pathogenesis and since a unilateral vertebral artery obstruction is unlikely to cause postural symptoms without any effect upon the hearing, brain stem and cerebellum, the next most plausible contributing mechanism might be the periarterial neural plexus.

The patients affected by the B.P.P.V. disease are mainly in the late forties, fifties and early sixties. Orthopedic and radiologic evidence indicates that bony, ostheoarthritic changes occur most commonly in this age group. The smallest bony deformities in the vertebral lateral foramina may interfere with the twisted arterial wall with a particular head movement. Could the effect then be periarterial or neural rather than circulatory?

Such considerations lead us to the following experiment. Three cats were operated under general anesthesia and the promontory of the right middle ear was exposed under the microscope. A fine hole was bored in the horizontal canal ampulla and a wire electrode inserted and fixed in position with dental cement. After the electrode was connected with an amplifier and recorder, a piece of ice was placed on the exposed bony labyrinth. Instantly, a signal was recorded (Fig. 1). Shortly after, a cotton pledget soaked in hot water was again placed on the labyrinth and a signal in the opposite direction was obtained. The neck on the same side was entered through a posterior saggital incision and with careful preservation of the vascular and neural structures, the lateral processes of the 2nd to 5th cervical vertebrae were exposed. The intervertebral spaces in the cat are so

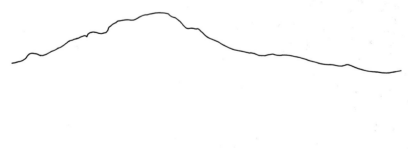

LABYRINTHINE RESPONSE

Fig. 1. Cold caloric stimulation (ice water) through the middle ear in cat.

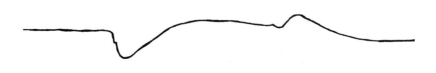

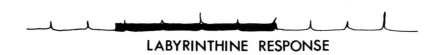

LABYRINTHINE RESPONSE

Fig. 2. Touching the surface of the vertebral artery.

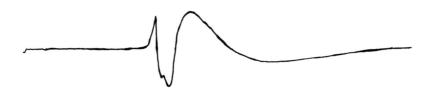

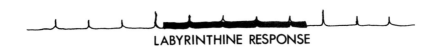

LABYRINTHINE RESPONSE

Fig. 3. Placing the KCl crystal on the vertebral artery surface.

narrow, that to make the vertebral arteries visible, parts of the lateral processes had to be removed. First the vertebral artery was only touched and a labyrinth response was obtained (Fig. 2). Repeated touching with a finger tip or with an instrument did not produce a response. Minutes later, however, another response was recorded. Eventually, a small crystal of potassium chloride was placed on the arterial wall and a differently shaped response was obtained (Fig. 3) and this could be reproduced instantly, as many times as the crystal was replaced on the vessel wall.

The experiment was later extended to dogs. Through a post-auricular incision, the tympanic bulla was exposed and opened and the oval window area visualized by drilling away part of the bony external canal. An electrode was introduced into the vestibule through the oval window and was fixed in position by a drop of tissue adhesive around it. The position of the electrode in the vestibule was confirmed by irrigating the middle ear with hot and cold water (Fig. 4). Exposure of the vertebral artery and nerve required sectioning of the sternomastoid and adjacent paravertebral muscles. By removing the transverse processes of two adjacent cervical vertebrae, an adequate length of the vertebral artery and nerve was exposed. The vertebral nerve in the dog consists of postganglionic sympathetic fibres arising from the stellate ganglion. In the human, these postganglionic sympathetic fibres form the plexus around the vertebral artery. The branches of the vertebral nerve travel along the branches of the vertebral artery much as they do in humans. The same experiments were then performed as in the cat. With simple touch a fatiguable labyrinthine signal was again obtained. Electrical stimulation on the arterial surface and of the vertebral nerve evoked a different type of impulse (Fig. 5 and 6). Finally, the potassium chloride produced the expected signal. The experiment was performed on 3 dogs with identical results.

Discussion

There is objective and undeniable evidence that without compressing the vertebral artery and through tactile or mechanical stimulation an ipsilateral labyrinthine impulse can be elicited. Chemical stimulation of the arterial wall creates a similar vestibular signal. The tactile stimulus can be reproduced after only about 15 minutes, whereas the chemical effect is reproducible immediately. All the different types of stimuli were applied to adjoining muscle and nerve elements. No labyrinthine response was seen except after electric stimulation of various neck muscles. These responses were entirely different from the labyrinthine responses following the vertebral arterial wall or vertebral nerve electrical stimulation in the dog.

If this experimental evidence is related to B.P.P.V. disease, the role of the vertebral artery can be confirmed. The pathogenesis of the instantaneous, short and fatiguable labyrinthine response however is not circulatory but neural. The impulse so created most likely affects all the vestibular receptors in the labyrinth, perhaps

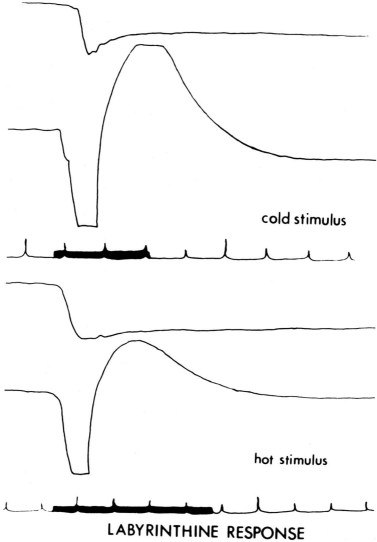

cold stimulus

hot stimulus

LABYRINTHINE RESPONSE

Fig. 4. Caloric stimulation through the middle ear in dog.

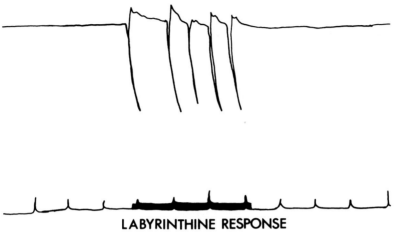

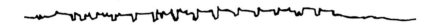

LABYRINTHINE RESPONSE

Fig. 5. Electrical stimulation of the vertebral artery.

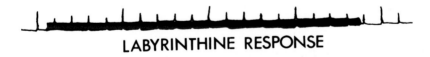

LABYRINTHINE RESPONSE

Fig. 6. Electrical stimulation of the vertebral nerve in dog.

with a predominance upon the ampullary end organs. This may be assumed because of the spinning or swerving sensations commonly reported. The resulting plane and direction of the nystagmus also suggests simultaneous excitation of the 3 ampullae. The fatiguability of the reaction is more comprehensible as a neural phenomenon rather than as a manifestation of an embarassed circulation. The responses in our animal experiments were recorded ipsilaterally. It is to be assumed that similar responses can be obtained from the contralateral labyrinth as well.

The post-traumatic postural vertigo is almost identical in symptoms to the B.P.P.V. disease. Naturally, it may occur in any age and often the short posture related dizzy attacks may be considerably prolonged. If the osteoarthritic bony deformities are the cause of the B.P.P.V., disarrangement of the cervical vertebral column suffered by a neck or 'whiplash' injury could explain the pathogenesis on the same basis.

The bony structural changes as the cause of the condition renders drug treatment of little value. The patient must be properly informed about the nature of his problem. When fear and uncertainty are eliminated, then there is more tolerance to the momentary discomfort. As an additional measure, an orthopedic collar around the neck provides the best prevention against the brief spell.

From the foregoing, it evolves that B.P.P.V. disease refers to the sudden, brief, fatiguable, spinning sensation upon certain head movement with no evidence of inner ear or CNS pathology. Since this condition is different from other types of postural vertigo a specific terminology with an acronym may be in order. Positioning Neurocervical Vertigo or P.N.V. is suggested to specify the condition when the recurring episodes are related to some cervical abnormality affecting the vertebral arterial surface.

Acknowledgements

Animal surgery was performed by Arthur Loewy, M.D., Arvind Kumar, M.D. and James Cambell, M.D. Assistance in electronic recording was provided by Lee R. Hamilton, B.S. and Raymond J. Mannarelli, M.A. The authors express appreciation for their valuable contributions.

References

Barany, R. (1920): Diagnose von Krankheitserscheinigungen im Bereiche des Otolithenapparates. *Acta Otolaryng.* 2, 434-437.

Barber, H.O. and Dionne, J. (1971): Vestibular findings in vertebro-basilar ischemia. *Ann. Otol. Rhinol.* 80, 805-811.

Biemond, A. and de Jong, I.M.B.V. (1969): On cervical nystagmus and related disorders. *Brain* 92, 437-458.

Dix, M.C. and Hallpike, C.S. (1952): The pathology, symptomatology and diagnosis of certain common disorders of the vestibular system. *Proc. Roy. Soc. Med.* 45, 341-354.

Frenzel, H. (1928): Rucknystagmus als Halsreflex und Schlagfeldverlagerung des labyrinthären Drehnystagmus durch Halsreflexe. *Z. Hals-Nasen-Ohrevheilk.* 21, 177-187.

Grahe, K. (1926): Beckenreflexe auf die Augen beim Menschen und ihre Bedeutung fur die Drehschwachreiz Prüfung des Vestibularapparates. *Z. Hals.-Nasen-Ohrenheilk.* 13, 613-616.

de Kleijn, A. (1921): Tonische Labyrinth und Hals Reflexe auf die Augen. *Pflugers arch.* **186**, 82-97.

Magnus, R. and Storm van Leeuwen, W. (1914): Die acuten und die dauerden Folgen des Ausfalles der tonischen Hals une Labyrinthreflexe. *Pflügers Arch.* **159**, 157-217.

Nylen, C.O. (1950): Positional nystagmus. *J. Laryngol. & Otol.* **64**, 295-317.

Pfaltz, C.R. and Richter, R.H. (1961): Disturbances of the cereblar circulation provoked by movements of the head. Motion Picture. VIIth Int. Congr. of Otolaryng., Paris.

Schuknecht, H.F. (1962): Positional vertigo: clinical and experimental observations. *Tr. Am. Acad. Ophth. & Otol.* **66**, 319-331.

3. Positional nystagmus elicited by industrial solvents

L.M. ÖDKVIST, B. LARSBY, R. THAM, S.R.C. LIEDGREN, G. ASCHAN

Linköping University, Department of Otolaryngology, University Hospital, Linköping, Sweden

Introduction

Ethyl alcohol as a vertigogenic drug elicits a positional nystagmus in man and other mammals. (Aschan, 1958, 1970).

People exposed to industrial solvents complain not only of fatigue and headache but also of nausea and vertigo (Browning, 1965; Goldie, 1960). The neurological symptoms that may be caused by the solvents are always very vague, and most clinical examinations fail to show any obvious pathological signs. Psychophysiological functions may be disturbed. (Gamberale and Hultengren, 1972, 1973). Exposed people may develop neurasthenia, personality changes, and intellectual reduction. (Axelsson *et al.,* 1976). All these findings are, however, vague, so there is a need for neurophysiological methods to estimate any influence on the nervous system. In order to unveil an influence by solvents on the vestibular system in analogy with positional alcohol nystagmus (PAN) an animal experimental series was started, administrating industrial solvents to rabbits.

Methods

Rabbits, bodyweight 2–4 kg, were mounted in a test box on a Stille rotatory platform. The box could be darkened by lid closure. Electrodes for nystagmography were attached (Aschan, 1970). Throughout the experiments the animals were tested for spontaneous nystagmus and nystagmus in lateral positions. Rotatory accelerations of $5°/\text{sec}^2$ up to a speed of $75°/\text{sec}$ were used to test for rotatory nystagmus. After 60 seconds of constant speed an analogous deceleration followed. The hydrocarbon industrial solvents xylene, styrene, methylchloroform and trichloroetylene were administered in four different series. (Fig. 1).

ETHANOL

PROPANOL

XYLENE

STYRENE

METHYLCHLOROFORM

TRICHLOROETHYLENE

Fig. 1. The chemical formula for the two alcohols and the four hydrocarbons that were used in the investigation.

As inhalation has failed to give stable blood concentrations in rabbit experiments the solvents were administered intravenously dissolved in a lipid emulsion (Larsby *et al.*, 1976; Ödkvist *et al.*, 1977). An infusion pump was connected to a polyethylene catheter introduced via an ear vein into the jugular vein. For comparison some additional rabbits were infused with ethanol or propanol. Arterial and central venous blood samples were collected. In some experiments cerebrospinal fluid (CSF) was collected from a fine catheter introduced suboccipitally. The solvents were estimated by gas chromatography.

Xylene and styrene were estimated by a head-space method using a flame ionization detector. Methylchloroform and trichloroethylene were determined using electron capture detection. (Tham *et al.*, 1977).

Results

For all solvents examined there was a good correlation between arterial blood levels and different speeds of infusion. After the infusion was started, a rapid rise of the arterial blood level during the first 10–20 minutes was followed by a slower increase to a steady state. Methylchloroform given with a speed of 9 mg/min reached this level in one hour. The three other solvents needed a longer time to reach a steady state.

The concentration of the solvents in the central venous blood rapidly levelled with the arterial blood.

The CSF solvent concentration mirrored the blood level, but was lower, the ratio being 0,3 for the methylchloroform and 0,05–0,1 for the other solvents.

During the intoxication by the solvents a positional nystagmus was often seen in lateral positions. The beat direction was to the left in right lateral position and vice versa. When infused with ethanol or propanol the beat direction was to the right in right lateral position.

The incidence of the positional nystagmus evoked by the solvents is related to the arterial blood concentration which is shown in Fig. 2. The minimum concentrations giving a positional nystagmus are approximately for xylene 30 ppm, trichloroethylene 30 ppm, styrene 40 ppm and methylchloroform 70 ppm.

Ethyl alcohol inhibits the nystagmus responses to rotatory acceleration. The responses are remarkably facilitated by xylene intoxication with regard to all its various parameters (Fig. 4). Neither methylchloroform nor trichloroethylene had any distinct effect on the rotatory responses. Styrene intoxication made the rotatory nystagmus reverse, i.e. beat to the left during clockwise rotation and vice versa. (Fig. 4). This effect as well as the alcohol and xylene effects ceased a short time after the infusion was ended.

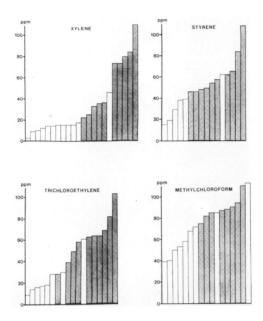

Fig. 2. Incidence of positional nystagmus elicited by the four tested industrial solvents. Each bar represents one rabbit experiment. An empty bar indicates absence of nystagmus and a filled one a rabbit that showed a positional nystagmus. The height of the bars indicates the blood concentration of the solvent 30 minutes after the start of the infusion, expressed in parts per million (ppm).

Discussion

Ethyl alcohol as well as propanol gives rise to a positional nystagmus as do the tested hydrocarbons, which however, evoke a different beat direction. The theory (Money and Myles, 1974) that the specific weight of the administered alcohol should offer the explanation for the direction of the nystagmus, due to the cupular buoyancy effect, cannot be valid for the solvents. This theory has to be called in question. (Greven *et al.,* 1977, Ödkvist *et al.,* 1977). The direction of the positional nystagmus is, as Fig. 3 shows, not related to the specific weight of the administered drug, but it seems as if its chemical properties determine the action on the vestibular system.

The different effects by alcohol, styrene and xylene on positional nystagmus and on the rotatory responses indicate that it cannot possibly be a simple effect on the peripheral vestibular system. The

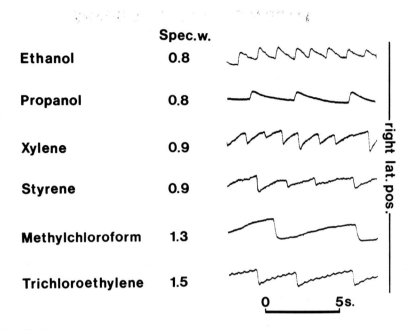

Fig. 3. Electronystagmographic recordings from rabbits intoxicated with the two alcohols with respect to the four hydrocarbons. The examples are chosen from rabbits in a right lateral position. The specific weight for the compounds are given. The hydrocarbons elicit a positional nystagmus with a beat direction the opposite of PAN.

underlying mechanisms have to be located in the central vestibular pathways.

Our experimental model thus seems to offer a way of evaluating some effects of solvents on the central nervous system. By future neurophysiological direct recordings in the central pathways it may be possible to develop the model even further.

The results from our rabbit experiments offer information concerning solvent effects on mammals but how close the human reactions come is not yet known. Experiments in man will be necessary. It is known that man is ten times as sensitive to alcohol compared to rabbit as far as positional nystagmus is concerned. (Aschan *et al.*, 1977). The corresponding man/rabbit ratio for solvents is not known. It is furthermore not yet possible to predict the correlation between the acute findings and the chronic effects of poisoning with industrial solvents.

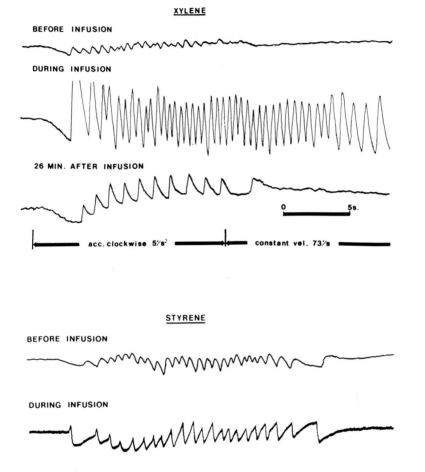

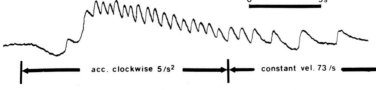

Fig. 4. Electronystagmographic recordings from two experiments using rotatory acceleration before, during and after intoxication. The response is exaggerated by xylene and reversed by styrene. The direction and the time of acceleration and constant speed is indicated below.

Acknowledgement

This research was supported by Arbetarskyddsfonden (Swedish Work Environment Fund), project 75–34 and Swedish Medical Research Council (MFR), project 14x–4503.

The authors wish to thank laboratory engineer Håkan Barreng and Irja Bunnfors for technical assistance.

References

Aschan, G. (1958): Different types of alcohol nystagmus. *Acta Otolaryngol.* Suppl. 140.

Aschan, G. (1970): Studies on the ascending vestibulo-ocular reflex arc. *Wenner-Gren Symposium* No. **15**, Pergamon Press, Oxford and New York.

Aschan, G., Bunnfors, I., Hydén, D., Larsby, B., Ödkvist, L.M. and Tham, R. (1977): Xylene exposure. Electronystagmographic and gas chromatographic studies in rabbits. *Acta Otolaryngol.* In press.

Axelsson, O., Hane, M. and Hogstedt, C. (1976): Neuropsychiatric illhealth in workers exposed to solvents – a case control study. *Läkartidningen* **73**, 322-325.

Browning, E. (1965): Xylene. *In Toxicity and Metabolism of Industrial Solvents,* pp. 77-89, Elsevier.

Gamberale, F. and Hultengren, M. (1972): Toluene exposure. II. Psychophysiological findings. *Work-environ-health* **9**, 3, 131-139.

Gamberale, G. and Hultengren, M. (1973): Methylchloroform exposure. I. Psychophysiological functions. *Work-environ.-health* **10**, 82-92.

Goldie, I. (1960): Can xylene (xylol) provoke convulsive seizures? *Ind. Med. Surg.* **29**, 33-35.

Greven, A.J., Oosterveld, W.J. and Samson, G. (1977): The influence of heavy water on the vestibular system. A study of heavy water nystagmus. *Adv. Oto-Rhino-Laryng.* **22**, 152-159.

Larsby, B., Ödkvist, L.M., Hydén, D. and Liedgren, S.R.C. (1976): Disturbances of the vestibular system by toxic agents. *Acta Phys. Scand. Suppl.* **440**.

Money, K.E. and Myles, W.S. (1974): Heavy water nystagmus and effects of alcohol. *Nature* **247**, 404-405.

Money, K.E., Myles, W.S. and Hoffert, B.M. (1974): The mechanism of positional alcohol nystagmus. *Can. J. Otolaryngol.* **3**, 302-313.

Ödkvist, L.M., Larsby, B. and Liedgren, S.C.R. (1977): Influence of industrial solvents on the vestibular system. XI World Congress in Otorhinolaryngology. Buenos Aires, Argentine.

Tham, R., Larsby, B., Hydén, D., Aschan, G. and Ödkvist, L.M. (1977): Pharmacokinetics of solvents in the experimental animal model. International symposium on the control of air pollution in the working environment Stockholm (Sweden).

4. Tilted-head mice with genetic otoconial anomaly. Behavioural and morphological correlates

D.J. LIM*, L.C. ERWAY**, D.L. CLARK†

*Department of Otolaryngology, Ohio State University College of Medicine, Columbus, Ohio, U.S.A.

**Department of Biology, University of Cincinnati, Cincinnati, Ohio, U.S.A.

†Department of Anatomy, Ohio State University College of Medicine, Columbus, Ohio, U.S.A.

Introduction

Many mutations in the house mouse (*Mus musculus*) are known to affect the inner ear (Deol, 1968). Among the mutants, tilted-head (*th*) was first discovered by Larsen (1959) and is known to have an otoconial deficiency or deformity (Erway *et al.*, 1971). This mutant is similar to the pallid mouse (*pa*) in having head-tilting behavior and a deficiency of otoconia (Lyon, 1951; Lim and Erway, 1974) but differs in having abnormal otoconia. Due to this selective pathology involving, as far as we know, only the gravity receptors, these animals serve as an excellent model for testing the function of the gravity receptor organs. Since the number of otoliths can be well defined in the tilted-head mouse, we have attempted to correlate the behavioural and physiological data with morphological findings in this mutant mouse.

Material and Methods

Eighteen random-bred mice were studied from a stock segregating for tilted-head (*th*) and leaden (*ln*) coat color (*th* and *ln* are located 2 map units apart on chromosome 1). The leaden phenotype (*ln/ln*) is a convenient marker for the tilted-head genotype (*th/th*). However, due to crossing-over, three leaden individuals (#2, 9 and 34 in Table I) had normal otoliths, indicative of homozygosity for leaden and heterozygosity for tilted-head (*ln th/ln +*). They served as controls, while the remaining 15 were double homozygotes (*ln th/*

ln th) and exhibited various degrees of behavioural and morphological defects.

The *swimming test* was conducted in a tank of water. Swimming behaviour was recorded by cinephotography and classified as normal, near normal, vertical, near vertical, or underwater circler (totally disoriented) on the basis of three independent trials. The *air-righting reflex* was recorded by stroboscopic photography, 1/30 sec per flash. The exposure number in which the mouse had righted itself was identified and averaged for six to eight trials per mouse (Fig. 1).

For the *morphological study,* the animals were sacrificed by intra-cardiac perfusion with 0.12 mole phosphate-buffered 1% paraformal-dehyde-1.5% glutaraldehyde mixture. The specimens were post-fixed in 0.1 mole *s*-collidine-buffered 1.33% osmium. They were dissected

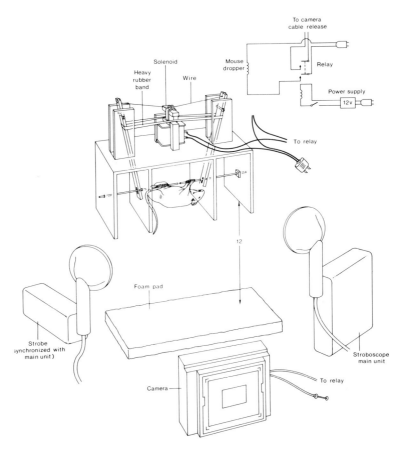

Fig. 1. A set-up for righting reflex measurement by stroboscopic photographs.

TABLE I

Morphology and Behavioral Data from 18 Tilted-Head Mice

Percentage of Sensory Area Covered by Crystals in Gravity Receptors (number of crystals)

TH No. (Swimming behavior)*	LEFT			RIGHT			BOTH	Direction** of	
	Saccule % Covered (No.)	Utricle % Covered (No.)	Mean % Covered (No.)	Saccule % Covered (No.)	Utricle % Covered (No.)	Mean % Covered (No.)	Mean % Covered (No.)	Head Tilt (side down)	Righting
2 (N)	100.0 (N)*	100.0 (N)	100.0 (N)	100.0 (N)	100.0 (N)	100.0 (N)	100.0 (N)	–	R
3 (N)	24.2 (3)	20.4 (1)	22.3 (4)	21.7 (3)	23.2 (1)	22.4 (4)	22.4 (8)	R	R
4 (NV)	7.1 (1)	0.0 (0)	3.6 (1)	10.6 (1)	0.0 (0)	5.3 (1)	4.5 (2)	L	R
5 (NN)	18.5 (16)	26.3 (7)	22.4 (23)	22.0 (13)	36.2 (9)	29.1 (22)	25.8 (45)	–	–
8 (V)	17.2 (4)	15.4 (1)	16.3 (5)	10.4 (1)	0.0 (0)	5.2 (1)	10.8 (6)	–	R
9 (N)	100.0 (N)	100.0 (N)	100.0 (N)	100.0 (N)	100.0 (N)	100.0 (N)	100.0 (N)	–	L
11 (NV)	12.6 (2)	14.3 (3)	13.5 (5)	13.2 (4)	25.6 (1)	19.4 (5)	16.5 (10)	–	L
12 (NV)	15.9 (2)	0.0 (0)	8.0 (2)	22.9 (3)	0.0 (0)	11.5 (3)	9.8 (5)	L	R
13 (C&V)#	13.2 (2)	0.0 (0)	6.6 (2)	15.6 (4)	0.0 (0)	7.8 (4)	7.2 (6)	L	R
14 (V)	23.9 (1)	0.0 (0)	12.0 (1)	15.3 (2)	0.0 (0)	7.6 (2)	9.8 (3)	–	L
16 (NV)	18.7 (1)	0.0 (0)	9.3 (1)	14.5 (1)	0.0 (0)	7.2 (1)	8.3 (2)	R	R
17 (C)	0.0 (0)	0.0 (0)	9.0 (0)	11.7 (1)	0.0 (0)	5.9 (1)	3.0 (1)	L	R
21 (C&V)#	0.0 (0)	0.0 (0)	0.0 (0)	11.1 (1)	0.0 (0)	5.5 (1)	2.8 (1)	–	L
23 (C)	6.3 (2)	0.0 (0)	3.1 (2)	13.0 (2)	12.4 (1)	12.7 (3)	7.9 (5)	–	R
25 (NV)	11.9 (2)	0.0 (0)	5.9 (2)	8.6 (2)	0.0 (0)	4.3 (2)	5.1 (4)	L	L
32 (N/A)	0.0 (0)	0.0 (0)	0.0 (0)	10.3 (1)	0.0 (0)	5.1 (1)	2.5 (1)	N/A	R
34 (N)	100.0 (N)	100.0 (N)	100.0 (N)	100.0 (N)	100.0 (N)	100.0 (N)	100.0 (N)	–	R
36 (V)	8.7 (2)	0.0 (0)	4.3 (2)	12.8 (5)	0.0 (0)	6.4 (5)	5.4 (7)	–	R

*N: normal; NN: near normal; V: vertical; NV: near vertical; C: underwater circler; N/A: not available.

**R: right; L: left; –: right and left equally; N/A: not available.

These mice were basically underwater circlers, although they also exhibited vertical swimming.

in 70% alcohol during the dehydration process. Each gravity receptor organ was stereoscopically photographed (Wild) to localize the areas in which otoconia were present, and the number and size of crystals were recorded. The areas of the sensory epithelia and the corresponding crystal areas were mapped on tracing paper and measured using a planimeter. After being photographed, the inner ear tissue was processed for either scanning electron microscopy (SEM) and x-ray analysis (EDAX-707) following critical-point drying using CO_2 or embedded in Epon® for light and transmission electron microscopy (TEM) to evaluate the sensory epithelium of the gravity receptors.

Results

Morphology of the Gravity Receptors

The otoconia of the 18 animals included in this study showed varying amounts of otoconia, ranging from one crystal covering 2.5% of the sensory area to normal (Fig. 2). Many animals had 1–45 gigantic abnormal crystals (Table I). Since crystal size varied, the percentage of the sensory epithelium covered by abnormal crystals was calculated (Table I). Of the 30 *th* ears examined, 19 contained crystals (otoconia) only in the saccule. The mean area of sensory epithelium was as follows: right utricle, 0.107 ± 0.040 mm^2; right saccule, 0.161 ± 0.044 mm^2; left utricle, 0.106 ± 0.032 mm^2; left saccule, 0.142 ± 0.029 mm^2.

The abnormal crystals were larger in cases where only a few crystals were formed and smaller where multiple crystals occurred. The long axis of some crystals measured about 0.25 mm. They were butterfly shaped, with 'wings' that are layered or petaled by crystallites (Fig. 3). The crystals are found to be made of calcium when examined with the x-ray analyzer.

The decalcified and thin-sectioned crystal shows subunits of crystallites that are demarcated by uneven condensation of an organic substance somewhat resembling the fast and slow growth zones of the fish otolith (Lim, 1974). The crystals are covered by a gelatinous gluey substance and adhere to the gelatinous layer of the otolithic membrane.

The sensory epithelium and the peripheral nerves of the gravity receptors appear normal in both light and electron microscopy (Fig. 4), and the vestibular nuclei also appear normal on the light microscopic level.

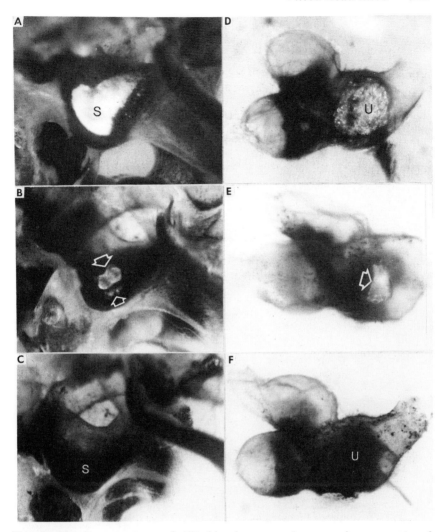

Fig. 2. Gravity receptors of tilted-head mouse show varying amounts of otoconia. About x 38. A: Normal otoconia in saccule (S). B: One large (big arrow) and one small (small arrow) giant crystal in saccule. C: Absence of otoconia in saccule (S). D: Numerous abnormal crystals in utricle (U). E: One giant crystal (arrow) in utricle. F: Absence of otoconia in utricle (U).

Swimming test

The normal swimmer is defined as one which assumes a horizontal position during swimming and the vertical swimmer as one which assumes a vertical position. Both maintain their heads above water.

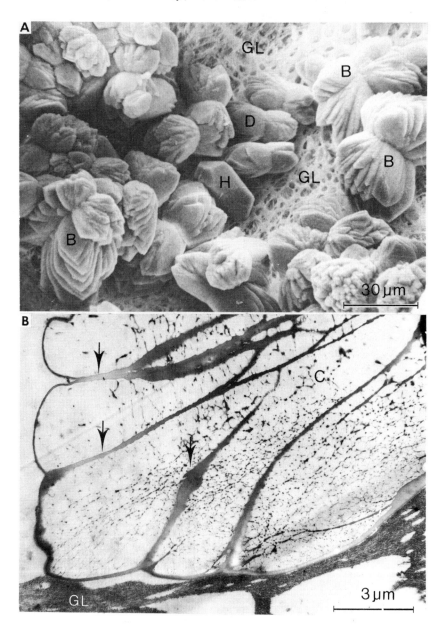

Fig. 3A. SEM micrograph shows numerous abnormal otoconia in the utricle of a tilted-head mouse. The crystals are mainly butterfly shaped (B), but a few are dumbell shaped (D) or hexagonal (H). The gelatinous layer (GL) of the otoconial membrane is well developed. B. TEM micrograph of EDTA-decalcified abnormal crystal shows that subunits (crystallites) are demarcated by dense organic substance (arrows). The crystal is attached to the gelatinous layer (GL) of the otoconial membrane.

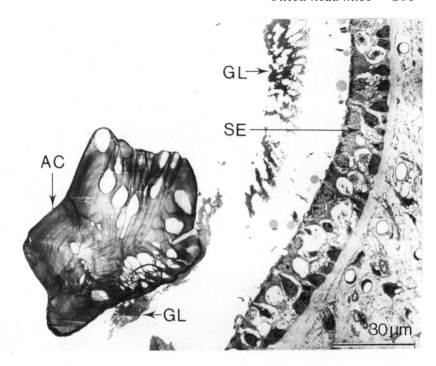

Fig. 4. TEM micrograph shows normal appearing sensory epithelium (SE) and well-developed gelatinous layer (GL) of the otoconial membrane in a tilted-head mouse. The abnormal crystal (AC) contains dense but lobulated organic substance and is partly attached to the gelatinous membrane, which is separated from the sensory epithelium. This separation is interpreted as an artifact.

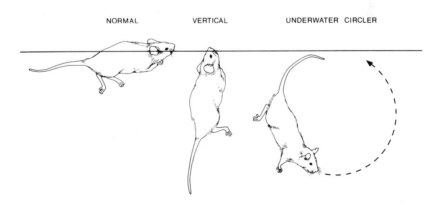

Fig. 5. Swimming behaviour is classified as: A—normal swimmer, B—vertical swimmer, C—underwater circler.

Some which were neither true vertical nor true horizontal swimmers are defined as near vertical or near normal. The underwater circler is defined as one which appears to lose orientation and circles underwater, possibly drowning if not rescued (Fig. 5).

Of the 18 animals that completed all the other tests and for which morphological data are available, 17 have swimming data. Of these 17, 5 were classified as normal (1 near normal), 8 as vertical (5 near vertical), and 4 as underwater circler.

When the swimming data are compared with morphological findings, normal swimmers are observed to have otoconia in all gravity receptors. By contrast, all but two of the vertical swimmers had otoconia exclusively in the saccules, and the two exceptional mice exhibited both vertical and circling behaviour. Three of the four underwater circlers had pronounced left-right asymmetry.

Air-righting reflex

One animal (#32) completely failed to right in eight trials, and the rest righted at varying distances (or times) from the beginning of the fall (Fig. 6). Most of the normal and near normal swimmers righted

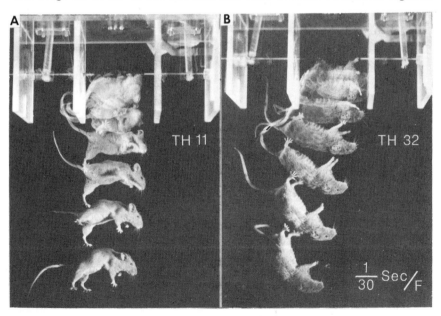

Fig. 6A. This tilted-head animal righted at the 7th exposure (6/30 sec), which is considered slower than normal, and is shown to have some otoconia in all gravity receptors. B. This tilted-head animal failed to right and is shown to have no otoconia in all gravity receptors.

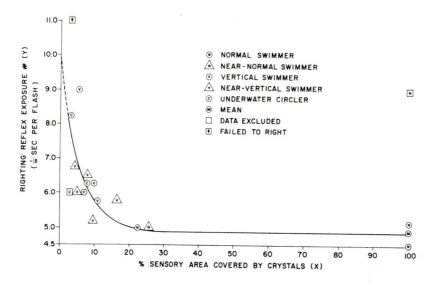

Fig. 7. Correlation between righting time and the averaged percentage of sensory area covered by crystals. The data for three animals are not included, two that deviated too much from the others and one that failed to right. The dotted line indicates the best fit curve extrapolated to its intercept even though we have no data for this area.

at about 5 exposures (4/30 sec), and one righted in the 9th exposure (8/30 sec). Because this animal deviated from the rest it was not included in the statistical analysis. The vertical, near vertical and underwater circlers showed delayed air-righting ability, as shown in Fig. 7. When the time required to right is compared with the average percentage of all sensory organs covered by otoconia, the animals which had crystals covering 20% or more righted normally. However, below 20% there appears to be a prolongation of time required for righting, increasing exponentially in relation to the otoconial deficiency. The one animal (#32) that failed to right in every trial possessed only one large abnormal crystal in the right saccule. Two other animals (#17, #21) with essentially the same condition did right themselves.

Statistical analysis of the righting reflex was accomplished in two steps because the data are modelled as a decaying exponential curve. The first step was to estimate the asymptotic value. The second step was to incorporate this value into the exponential model and then evaluate the coefficients. Step one was accomplished by using a linear regression analysis. Step two used all the raw data plus the mean of the data obtained from the animals with sensory areas 100% covered by otoconia, and the best fit curve is derived by polynomial regression analysis. The significance of the regression analysis is demonstrated by an extremely significant ($p<.001$) $F_{(2, 11)}$ value of 108.9.

Discussion

The only known primary pathology of the tilted-head mouse is confined to otoconia malformation or deficiency of varying magnitudes, affecting some or all of the gravity receptors (Erway *et al.,* 1971; McGraw, 1973; Coccia, 1975). The sensory epithelium of all vestibular organs and nerve fibres innervating sensory cells showed no obvious pathology when examined by light and electron microscopy in the present study, confirming earlier reports. Vestibular nuclei also showed a normal appearance in preliminary observations using light microscopy.

The gelatinous layer of the otoconial membrane described earlier in the pallid mouse (Lim and Erway, 1974) also was observed in the tilted-head mouse. The large crystals are often glued to this membrane, which would indicate that even a single crystal can exert a uniform stimulus to a larger area, if not to all, of the sensory epithelium that is covered by this gelatinous membrane.

Our study showed that the malformed crystals have a definite shape which resembles a butterfly, with wings made of layered or petaled subunits of crystallites. In some respects, these crystals are similar to those observed in the 'immature crystals' found in newborn rats (Ross and Peacor, 1975). Our x-ray study revealed that they are organic crystals made of calcium, in agreement with Ross and Peacor. Uneven distribution of organic matrix coincided with subunits of crystallites. This indicates that the crystal is formed either by cyclic deposition of calcium and organic substance or by the aggregation of the crystallites. The former is similar to the fish otolith, which possesses age (or seasonal) rings that are made up of alternate bands of calcium-rich zones and organic-substance-rich zones (Lim, 1974). The latter process is observed in the otoconia of ethacrynic acid-intoxicated animals, which aggregate by fusion (Lim, 1973). Since the developmental morphology of the abnormal crystals is not complete, we cannot determine in which way the unusual crystals are formed.

Erway *et al.* (1971) observed that manganese supplementation during the critical time of otoconia formation in pallid mice can prevent or reduce the otoconia dysgenesis (deficiency), but manganese supplementation only slightly enhances the number of abnormal crystals in tilted-head mice, never approaching normal otoconia.

Shrader *et al.* (1973) provided evidence that manganese is involved in the biosynthesis of mucopolysaccharides related to otolith formation, but no evidence is available as to whether the mucopolysaccharide is normal in the otoconial membrane of the tilted-head mouse.

Erway *et al.* (1971) and McGraw (1973) found that the development of the body-righting reflex is delayed in tilted-head mice as compared to normal mice. It is known that the righting reflex is related to gravity receptor function, so its delayed development is considered to be the result of otoconial deficiency in this genetic mutant. Whereas body-righting was only delayed in development, the physiological delay in the air-right reflex persists in the adult. Despite this statistically significant delay, perhaps related to inefficiency of the macular system, those mutants with any potential for saccular input did air-right themselves. Only one tilted-head mutant in this study (#32), possessing a single saccular crystal, could not air-right itself, but numerous pallid mice, which often lack otoconia, completely failed this same test (unpublished data). Therefore, tilted-head mice provide strong evidence that the presence of otoconia in the saccule only enables mice to maintain a vertical position in the water and to air-right themselves. These observations may provide a basis for distinguishing between the equilibratory functions of utricular and saccular otoconia. Although most of the animals tested have equal distribution of otoconia in the right and left gravity receptors, there were a few that had asymmetry. There appears to be no correlation between morphological asymmetry of otoconia and the direction of head-tilt in the direction of turning during the righting reflex, which is in agreement with earlier reports (Lyon, 1951; Erway *et al.*, 1971).

Swimming behaviour correlated well with the morphological findings. Vertical swimming behaviour correlates with the presence of saccular otoconia combined with the absence of (or decreased) utricular otoconia. Vertical and underwater circling correlate with asymmetry between right and left otoconia.

Acknowledgement

This study was supported in part by research grants from NASA (NGR 36-008-211) and from The Deafness Research Foundation. The authors wish to acknowledge the invaluable assistance of Ilija Karanfilov, Jonathan Darby, Joan Osborne, Laurence Owens, Scott Gordon, Steven McBride, Nancy Sally and Katherine Adamson.

References

Coccia, M.R. (1975): The influence of the otoliths on semicircular canal induced nystagmus. Ph.D. dissertation, The Ohio State University, Columbus, Ohio.

Deol, M.S. (1968): Inherited diseases of the inner ear in the light studies on the mouse. *J. Med. Genet.* **5**, 137-155.

Erway, L.C., Fraser, A.S. and Hurley, L.S. (1971): Prevention of congenital otolith defects in pallid mice by manganese supplementation. *Genetics* **67**, 97-108.

Larsen, M.M. (1959): Personal Communication. Mouse News Letter **20**, 49.

Lim, D.J. (1973): Formation and fate of the otoconia. *Ann. Otol. Rhinol. Laryngol.* **82**, 23-36.

Lim, D.J. (1974): The statoconia of the non-mammalian species. *Brain Behav. Evol.* **10**, 37-51.

Lim, D.J. and Erway, L. (1974): Influence of manganese on genetically defective otolith. *Ann. Otol. Rhinol. Laryngol.* **83**, 565-581.

Lyon, M.F. (1951): Hereditary absence of otoliths in the house mouse. *J. Physiol.* **114**, 410-418.

McGraw, R.H. (1973): The tilted-head mouse: A study in vestibular equilibrium physiology. M.S. Thesis, University of Cincinnati, Cincinnati, Ohio.

Ross, M.D. and Peacor, D. (1975): The nature and crystal growth of otoconia in the rat. *Ann. Otol. Rhinol. Laryngol.* **84**, 22-37.

Shrader, R.E., Erway, L.C. and Hurley, L.S. (1973): Mucopolysaccharide synthesis in the developing inner ear of manganese-deficient and pallid mutant mice. *Teratology* **8**, 257-266.

5. Neurotological studies on methylmercurial intoxication in Macaca irus.

M. AOYAGI*, I. KATO*, Y. SATO**, K. MIZUKOSHI**, T. SATO†, H. INO**

*Department of Otolaryngology, Yamagata University

**Department of Otolaryngology, Niigata University

†Department of Neuropathology, Brain Research Institute, Niigata University

Methylmercury Intoxication

In 1965 some of the inhabitants in the riverside area of the Aganogawa River in Niigata, Japan, complained of a strange illness subsequently diagnosed as chronic poisoning by organic mercury compounds, generally well known as the Minamata disease. In these patients dysequilibrium as well as sensory disturbances and visual field impairment were frequently observed (Mizukoshi et al., 1975).

Therefore, we have attempted to determine whether or not neurotological signs similar to those observed in patients could be reproducible in animals and to assess the toxic level of methylmercury from the neurotological point of view.

Experimental Design

Five cynomolgus monkeys of both sexes weighing between 2.1 and 3.5 Kg were used in the present experiment. They were divided into three groups, i.e., the subacute group, the subchronic group and the subclinical group depending upon the doses and duration of methylmercury compound administered.

Methylmercury compounds were given orally by a stomach tube or by addition to the diet. Blood and hair samples for Hg determination were collected regularly once a week.

Examination Procedures

Neurological examination and electronystagmographic (ENG) tests were performed one or two times a week. The ENG test was performed in the following manner:

1. Spontaneous nystagmus
2. Positional nystagmus
3. Experimental nystagmus
    (1) Caloric nystagmus
    (2) Visual suppression test
    (3) Optokinetic nystagmus

Recording Procedure

Platinum needle electrodes were used to record eye movements. Test trials took place in total darkness. Mental alertness was maintained by the use of methanphetamine at least 30 minutes before testing.

Optokinetic nystagmus was elicited by rotating stripes of light projected on a white screen.

Caloric stimuli consisted of 20 ml of water at temperatures of 28°C and 48°C irrigated over a 20 sec period. During the maximum intensity of caloric nystagmus, the visual suppression test was performed. At the maximum intensity the screen placed about 50 cm in front of the monkey was illuminated from behind the animal for 10 sec (Kato et al., in press). The amounts of visually induced suppression in slow-phase velocity were determined during the first half of the period in light, and percent reduction in slow-phase velocity was established according to the formula described by Takemori and Cohen (1974).

ENG Findings

One of the most striking ENG findings in all three groups was that spontaneous and positional nystagmus were the earliest signs appearing prior to the onset of such clinical symptoms as diarrhea and hyperreflexia of tendon reflexes. Even in the subclinical group, which did not show any detectable clinical signs and symptoms nor microscopic pathological findings, the only abnormal signs were spontaneous and positional nystagmus. Optokinetic nystagmus and caloric nystagmus remained unchanged until severe neurological symptoms appeared. Hyperexcitability of optokinetic after nystagmus and caloric nystagmus, i.e., the secondary and third phase, however, were recognized a few months before severe neurological symptoms could be detected.

Loss of visual suppression of caloric nystagmus was observed prior to pathological findings of optokinetic nystagmus and manifestations of cerebellar ataxia.

Comment

The Table summarizes the relationship between the dosages adminis-tered and other signs and symptoms. In the subacute and subchronic groups, the dose levels at the onset of neurotoxic symptoms are generally in good agreement with the experiment by Ikeda (1973).

Methylmercury Intoxication in Macaca irus

	NO.	Nystagmus		Severe Neurol. Symptoms		Neuropathological Findings	
		Total Hg mg/Kg	days	Total Hg mg/Kg	days	light microscopic	light microscopic
Subacute	8	1.2	7	14.3	67	++	+++
	13	2.6	7	12.9	58	+++	+++
Subchronic	10	1.7	14	11.3	105	++	+++
Subclinical	9	9.0	171	-	-	-	-
	12	5.7	248	-	-	-	-

As illustrated in the Table the subclinical group, on the other hand, showed neither neurological signs and symptoms nor microscopic findings. Only by using electron microscopy could fine structural damage be observed (Sato and Ikuta, 1977). In this group, however, spontaneous and positional nystagmus was definitely detected as shown in the Table.

Hence, it can be deduced that the ENG test is one of the most sensitive measures for detecting functional disturbance in methyl-mercury intoxication.

References

Ikeda, Y., Tobe, F., Kobayashi, K., Suzuki, S., Kawasaki, T. and Yonematu, H. (1973): Long-term toxicity study of methylmercuric chloride in monkeys. *Toxicology* 1, 361-375.

Kato, I., Aoyagi, M., Sato, Y., Kawasaki, T. and Mizukoshi, K.: Visual suppression in vertebrate. *Brain Research* (in press).

Mizukoshi, K., Nagaba, M., Ohno, Y., Ishikawa, K., Aoyagi, M., Watanabe, Y., Kato, I. and Ino, H. (1975): Neurological studies upon intoxication by organic mercury compounds. *ORL*, 37, 74-87.

Sato, T. and Ikuta, F. (1977): Neuropathology of methylmercury intoxication in Niigata and chronic effects in Monkeys. *Neurotoxicology*, pp. 261-269 (Raven Press, New York).

Takemori, S. and Cohen, B. (1974): Loss of visual suppression of vestibular nystagmus after flocculus lesions. *Brain Research* 72, 213-224.

6. Positional nystagmus of the persistent type

K. ZILSTORFF, J. THOMSEN, N.J. JOHNSEN

University ENT Department, Rigshospitalet Copenhagen, Denmark

Introduction

The occurrence of positional nystagmus in individual cases was first described by Barany 1906, 1913 and 1921. The case in 1913 was – in contrast to the cases described in 1906 and 1921 – persistent and due to multiple sclerosis (Barany, 1921).

The most widely used classification of different types of positional nystagmus is that of Nylén. He mentioned his classification for the first time in 1924 and published the three main types of positional nystagmus in 1953.

Type I, direction changing positional nystagmus, Type II, direction fixed positional nystagmus, and Type III, irregular positional nystagmus, characterized by variations in its behaviour.

Aschan *et al.* (1957) took note of the duration of nystagmus stating that in their type I and II the nystagmus was persistent. In the persistent type Aschan *et al.,* found the position of the head to be a determining factor and not the movements of the head to the position.

Dix and Hallpike (1952) and Cawthorne (1954) described 2 types of positional nystagmus, peripheral and central.

According to Kornhuber (1969) there are only two clearcut types of positional nystagmus, one: positional nystagmus in the narrower sense or positional of the central type. Two: positioning or positional nystagmus of peripheral origin, also called benign paroxysmal posional nystagmus.

We have adopted the last classification and registered a positional nystagmus of the persistent or central type, if the nystagmus has no latent period, lasting as long as the position was maintained and if the nystagmus was constant by repetition of the positional tests, the nystagmus often being irregular, sometimes with dissociation of the movements of the two eyes, with low frequency and high amplitude and no accompanying vertigo. The direction of the nystagmus, change of direction and occurrence in one or more positions we find of less importance.

Material, Methods and Results

A total of 10.730 patients were referred to routine neuro-otologic examination at the University ENT department, Rigshospitalet, from the neurologic and neurosurgical departments during the years 1970-1975. The examination included examination for positional nystagmus using Frenzels glasses, in the following positions: right and left lateral position, suppine position and head hanging position. Electronystagmography was not performed. The same physician (Zilstorff) performed all the examinations. A total of 124 patients had positional nystagmus of the persistent type. The age and sex distribution is given in table I, no difference between men and women could be noted. 21 patients (17%) were below 15 years of age.

TABLE I
Age Distribution of 124 Patients with Persisting Positional Nystagmus
and 173 Patients with Persisting Spontaneous Nystagmus

	0−15 Year	16−30 Year	31−50 Year	51−70 Year	70 Year	TOTAL Male	Female
PN	21	16	33	48	6	65	59
%	17%	13%	27%	38%	5%	52%	48%
SN	32	15	61	59	6	90	83
%	19%	9%	35%	34%	3%	52%	48%

In contrast 111 patients in our material had a positional nystagmus of the non-persistent (peripheral) type. None of these patients had central neurological disease.

Table II shows the distribution of positions in which was elicited. In 82 cases (66%), the nystagmus was found in the head hanging position, and in 52 cases positional nystagmus could only be elicited in this head hanging position.

33 patients exhibited a vertical positional nystagmus, this type being evenly distributed in the different positions.

The clinical diagnosis in the 124 patients with positional nystagmus is given in table III. Positional nystagmus is, overall, a rare symptom, being found in this material only in about 1%. It is to be noted that 53 patients (43%) suffered from intracranial tumors, all diagnosed by operation and verified histologically. The remaining patients were

TABLE II

Distribution of Positions in which Nystagmus was elicited in 124 Patients with
Persisting Positional Nystagmus

Position	Number
Lateral (left and/or right)	54 (44%)
Suppine	45 (36%)
Head hanging	82 (66%)

In 52 cases (42%) Persisting Positional Nystagmus on *Hanging Head* was the only finding.

TABLE III

Distribution of Diagnosis in 124 Patients with Persisting Positional Nystagmus
in Relation to Total Number of Patients Examined

Diagnosis	Positional nystagmus		Total number of patients examined	
	Number	%	Number	% with PN
Infratentorial tumor	34 53	28% 43%	168	20%
Supratentorial tumor	19	15%	858	3%
Encephalopathia	14	11%	1070	1%
Epilepsia	11	9%	616	2%
Multiple sclerosis	12	10%	194	6%
Head trauma	9	7%	1172	1%
Intracranial vascular disease	15	12%	536	3%
Other	10	8%	6116	0.1%
Total	124		10730	1%

fairly evenly distributed among the diagnoses: encephalopathia, epilepsia, multiple sclerosis, head trauma and intracranial vascular disease. Special emphasis has to be made on the infratentorial tumors, since among the 168 patients examined in this 6 year period from 1970–1975, with this diagnosis, 20% exhibited positional nystagmus of the persistent type. The other diagnoses mentioned were not represented in any percentage significantly different from that of the total material. Nevertheless, 6% of a total of 198 patients with multiple sclerosis did exhibit this symptom.

It is noteworthy however that in young patients below 15 years of age as shown in table IV 17 out of 21, that is 80%, suffered from intracranial tumors, 57% being infratentorial.

Table V shows some of the co-existing oto-neurologic findings in the 124 patients with positional nystagmus, none of the symptoms,

TABLE IV
Age Group 0–15 Year

	Infratentorial tumors	Supratentorial tumors	Total tumors
PN (N =21)	12 = 57%	5 = 23%	17 = 80%
SN (N =32)	4 = 12%	5 = 18%	10 = 30%

TABLE V
Additional Vestibular Symptoms in 124 Patients with Persisting Positional Nystagmus

Directional preponderance	14	11%
Hyporeactivity	16	13%
Gaze nystagmus	6	5%
Optokinetic nystagmus	14	11%
Hearing loss (sensorineural type)	9	7%
Hyperreactivity	4	3%
Without additional vestibular symptoms	61	50%

directional preponderance, hyporeactivity, gaze nystagmus, opto-kinetic defects, or hyperreactivity occurred with significantly high frequency. It has to be noted that 7 of the 9 patients with sensori-neural hearing loss, had an acoustic neuroma.

Furthermore, it is remarkable, that 61 patients (50%), had persistent positional nystagmus as the only oto-neurologic finding, indicating intracranial disease.

Discussion

The role of electronystagmography in the examination for positional nystagmus is questionable. Several authors have demonstrated a very high frequency, up to 80%, of positional nystagmus in normals, using ENG. However, without ENG, but with Frenzel's or Bartel's glasses, the occurrence of positional nystagmus in normals is rare, (Mulch and Lewitzki, 1977). We therefore share Kornhuber's opinion (1969) that examination with Frenzel's glasses at the present time represents the best method for differentiating between physiological and pathological nystagmus. We therefore feel that our material can also serve as a normal material even though derived from neurological and neurosurgical departments, since positional nystagmus of the persistent type was only present in about one per cent of the patients. Experimental persistent positional nystagmus may be due to different lesions in the posterior fossa, especially in the nodulus (Fernandez, 1960; Grant *et al.,* 1964) or the vestibular nuclei (Uemura *et al.,* 1972). Also intoxication by alcohol, barbiturates, etc. may cause positional nystagmus.

Aschan *et al.* (1964) state that electric stimulation in the nodulus of rabbits results in a nystagmus, that was always influenced by position, whereas nystagmus provoked by stimulation in the vestibular nuclei was spontaneous, i.e. not influenced by the position of the head. The direction of spontaneous nystagmus after stimulation depended very much upon which nucleus and which part of the same nucleus was stimulated.

In clinical cases it is usually difficult to correlate the nystagmus-findings with the structural changes within the central nervous system. What is primary and what is secondary, due to pressure, oedema, vascular changes etc.?

Though positional nystagmus is a sign or index of an organic lesion, its localizing value is still very much in question. The location of the lesion must largely depend on associated signs and symptoms. However, based on our findings the presence of positional nystagmus of the persistent type, is most indicative of an intracranial tumor or multiple sclerosis. The persistence of the nystagmus in the position and the constant occurrence by repetition of the position is according to our experience, essential. In all cases we found it the result of a central lesion. Thus persistent positional nystagmus is the same as central positional nystagmus.

As mentioned, the majority of the cases with positional nystagmus was elicited in the head hanging position, and in 42% of the total cases this was the only nystagmus finding. Similar observations have been reported by Nylén (1931). However, one must be sure that the nystagmus is really due to head position and not to neck torsion, since in the latter case the nystagmus is secondary to ischemia of the brainstem, caused by compression of the vertebral arteries.

Finally, we wish to emphasize the significance of persistent positional nystagmus in children below 15 years of age. In the 6 year period a total of 876 children were examined, as seen from table VI. 21 presented positional nystagmus of the persistent type and 17 of these had an intracranial tumor, especially infratentorial, verified by operation. The diagnostic specificity of the test is 81% (95% confidence limits: 58–95) and the diagnostic sensitivity 91% (95% confi-

TABLE VI
Diagnostic Value of Persisting Positional Nystagmus in Children
with Intracranial Tumors

	+ Tumor	− Tumor	Total
+ PN	17	4	21
− PN	73	782	855
	90	786	876

Diagnostic specificity: 17/21 = 81% (95% confidence limits: 58−95)
Diagnostic sensitivity: 782/855 = 91% (95% confidence limits: 89−94)

dence limits 89−94). This means that if a child exhibits persistent positional nystagmus he has a 81% chance of having an intracranial tumor, while on the contrary, if he does not exhibit persistent positional nystagmus, he has a 91% chance of not having a tumor.

References

Aschan, G., Bergsted, M., Drettner, B., Nylén, C.O. and Stahle, J. (1957): The Effect of Head Movement on Positional Nystagmus. *Laryngoscope* **67**, 884-893.

Aschan, F., Ekvall, L. and Grant, G. (1963): Nystagmus Following Stimulation In The Central Vestibular Pathways Using Permanently Implanted Electrodes. *Acta Oto-laryng. (Stockh.) Suppl.* **192**, 63-77.

Baràny, R. (1921): Diagnose von Krankheitserscheinungen im Bereiche des Otolithenapparates. *Acta Otolaryng. (Stockh.)* **2**, 434-437.

Cawthorne, T. (1954): Positional Nystagmus. *Ann. Otol.* **63**, 481-484.

Dix, M.R. and Hallpike, C.S. (1952): The pathology symptomathology and diagnosis of certain common disorders of the vestibular system. *Proc. Roy. Soc. Med.* **45**, 341-354.

Fernandez, C. (1960): Interrelations between flocculonodular lobe and vestibular system. pp. 285-296 in: G.L. Rasmussen and W.F. Windle, Eds. Neural mechanisms of the auditory and vestibular systems. Springfield: C.C. Thomas.

Grant, D., Aschan, G. and Ekvall, L. (1964): Nystagmus produced by localized cerebellar lesions. *Acta Otolaryng. (Stockh.) Suppl.* **192**, 78-84.

Kornhuber, H.H. (1969): Physiologie und Klinik des vestibulären Systems. *Arch. Klin. exp. Ohr.-Nas.-, u. Kehil.-Heilk,* **194**, 111-148

Mulch, G. and Lewitzki, W. (1977): Spontaneous and Positional Nystagmus in Healthy Persons demonstrated only by Electronystagmography. *Arch. Oto-Rhino-Laryng.* **215**, 135-145.

Nylén, C.O. (1931): A clinical study on positional nystagmus in cases of brain tumor. *Acta Otolaryng. (Stockh.) Suppl.* **15**.

Uemura, T. and Cohen, B. (1972): Vestibulo-ocular reflexes: Effects of vestibular nuclear lesions. pp. 515-528. In: A. Brodal and O. Pompeiano, Eds., Basic Aspects of Central Vestibular Mechanisms, Progress in Brain Research, vol. **37**, Amsterdam: Elsevier.

7. Study of positional nystagmus in patients with multiple sclerosis

J.T. BENITEZ**, K.R. BOUCHARD**, S. GONZALEZ†

**Division of Otoneurology, William Beaumont Hospital

†Director, Multiple Sclerosis Clinic, Wayne State University

Introduction

Multiple sclerosis is a disorder of the central nervous system. Vestibular dysfunction in patients with this disease should be of the central type. The purpose of this communication is to report on the nature of positional nystagmus observed in the course of an electronystagmographic investigation in cases with established diagnosis of multiple sclerosis.

Material and Methods

Thirty-four patients with multiple sclerosis were neurologically examined by one of the authors (S.G.) at the Multiple Sclerosis Clinic of Wayne State University. They were seen during a period of remission and they ranged in age from 21 to 50 years with a median age of 34. Thirteen were male and 21 were female. Each patient was evaluated in accordance with the study of Rose *et al.* (1970). A group of 17 volunteer individuals with no evidence of otoneurological disease, was used as electronystagmographic control. They ranged in age from 17 to 30 years, with a median age of 23.5. Certain cases of known peripheral disorders were also evaluated for comparative purposes.

Positional testing was performed as part of a battery of tests for vestibular function. Positions tested included supine, sitting up, right ear and left ear down without rotation of the neck, and head hanging.

Recordings were made with horizontal and vertical leads on a 6-channel Beckman Dynograph. Direct nystagmus was recorded in AC with a time constant of 5 seconds and also in DC in another channel. The nystagmus intensity was measured by electronic differentiation

*This study supported in part by NIH grants NB-03953-07 and 07862-02.

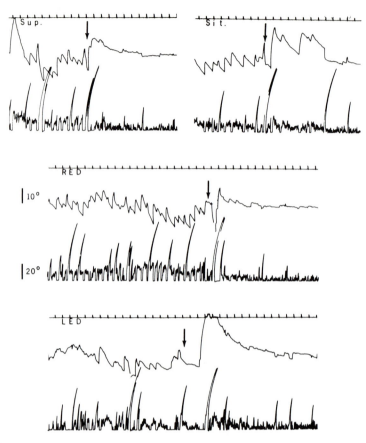

Fig. 1. Nystagmograms of a 23-year-old patient with multiple sclerosis, on supine, sitting, right ear down and left ear down positions. The event marker (top) shows 1-sec. intervals; the upper tracing the direct nystagmus; the lower tracing the nystagmus velocity in degrees per second. Calibrations are shown for both channels. There is direction-fixed nystagmus to the right in all positions. It is suppressed by optic fixation (arrows). Paper speed 5 mm/sec.; time constant of direct channel 5 sec.

by the method of Henriksson (1955). Each position was maintained for 60 seconds recording with eyes closed in semi-darkness, and also with eyes open in light with optic fixation.

Findings

Horizontal positional nystagmus (5°/sec or greater) was found in 30 patients. It was direction-fixed in 23 (77%). In all of these 23

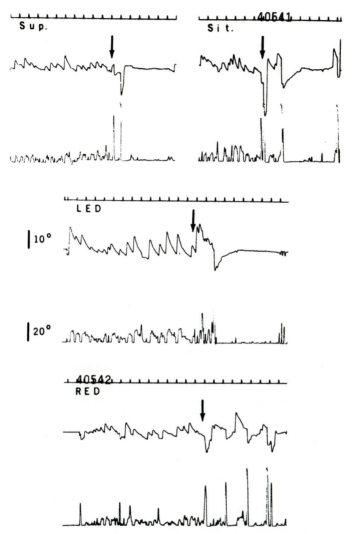

Fig. 2. Nystagmograms of a 35-year-old patient made 12 days after transverse fracture of the left temporal bone. Positions tested and calibrations are the same as Fig. 1. There is direction-fixed nystagmus to the right in all positions. It is suppressed with optic fixation (arrows), as in the patient with multiple sclerosis of Fig. 1. Paper speed 5 mm/sec.; time constant of direct channel 5 sec.

patients, the nystagmus was suppressed by optic fixation. Three of them, in addition, presented vertical nystagmus. Direction-changing positional nystagmus was found in seven patients (23%); one of them was paroxysmal. This was the only case in which the nystagmus was enhanced by optic fixation. The remaining six patients with direction-changing nystagmus showed suppression by optic fixation.

The direction-fixed positional nystagmus found in 23 patients beat to the right in 16 and to the left in seven patients. There was no nystagmographic difference between the tracings of direction-fixed positional nystagmus in the patients with multiple sclerosis and patients with known vestibular labyrinthine lesions.

Fig. 1 shows nystagmograms of a 23-year-old female patient with multiple sclerosis for seven years. The history revealed that for one year prior to examination, she had had episodes of vertigo, episodes of blindness in the left eye, diplopia, nausea (particularly developed by movements) and urgency of urination. She also had difficulty with her gait and weakness of the left arm and left leg and abnormal sensations affecting the left side of the face and also dysarthria. The neurological examination showed saccadic eye movements, truncal ataxia and bilateral cerebellar ataxia.

There was no Babinski and the sensory system was intact. The tracings showed nystagmus direction-fixed to the right in supine, sitting, right ear down and left ear down positions with the eyes closed. With eyes open in the light, the nystagmus was suppressed by optic fixation. These are usually characteristic findings of peripheral vestibular lesions. Fig. 2 shows for comparison nystagmograms of a 35-year-old patient tested twelve days after transverse fracture of the left temporal bone. The nystagmus throughout the positional testing was direction-fixed to the right. Greater velocity of eye movement was noted with the left ear down position. With eyes open in the light the nystagmus was suppressed by optic fixation. Thus, the findings observed in these cases of central and peripheral disorders were quite similar.

One of the patients with direction-changing positional nystagmus developed paroxysmal vertigo at the time of testing. The history revealed a 46-year-old female with multiple sclerosis for eight years. She had had paresis and ataxia for seven years with episodes of bilateral blurry vision for five years. There was progressive weakness of the left arm and left leg. The neurological examination showed bilateral gaze nystagmus, spastic ataxic gait and positive Romberg. The strength was diminished throughout but more so on the left side than on the right. There was bilateral cerebellar ataxia on both sides, more on the left than on the right. There was bilateral Babinski and dysarthria. There was no sucking reflex. Sensation was intact for all modalities. The patient also had urinary retention. Fig. 3 shows nystagmograms of the positional testing. On right ear down position,

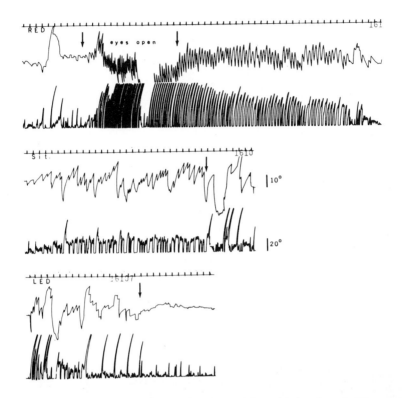

Fig. 3. Nystagmograms of a 46-year-old patient with multiple sclerosis. The event marker (top) shows 1-sec. intervals; the paper tracing the direct nystagmus; the lower tracing the nystagmus velocity in degrees per second. Calibrations are shown for both channels. There is paroxysmal nystagmus to the right on right ear down position. It is markedly enhanced by optic fixation with eyes open (arrows); on sitting up the nystagmus is to the left. With opposite position of the head, on left ear down position, the nystagmus is to the left. Optic fixation (arrows) suppressed the nystagmus in the two latter positions. Paper speed 5 mm/sec.; time constant of direct channel 5 sec.

there was paroxysmal nystagmus to the right which was enhanced by optic fixation with eyes open in the light. This indeed is a manifestation of a central lesion. On sitting, the nystagmus reversed to the left. On the left ear down position, the nystagmus was to the left. Fig. 4 shows nystagmograms of a 44-year-old female patient with positional nystagmus of the benign paroxysmal type for comparison. For four weeks she had had vertigo when lying down on her left side. On the left ear down position, the tracing showed nystagmus to the opposite ear (right). It was suppressed in the light by optic fixation. On sitting,

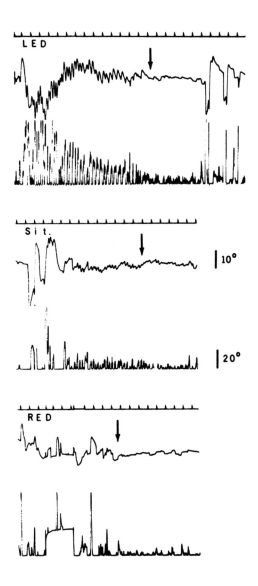

Fig. 4. Nystagmograms of a 44-year-old patient with positional nystagmus of the benign paroxysmal type. Positions tested and calibrations are the same as Fig. 3. There is paroxysmal nystagmus on left ear down position. It is suppressed by optic fixation with eyes open (arrow); on sitting up the nystagmus is to the left. There is no nystagmus on right ear down position. Arrows indicate optic fixation with eyes open. Paper speed 5 mm/sec.; time constant of direct channel 5 sec.

the nystagmus was also to the left. No nystagmus was detected during the right ear down position.

Horizontal positional nystagmus (5°/sec or greater) was found only in one of the normal subjects (6%) and it was direction-fixed. No vertical nystagmus was detected in the normal group.

Comment

We have shown that multiple sclerosis patients with direction-fixed positional nystagmus showed consistently a suppression of nystagmus by optic fixation, thus resembling a peripheral vestibular dysfunction. This finding is a disturbing phenomenon which is difficult to explain on the basis of the known sites of the pathologic lesions.

Clinically, the paroxysmal positional nystagmus found in one of the patients might have been interpreted as a peripheral dysfunction. However, recordings showed clearly marked enhancement of the nystagmus by optic fixation and a change of direction with opposite position of the head.

In contrast to this, a consistent finding has been observed in ten consecutive patients with positional nystagmus of the benign paroxysmal type examined recently at the Equilibrium Clinic of William Beaumont Hospital. These recordings have shown that the horizontal nystagmus beats to the opposite ear (affected ear undermost). This nystagmus was always suppressed by optic fixation. There was a change of direction of the nystagmus in three of these cases, however, only when they resumed the sitting position. This reversal of direction is in agreement with observations of Schuknecht (1974) and Barber and Stockwell (1976).

References

Barber, H.O. and Stockwell, C.W. (1976): *Manual of Electronystagmography.* The C.V. Mosby Company, St. Louis, Missouri.

Henriksson, N.G. (1955): An electrical method for registration of the movement of the eyes in nystagmus. *Acta Oto-laryng.* **45**, 25-41.

Rose, A.S., Kuzma, J.W., Kurtzke, J.F., Namerow, N.S., Sibley, W.A. and Tourtellotte, W.W. (1970): Cooperative study in the evaluation of therapy in multiple sclerosis; ACTH vs. placebo. *Neurology* **20**, 1.

Schuknecht, H.F. (1974): *Pathology of the Ear.* Harvard University Press, Cambridge, Massachusetts.

8. Four cases with polyphasic positional nystagmus

I. KATO*, Y. SATO**, M. AOYAGI*, K. MIZUKOSHI†, Y. WATANABE†, H. INO†

*Department of Otolaryngology, Yamagata University

**Department of Physiology, Toyama Medical and Pharmaceutical University

†Department of Otolaryngology, Niigata University

Introduction

The secondary phase of nystagmus is commonly recognized even in normal individuals when an appropriate stimulus is applied. However, the secondary phase of positional nystagmus induced by head position change is an unusual finding during routine tests.

Since we have encountered four cases of such peculiar findings, some comments are made on the generation of the secondary phase of positional nystagmus from the otoneurological point of view.

Method and Materials

The electronystagmographic (ENG) examination consisted of the following: (1) spontaneous nystagmus test, (2) provoked nystagmus test; gaze test, position test, (3) induced nystagmus test; caloric test. optokinetic test, eye tracking test. The method of the caloric pattern test by which amounts of visually induced suppression in the slow-phase velocity of caloric nystagmus are evaluated was described in detail in a previous report. (Kato *et al.*, 1977).

The ENG examination was performed on all patients with the room dimly illuminated and eyes closed. All subjects were spoken to or required to do mental arithmetic in order to maintain mental alertness. Eye movements were recorded with a San-ei ENG apparatus (4 channels) with a rectilinear pen linkage.

Electrodes were placed lateral to the outer canthi to record horizontal eye movements and above and below the right eye to record vertical eye movements.

The four cases listed in the Table were as follows: the first case was diagnosed as chronic myeloid leukemia, and progressive multifocal leucoencephalophthy attributed to the leukemia was deeply

ENG findings

ENG Case	Spontaneous Nystagmus	Positional Nystagmus*	OKN	ETT	Caloric Nystagmus	Gaze Nystagmus
1	←——— 40/30″	Type 1 (geotropic) 2nd-4th phase	diminished	ataxic	exaggerated 2nd-4th phase FFS	bilat. rebound nystagmus
2	———→ 44/30″	Type 1 (apogeotropic) 2nd-3rd phase	diminished	saccadic	exaggerated 2nd-3rd phase FFS	bilat. rebound nystagmus
3	———→ 30/30″	Type 1 (geotropic) 2nd phase	diminished	saccadic	normal 2nd phase FFS	bilat.
4	←——— 25/30″	Type 1 (geotropic) 2nd phase	not done	saccadic	exaggerated 2nd phase FFS	bilat. rebound nystagmus

suspected. The pathological diagnosis, however, has not, as yet, been adequately established. The second case was Marie's Ataxia evaluated by detailed clinical data. The third case was diagnosed as a Fourth ventricular tumor which was later confirmed as hemangioblastoma by surgery. The fourth case was verified as hemangioblastoma of the cerebellum extending from the paramedian portion on the right side up to the near lateral end of the left cerebellar himisphere.

ENG Findings

As presented in the Table, ENG findings were similar in all four cases. Positional nystagmus of direction-changing Type (Nylén's type 1, Nylén, 1950) was common, and was subsequently followed by rhythmic phases from the secondary to the fourth phase depending upon the patient being held in the same head position. The number of rhythmic phases induced by the head position changes coincided with that of postcaloric nystagmus in all patients, though the number of the phases differed with each patient.

Mechanism of Polyphasic Positional Nystagmus

The secondary phase of nystagmus is taken as a basic pattern common to nystagmus response induced by vestibular and optokinetic stimuli (Mizukoshi, 1961; Morimoto *et al.*, 1963; Jung and Kornhuber, 1964; Takemori, 1974; Robinson, 1976). Thus viewed, it appears possible that a secondary phase of positional nystagmus occurs as a basic pattern of the nystagmus response. If the central inhibitory mechanism controlling the vestibulocular system functions normally, the secondary phase of positional nystagmus will be inhibited. In extreme disturbance of the central controlling system however, shown by animal experiments Mizukoshi (1961), nystagmus will be released and the secondary phase of positional nystagmus will appear, and as a reaction there will appear a third phase and fourth phase.

In the present cases ENG findings related to the cerebellar lesions were observed such as rebound nystagmus (Hood, Kayan and Leech, 1974), and Failure of Fixation-Suppression of Caloric Nystagmus (FFS) (Coats, 1970) which was reproduced in animal experiments (Takemori and Cohen, 1974), while on the other hand, cerebellar signs were found in all cases. Moreover, the common lesion in all four cases was attributed to the cerebellum. Hence, there seems to be a sound basis for speculation that the cerebellum plays an important role in the production of the alternating rhythmic phases.

References

Coats, A.C. (1970): Central electronystagmographic abnormalities. *Arch Otolaryngol.* **92**, 45-53.

Hood, J.D., Kayan, A. and Leech, J. (1973): Rebound nystagmus. *Brain* **96**, 507-526.

Jung, R. and Kornhuber, J.N. (1964): Results of electrobystagmography in man: the value of optokinetic, vestibular, and spontaneous nystagmus for neurological diagnosis and research. *In: 'The Oculomotor System.'* Edited by M.B. Bender, New York: Harper and Row, 428-292.

Kato, I., Kimura, Y., Aoyagi, M., Mizukoshi, K. and Kawasaki, T. (1977): Visual suppression of caloric nystagmus in normal individuals. *Acta Otolarygol.* **83**, 245-251.

Mizukoshi, K. (1967a): Some observation on the optokinetic nystagmus (in Japanese). *Jap. Journ. Otol. Tokyo* **64**, 23-49.

Mizukoshi, K. (1961b): Some observation on the optokinetic nystagmus (in Japanese). *Jap. Jour. Otol. Tokyo* **64**, 207-240.

Morimoto, M., Mizukoshi, K., Otani, T., *et al.* (1963): On the secondary phase of nystagmus. *Acta Oto-laryng. Suppl.* **179**, 32-41.

Nylén, C.O. (1950): Positional nystagmus. A review and future prospects. *J. Laryng.* **64**, 295-318.

Robinson, D.A. (1976): How signals are processed in the vestibulo-ocular reflex. Proceedings, V extraordinary meeting of the Barany Society, 130-141.

Takemori, S. (1974): The similarities of optokinetic after-nystagmus to the vestibular nystagmus. *Ann Otol.* **83**, 230-238.

Takemori, S. and Cohen, B. (1974): Loss of visual suppression of vestibular nystagmus after flocculus lesions. *Brain Research* **72**, 213-224.

9. Positional nystagmus and positioning nystagmus

T. SEKITANI, T. KOBAYASHI, K. KANESADA, S. HONJO

Department of Otolaryngology, Yamaguchi University School of Medicine, Ube City, 755 Japan

Introduction

According to Nylén (1954), positional nystagmus is one of the most positive, objective and easily demonstrated signs of disturbance in the human vestibular system.

Evaluation of the clinical diagnostic significance of positional nystagmus is aimed at clarifying questions such as the relationship between types of positional nystagmus and localization of disease, occurrence of positional nystagmus and positioning nystagmus in the various diseases; and a factor which has an even greater significance, the positioning test or the positional test.

This paper presents the results of positional and positioning tests performed as part of the routine otoneurological examination on patients with vertigo, disequilibrium or other otologic diseases at Yamaguchi University Hospital during 1975 (January) to 1976 (September).

Observation of the positional nystagmus (Abbr.: P.N.) was carried out with the eyes open in a dimly lit room and behind Frenzel glasses, simultaneous recordings being made with ENG (both horizontal and vertical leads).

Results and Comments

The 310 patients were examined by routine otoneurological examination (Table 1).

Of these, 171 cases showed positive findings with the positional test. In other words, 55.2% of the total patients examined showed some kind of positional and/or positioning nystagmus.

105 of these 171 cases showed positive findings on both positional and positioning testing, 46 cases (26.9%) on positional alone and 20 cases (11.7%) on positioning alone.

TABLE 1
310 examinations from April 1975 to September 1976
171 cases, positive positional nystagmus

Positive of:	No. of cases		Groups
Positional + positioning	105	61.4%	A
Positional	46	26.9%	B
Positioning	20	11.7%	C
	171		

The localization of the lesion in the 171 cases is given in Table 2. 42 cases were due to central lesions; 9 to cervical lesions; 100 to peripheral lesions and 20 despite careful otoneurological or neurological study remained of 'unknown etiology'.

TABLE 2
Disease entity in 171 with Positive Positional Nystagmus
and/or Positioning Nystagmus

Central lesion	42
Cervical lesion	9
Peripheral lesion	100
Unknown	20
	171

The 105 cases in Group A with both positional or positioning nystagmus have been classified in Table 3 according to Nylén's 3 Types. Thus, positional nystagmus Type I, direction-changing was seen in 13 cases (12.4%): Type II, direction-fixed, in 45 cases (42.9%); and Type III, irregular in direction, in 47 cases (44.7%).

With respect to the positioning test, Type I occurred in 5 cases (4.8%), Type II in 43 cases (41.0%) and Type III, in 57 cases (54.2%).

The direction-changing nystagmus was noted using the positioning test less than with the positional test, thus showing an increase in the irregular type.

There was no marked difference in Type II between the positional test and positioning test; i.e., 45 cases vs. 43 cases, 42.9% and 41.0% respectively. Such findings are significant.

Table 3 shows the number of occurrences of positional nystagmus and the relationship between classified type and localization of disease, among cases of Group A.

First, central lesions showed every type of positional nystagmus; 12 cases showing irregular type (48%); 10 as direction-fixed, and 3 as direction-changing.

TABLE 3

Type of Positional Nystagmus and Disease Entity
— In Patients with Positive Findings in the Positional and Positioning Tests —

	Direction-changing	Direction-fixed Horizontal	Irregular
Central	3	10	12
Cervical	0	3	2
Peripheral	10	28	23
Unknown	0	4	10
	13	45	47

Nyléns Type II, direction-fixed nystagmus, was seen in a rather higher percentage in cases with a central origin.

In those with a peripheral lesion, 28 showed a direction-fixed nystagmus (45.9%). However, 23 showed an irregular type (37.7%).

When comparing differences between the central origin group and the peripheral group, 'irregular P.N.' was seen in 48% and 37.7%, respectively.

In the group with symptoms of cervical origin and those with unknown lesion, there were no cases of direction-changing nystagmus. One of the remarkable findings was that a considerable number of patients with unknown origin vertigo showed irregular type (71.4%). This means that some of these unknown cases will have a 'not detectable origin' in the central region.

Table 4 shows the type of positional nystagmus in each test, i.e., the positional and the positioning and localization of disease in group A with central origin.

TABLE 4

Type of Positional Nystagmus in Each Test and Disease Entity (Group A)
Central Lesion (25 Cases)

	Direction-changing		Direction-fixed	Irregular
	Upward	Downward		
Positional nystagmus	2	1	9 (36%)	13 (48%)
Positioning nystagmus	2	0	7 (28%)	16 (64%)

With the positional test, there was direction-fixed P.N. in 10 cases, (40%) and an irregular P.N. in 12 cases (48%).

The positioning test yielded slightly different findings of P.N., i.e., some patients with a direction-fixed type in the positional test showed a different type to irregular P.N. with the positioning test.

The number of cases with an irregular P.N. in the positional test increased after the positioning test (from 48% to 64%).

In the cervical origin vertigo cases, there was no marked change or difference between positional test and positioning test. There was no Type I, direction-changing P.N. in this group.

In the group with peripheral lesions (61 cases), the number of cases with direction-fixed positional nystagmus in the positional test increased with the positioning test (from 45.9% to 52.2%), while on the contrary, the number of direction-changing nystagmus decreased with the positioning test from 16.4% to 5.0%.

In the group of unknown origin vertigo (14 cases), direction-fixed P.N. with the positional test was changed to irregular P.N. with the positioning test in two out of 4 patients.

Thus there is a tendency for the positioning test to yield a higher manifestation of irregular nystagmus in a central lesion case, and higher manifestation of direction-fixed nystagmus in those with peripheral lesions.

Of significance was the marked decrease in direction-changing nystagmus after the positioning test in those with peripheral lesions.

OKP-ETT Abnormality and Positional Nystagmus

Evaluation of occurrence of abnormal findings in optokinetic nystagmus (optokinetic pattern test, OKP) and eye tracking test (ETT) in those with positive positional nystagmus was made.

Most of the cases were those with positive findings both in the positional and positioning tests.

The results are shown in Table 5. The numbers are expressed as percentages, and show that there are differences between each disease entity. The relationship between the type of P.N. and OKP-ETT abnormality is also shown.

Regarding the data of the Type III group of positional nystagmus, those with central lesions showed an abnormal OKP and/or ETT of 79.2%, and 66.7% of those with central lesions showed abnormalities in both OKP and ETT.

In those with peripheral lesions, 50.0% showed abnormal findings in either OKP or ETT, but in only 39.1% was this so in both tests. Our findings suggest that a combination of the positional test and OKP or ETT tests will provide more pertinent information for an accurate clinical diagnosis.

TABLE 5
Relationship Between Positional Nystagmus (Types) and OKP-ETT Abnormality
– % Expression in Group A –

OKP and/or ETT Abnormality in:

| | Type I | | Type II | Type III |
	Up-	Down-		
Central	33.3 (33.3)	0	70.0 (60.0)	79.2 (66.7)
Cervical	0	0	16.7 (0)	50.0 (50.0)
Peripheral	50.0 (33.3)	12.5 (0)	28.6 (14.3)	50.0 (39.1)
Unknown	0	0	50.0 (25.0)	35.0 (10.0)

( ): Abnormal OKP and ETT.

Conclusions

(1) Positional nystagmus in the wide sense as determined by the positional and positioning tests was seen in 55.2% of all patients otoneurologically examined at Yamaguchi University Hospital (171 cases among 310).

(2) The positioning test elicits irregular type positional nystagmus much more than does the positional test. This tendency was relatively higher in those with central lesions than in those with peripheral lesions.

(3) Direction-fixed positional nystagmus occurred in a high percentage in those with central lesions, though textbooks describe 'direction-fixed as being of high incidence in those with peripheral lesions'.

(4) Direction-changing nystagmus was an unexpectedly frequent occurrence in those with peripheral lesions.

The interpretation of positional nystagmus as seen in each patient is at variance with certain statements which appear in textbooks. Positive findings strongly suggest the necessity of further examinations and follow-up.

Caloric Nystagmus

1. Quantification of compensatory eye movements caused by vestibular and optovestibular stimulation in normal humans and in patients with labyrinthine and brain stem diseases

J. CORVERA, R. ROMERO

Department of Otolaryngology, Hospital General, Centro Medico Nacional, I.M.S.S., Mexico City

Introduction

The optomotor responses to vestibular and optokinetic stimuli has always been difficult to measure. The criteria for abnormality has been based most of the time on the symmetry of responses or in the comparison of the magnitude of certain parameter of the reaction with a value obtained by statistical determination in a set of normal individuals. So far, no clinical method has been devised to compare the magnitude of the optomotor response directly with the magnitude of the stimulus.

This is probably due to the choice of parameters. Measurement of the duration of the poststimulatory nystagmus is, in fact a measure of an artificial situation, since, in normal conditions, no stimulus exists that could elicit such a response. Normal accelerations are always brief, and are followed very soon by an acceleration in the opposite sense when the movement is stopped.

Measurement of the speed of the slow component is also artificial. Teleologically speaking, the vestibule needs to know two things: First, the direction of an abrupt acceleration, to prepare the body and limbs for the probable impact, and second, the magnitude of the angular displacement of the head during slower movements in order to make compensatory eye movements and minimize the slipping of the image of the external environment on the retina. In both cases, acceleration and speed are incidental to the basic needs namely direction and displacement.

The vestibule must achieve its aims with the only information it can get: Acceleration and time. With this data, speed and displacement are accurately calculated, since the quotient of acceleration and time is velocity, and the quotient of velocity and time is displacement.

In the present paper, we will present a method that attempts to assess in quantitative terms the optomotor response to vestibular and optovestibular stimuli. For this purpose the parameter of the response is taken to be the angular displacement of the eyes in relation to the skull, and the parameter of the stimulus the angular displacement of the skull, oscillating with a fixed frequency.

The quantitative relationship between stimulus and response in normal humans will be presented, as well as alterations that occur in some diseases of the inner ear and the vestibulo-optomotor neurological mechanism in the brain stem.

Methods

Selection of Cases

1. Normals. Twenty-five volunteers, aged between 20 and 32 years, with no history of ear disease or vertigo were selected. The group was formed by medical residents and students, 17 males and 8 females, all with normal eardrums. Cochlear and vestibular testing, including Hallpike bithermal caloric tests, gave normal results.

2. Patients with unilateral labyrinthine disease. 18 patients were studied. Seven suffered from unilateral Méniére's disease, 7 had vestibular neuronitis, 3 had labyrinthitis due to middle ear infection, and one had iatrogenic deafness and vestibular ear paralysis after a stapedectomy procedure.

None showed nystagmus with eyes open, but 5 had contralateral nystagmus with eyes covered.

A complete neurological and neurotological evaluation revealed no evidence of disease of the central nervous system or the contralateral ear.

3. Patients with bilateral labyrinthine disease. Thirteen cases were selected, 9 with bilateral Méniére's disease, 3 with aminoglucosidic ototoxicity and one with bilateral serous labyrinthitis secondary to otomastoiditis. Again, complete examination excluded neurological disease. Age bracket was 18—35 years. The caloric test in all cases showed depressed responses of both ears, but no case of abolished responses was included.

The bilaterality of the lesions was further insured by selecting cases with bilateral end organ deafness due to the same disease that affected the vestibules.

4. Patients with brain stem disease. Twenty-four cases were selected, the diagnosis was made on neurological studies, as follows: 8 cases of cerebral cysticercosis with posterior fossa localization, 4 cases of multiple sclerosis, 7 posterior fossa tumours, 2 cases of pontocerebellar atrophy, and 3 cases of brain stem infarction. In all cases, there was brain stem involvement, but other structures of the posterior fossa, especially the cerebellum, were also affected.

No evidence of ear disease was found. No case was used if there was conjugate or bilateral paresis of the eyes. In case of unilateral paresis, the tracing corresponding to the normal eye was used.

Testing Procedures

1. Stimulation. Vestibular and optovestibular stimulation were performed using the alternate rotating chair described by Greiner and Conraux (1961). This chair is suspended by a steel rod, and acts as a torsion pendulum, oscillating in the vertical axis with a 20 second period. This produces an angular acceleration that varies sinusoidally. From the initial angular displacement of any isolated oscillation, both the maximum speed and acceleration can be determined.

Three tests were performed on each patient:

(a) Stimulation with covered eyes. This is a test of the oculomotor reactivity to an isolated vestibular stimulus, and will be referred to as 'vestibular stimulation' (VS). It is important that the eyes should be covered, and not closed.

(b) Stimulation with open eyes, looking at the stationary surroundings. This has received the name of 'vestibular stimulation with spatial fixation'. We prefer the term 'opto vestibular stimulation' (OVS), since the vestibular stimulus is combined with an optokinetic stimulus, caused by the illusion that the room rotates around the patient. In this test, the patient is rotated with eyes open, so that he can see the room in which the rotatory chair is installed.

Both vestibular and optokinetic stimuli would produce nystagmus to the same side. A clockwise rotation produces a vestibular stimulation that will cause a right beating nystagmus; at the same time, the optical image, moving apparently to the left, will originate an optokinetic nystagmus to the point where the image appears, that is, to the right.

(c) Stimulation with eyes fixed on an optical target that moves synchronously with the patient. This will be referred to as 'vestibular stimulation with optic fixation' (VSOF). In this test, the patient is rotated with eyes open, looking at a small white cross painted on a black curtain, placed 30 cm in front of the patient. The curtain is fixed to the rotating chair and blocks the view of the room. In this way, the vestibular nystagmus will be inhibited, due to the fact that a right vestibular nystagmus, for instance, will produce an optical illusion of objects circling to the right, and thus, an optokinetic nystagmus to the left.

2. Recording. The eye movements were recorded by electro-oculographic technique with a six channel Grass polygraph, using DC coupling. Each eye and a bitemporal lead were directed to three separate channels.

The bitemporal lead was used, on some occasions, to feed an integration circuit. Eye blinks were monitored by electrodes above and below the right eye leading into a fifth channel. To monitor the angular displacement of the subject, a photovoltaic cell was located in front of a circular tubular structure that surrounds the base of the chair, and in which alternate black and white bands were painted, with a breadth equivalent to 10 degrees each. The photocell registered the different light reflectance of the bands, by generating a fluctuating electric current that was recorded in the sixth channel of the polygraph, as a distorted sinusoidal wave in which the distance between cusps was equivalent to 20 degrees of the rotatory movement of the chair.

3. Parameter of response. The parameter of stimulation was the angular displacement of the rotatory chair in each semiperiod. The parameter of response was the cumulative eye position for the same semiperiod.

The term 'cumulative eye position' (CEP) was used by Meiry (1971) to describe the total compensatory travel of the eyes relative to the skull, caused by vestibular, optokinetic and other reflexes. The CEP is then the sum of all segments of slow phase motion put end to end thus eliminating the effects of the saccades corresponding to the fast phases of nystagmus. The magnitude in degrees is obtained by referring to the calibration.

The CEP can be obtained by 'geometric' methods, actually drawing the segments end to end (Fig. 1) or by computing by means of the integrator channel in the polygraph.

Evaluation

1. Normals. CEP were determined for semiperiods every 40 degrees of chair displacement, both with vestibular and optovestibular stimulation. No nystagmus could be observed during VSOF.

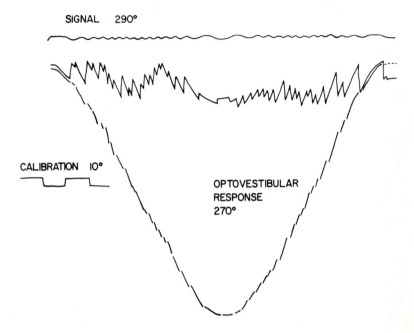

Fig. 1. Cumulative eye position. The first tracing corresponds to the movement of the chair; the second is the nystagmic response and the third shows the manual way in obtaining the cumulative eye position value.

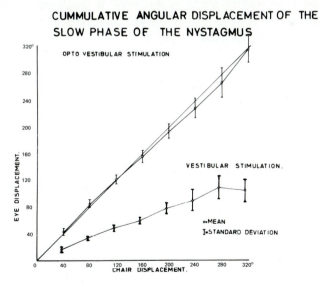

Fig. 2. Value of the vestibular and optovestibular responses in normal subjects.

Means and standard deviations were obtained for the 24 subjects in each measurement, and these values were used to plot the VS and the OVS against the stimulation values (Fig. 2).

To test symmetry of the responses, CEP of the first and fifth semiperiod were added (representing nystagmus to the left) and subtracted from the sum of the CEP of the second plus the fourth semiperiod (nystagmus to the right). These are strong stimuli, since chair displacements vary between 260 and 340 degrees. To test the symmetry under weak stimuli, the procedure was repeated with semiperiods $(11 + 15) - (12 + 14)$, corresponding to chair displacements between 60 and 140 degrees. The values obtained were a measurement of asymmetry; showing preponderance to the left when positive and to the right when negative. Mean and standard deviation were also calculated for these values.

2. *Patients with labyrinthine and brain stem disease.* Six CEP values were calculated for each patient, corresponding to VS, OVS and VSOF each to the right and to the left. For each pair a single full cycle of oscillation in the range between 120 and 260 degrees of chair displacement was used.

To facilitate the analysis of abnormalities, the CEP values were expressed as percentage of the stimulation values. For example, if a $250°$ semiperiod was measured, and the CEP was determined to be $125°$, it was expressed as 50%. In this way, it was easy to compare with another semiperiod in which the stimulation was different, for instance, $180°$ with a CEP value of $90°$ gives the same 50% value.

To the values for each condition, expressed in percentage, the mean and standard deviation were added.

Abnormalities for each test were determined in the following way:

(a) *Decrease or increase of optomotor reactions.* Arbitrarily, the CEP was considered abnormally high or low when the value exceeded plus or minus 30% of the expected response, this being the mean value obtained in normal subjects. This criterion was applied to VS and OVS; the appearance of nystagmus during VSOF was considered abnormal whatever its magnitude.

(b) *Asymmetry of response.* Independently of the decrease of responses they were considered asymmetrical when comparing the optomotor reaction to the left and to the right, the smaller value measured less than two-thirds of the larger.

Results and Discussion

Normal Subjects

1. Optovestibular stimulation. The responses are very precise. The CEP keeps a linear relationship with the stimulation at all amplitudes tested. Since the frequency of oscillation is kept constant at 0.05 Hz, the amplitude conditions the angular speed and acceleration. The gain of the system, defined as the quotient eye displacement over skull displacement, is 1.0, and the variation, represented by the standard deviation of the means, is very small (Fig. 2). This is in accordance with findings of other investigators (Meiry, 1971).

2. Vestibular stimulation. The CEP was found to be proportional to the angular displacement of the chair, and the variation was linear when such displacement was kept between 40 and 280 degrees. The gain was 0.4, and the standard deviation small.

It has been shown in respect of vestibular compensation that the gain varies with different stimuli; with oscillations of higher frequency (0.3 Hz), Zee, Yee, Cogan *et al.* (1976) found a 0.65 gain. The value of the gain appears to be determined, not by the sensitivity of the labyrinth, but by an active damping effect produced by the cerebellum, since in cerebellar diseases the gain can be found abnormally high. (Zee, Yee, Cogan *et al.*, 1976). Very little asymmetry was found in the responses. The responses with strong stimuli gave a mean asymmetry of $+4.18°$, equivalent to 2.46%, with a standard deviation of $18.3°$.

The weak stimulus gave slightly higher values, the mean asymmetry was found to be $+18.04°$, equivalent to 17.9%, with a standard deviation of $25.7°$.

3. Vestibular stimulation with optic fixation. No oculomotor responses were found with this test. It can be said that the CEP gain is zero in these circumstances.

Unilateral Labyrinthine Disease (Table 1)

1. Optovestibular stimulation. In view of the common concept that the vestibular organ has little or no influence on optically induced eye movements, it was surprising to find that it does alter the CEP resulting from optovestibular stimulation. The responses were found to be bilaterally depressed in two cases, contralaterally depressed (in relation to the diseased ear) in three cases and ipsilaterally depressed

TABLE 1
Unilateral Labyrinthine Disease

	Optovestibular Stimulation		Vestibular Stimulation		
Case	Contralateral	Ipsilateral	Contralateral	Ipsilateral	
1	99	78	35	33	
2	84	86	45	50	
3	63	73	0	13	
4	68	67	39	27	
5	119	107	17	40	
6	80	69	0	40	
7	65	71	0	0	
8	104	107	28	38	
9	85	85	5	19	
10	17	64	0	94	Vestibular nystagmus
11	74	93	9	18	
12	78	93	10	37	
13	77	70	0	38	Vestibular nystagmus
14	96	165	16	17	Vestibular nystagmus
15	98	90	22	35	
16	59	78	14	88	
17	96	103	50	62	Vestibular nystagmus
18	83	90	18	34	
$\bar{x}$	80.11	88.28	17.11	37.94	
s	22.49	23.47	16.34	24.02	

Note: The value of the response is expressed as a percentage of the stimulus.

in one. The depression has to be pronounced, since the 30% limit used to determine it, is about three times the standard deviation of the mean for normal subjects. Three patients showed asymmetrical responses with ipsilateral preponderance. In one of these, an increase of response was found. Note that, since the CEP is related to the slow phase of the nystagmus, a contralateral depression of CEP is equivalent to a contralateral preponderance of the nystagmus. The asymmetry, and the increase of response, are probably linked to the tonic activity of the vestibular system, since all of these cases had contralateral spontaneous nystagmus with eyes covered.

The depression and asymmetry of the optovestibular responses are also evident in the statistical treatment of the CEP values. The mean values are 80.11% for contralateral eye movements and 88.28% for ipsilateral eye movements. The probability of these values were tested with the chi square method, and a $P < .05$ was found.

2. Vestibular stimulation. The same depression and asymmetry

found for OVS was detected, but with a far larger magnitude. Only three cases could be considered within the normal range. In the rest, one had ipsilateral depression, five had bilateral depression and nine had contralateral depression.

Two patients showed ipsilateral increase of responses; in both, a contralateral nystagmus was present with eyes covered.

The statistical treatment shows marked asymmetry, the mean value of contralateral slow movements being less than half that of the mean value of ipsilateral CEP. The asymmetry is due to depression on one side and not an increase on the other, since the mean value of the ipsilateral CEP is still slightly below normal. This, and the high incidence of bilateral depression, suggests that the vestibular compensation after unilateral damage, acts by lowering the activity to the healthy side as well as by increasing the labyrinth's capacity to produce slow eye movements towards the diseased side.

3. Vestibular stimulation with optic fixation. Labyrinthine disease does not affect the capacity of the visual tracking system to suppress vestibular nystagmus, as shown by the fact that no nystagmic responses were evident under VSOF conditions although vestibular type nystagmus was present in five cases. It appears that vestibular nystagmus does not appear in VSOF unless it is of second degree with eyes open (Fig. 3).

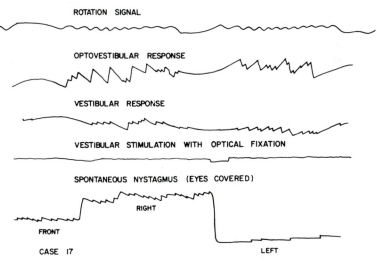

Fig. 3. A case of iatrogenic labyrinthine destruction. Note that in spite of a third degree spontaneous nystagmus with eyes covered, no nystagmus appeared when testing with optical fixation.

Bilateral Labyrinthine Disease (Table 2)

The findings were essentially similar in bilateral and unilateral disease, except that asymmetrical responses did not occur as frequently.

TABLE 2
Bilateral Labyrinthine Disease

	Optovestibular Stimulation			Vestibular Stimulation	
Case	Right	Left		Right	Left
1	65	67		20	20
2	91	88		23	22
3	76	61		36	21
4	89	106		0	0
5	50	61		14	18
6	103	120		9	40
7	79	98		7	9
8	96	87		8	13
9	92	95		12	62
10	63	64		31	25
11	59	77		21	29
12	116	110		34	34
13	118	110		26	42
$\bar{x}$	84.38	88		18.54	25.77
s	21.4	20.54		11.27	16.06

Brain Stem Disease (Table 3)

1. Optovestibular stimulation. Ten patients (42%) showed unilateral or bilateral depression of responses. This figure is slightly greater than the one corresponding to vestibular disease (35%). The mean depression is also similar and in no case was a significant increase of response found.

2. Vestibular stimulation. In only four cases was a distinct increase found. The percentage of cases with unilateral or bilateral diminution of responses was 70%, slightly lower than the 80% figure corresponding to vestibular disease, but the magnitude of the depression was clearly smaller, the means being 34.25 to the right and 28.33 to the left, compared to 18.54 and 25.77 in cases of bilateral labyrinthine disease.

3. Vestibular stimulation with optic fixation. More than 60% of the cases gave abnormal results, showing nystagmus, the CEP values of which were, in many cases, equivalent to the CEP values obtained during vestibular stimulation. This is equivalent to a hundred per cent loss of the capacity to suppress vestibular nystagmus by the eye

TABLE 3
Brain Stem Disease

Case	OVS Right	OVS Left	VS Right	VS Left	VSOF Right	VSOF Left
1	82	60	37	17	50	15
2	117	100	4	7	0	0
3	66	90	40	44	14	39
4	83	81	45	14	11	14
5	88	91	38	24	0	0
6	99	101	49	26	11	20
7	100	120	41	25	0	0
8	128	121	20	25	0	0
9	80	99	45	13	0	0
10	78	64	15	5	0	0
11	100	70	46	30	21	25
12	84	73	27	33	0	0
13	90	44	53	21	52	37
14	65	80	14	23	8	14
15	83	74	47	49	35	37
16	79	82	29	42	9	24
17	84	57	74	44	50	0
18	50	60	20	25	17	17
19	74	52	37	23	13	14
20	72	80	14	31	8	5
21	86	86	0	0	0	0
22	118	124	79	103	10	8
23	100	106	0	0	0	0
24	63	60	48	56	39	30
x̄	86.21	82.29	34.25	28.33	14.5	12.88
s	18.32	22.34	20.77	21.69	17.5	13.85

tracking mechanism. Clearly, although brain stem disease affects the vestibular pathway, it does much more damage to the descending connections regulating the oculomotor responses to visual stimuli. This is hardly surprising, since both eye tracking loss (Corvera, Torres-Courtney, López-Rios, 1973) and optokinetic nystagmus depression (Tos, Adser, Rosborg, 1972) have been reported in brain stem disorders. The test allows the quantitative determination of the functional loss by the formula VSOF/VS X 100 (Fig. 4).

Conclusion

By measuring rotatory, vestibular and optovestibular stimulation in terms of angular displacement, and the oculomotor responses as the sum of the slow compensatory movements of the eyes relative to the skull, the vestibulo-optomotor function can be quantitatively evaluated.

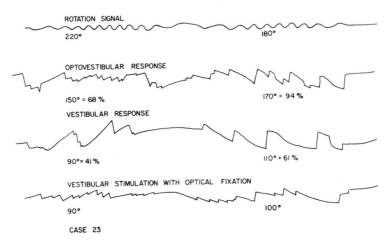

ROTATION SIGNAL

220°   180°

OPTOVESTIBULAR   RESPONSE

150° = 68 %   170° = 94 %

VESTIBULAR   RESPONSE

90°= 41%   110° = 61 %

VESTIBULAR   STIMULATION WITH OPTICAL   FIXATION

90°   100°

CASE 23

Fig. 4. A case of brain stem tumour. Note that the nystagmus produced when tested with optical fixation is of equal magnitude and better organized than the vestibular nystagmus with eyes covered. The optovestibular CEP is depressed to the right.

In normal humans, the oculomotor responses are very precise and stable; accordingly, the alteration of their magnitude in vestibular and neurological diseases have important clinical significance.

References

Greiner, C.F. and Conraux, C. (1961): Les conditions physiques de la stimulation vestibulaire. Ses applications aux examens par stimulation rotatoire alternée (pendulaire). *Confinia Neurologica* **21**, 438-446.

Meiry, J.L. (1971): Vestibular and propioceptive stabilization of the eye movements. *In* Bach-y-Rita and Collins, editors: The control of the eye movements. Academic Press, New York, pp. 483-496.

Zee, D.S., Yee, R.D., Cogan, D.C. *et al.* (1976): Ocular motor abnormalities in hereditary cerebellar ataxia. *Brain* **99**, 207-234.

Corvera, J., Torres-Courtney, C. and López-Rios, C. (1973): The neurotological significance of alterations of pursuit eye movements and the pendular eye test. *Ann Otol.* **82**, 855-867.

Tos, M., Adser, J. and Rosborg, J. (1972): Horizontal optokinetic nystagmus in cerebral disease. *Acta Neurol. Scandin.* **48**, 607-618.

2. On the role of the brain stem in the visual suppression of caloric nystagmus

T. KAWASAKI*, I. KATO**, M. AOYAGI**, Y. SATO*, Y. KOIKE**, H. INO†

*Department of Physiology, Toyama Medical and Pharmaceutical University

**Department of Otolaryngology, School of Medicine, Yamagata University

†Department of Otolaryngology, School of Medicine, Niigata University

Introduction

The visual signals mediated to the cerebellar flocculus via the mossy fiber (MF) pathway are assumed to be responsible for immediate adjustment of vestibulo-ocular reflex by vision, but those via the climbing fiber (CF) pathway are not (Ito, 1976 and Lisberger and Fuchs, 1974). Takemori and Cohen (1974) demonstrated that visual suppression (VS) of caloric nystagmus was lost after extirpation of the flocculus. VS of caloric nystagmus, therefore, might be lost after interruption of visual signals via MF, but not after interruption of those via CF. This study aimed at confirming this hypothesis and at discussing a possible pathway in the brain stem responsible for VS of caloric nystagmus.

The experiments were performed on cats prepared chronically. The control test was carried out more than one week before the left side of either the inferior olive (IO) or the superior colliculus (SC) was destroyed. The lesion of the left IO or SC was made electrolytically through a steel electrode by confirming a proper site with the light-guided evoked potentials under halothane or -chloralose anesthesia. Follow-up studies started from the fourth or the fifth postoperative day at a week interval. The lesion site was confirmed histologically after all the tests had been done.

VS After IO Lesion

The flocculus receives projections from the dorsal cap of the contralateral IO (Brodal, 1940). Visual signals are conveyed to the flocculus

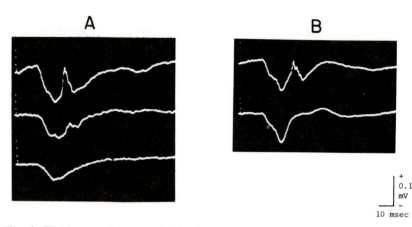

Fig. 1. Field potentials recorded in the flocculus following flash stimulation and averaged during 20 successive sweeps. A: different susceptibility of two components to stimulus frequency. The top trace is the field potentials at a stimulus frequency of 0.5 Hz; the second at 3 Hz; the third at 5 Hz. The second negative wave is reduced markedly at 5 Hz. B: the field potentials before (upper trace) and after (lower trace) the lesion of the inferior olive. The second negative wave is abolished in the lower trace.

via the caudal part of the dorsal cap (Alley *et al.*, 1975). If IO is the relay station of visual signals to the flocculus responsible for VS of caloric nystagmus, destruction of it should reduce or abolish VS of caloric nystagmus.

This possibility was tested in 12 cats. The lesion site was determined by monitoring of physiological evidence: (1) flash light induces field potentials in IO, (2) stimulation of the contralateral flocculus evokes field potentials antidromically in the same region as those induced by flash illumination are recorded (Alley *et al.*, 1975). Such a region wherein both ortho- and anti-dromical responses are recorded should be the caudal part of the dorsal cap of IO. This was confirmed by further evidence described below. Fig. 1 shows the visually induced field potentials recorded from the flocculus. The field potentials consist of two components, an early component with a latency of 20—25 msec and a later one with that of 30—40 msec. The first negative wave is preserved at the stimulus frequency of 5/sec, while the second is markedly reduced at rates above 3/sec (Fig. 1A). This different susceptibility of two components to the stimulus frequency is characteristic of MF and CF respectively in response to electrical stimulation of the optic disc (Maekawa and Takeda, 1976). The second negative wave is abolished after electrolytical destruction of the region wherein both ortho- and anti-dromical

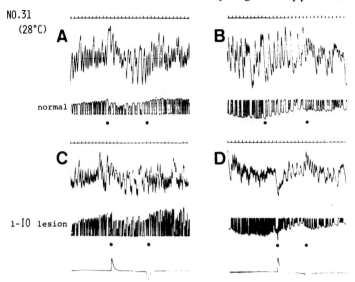

NO.31
(28°C)

Fig. 2. Visual suppression of caloric nystagmus and effect of a lesion of the left inferior olive. A and B: visual suppression of caloric nystagmus with quick phase toward left and right sides before the lesion of the inferior olive. C and D: effect of the lesion of the inferior olive on caloric nystagmus. Note that visual suppression of caloric nystagmus is observed in both left and right nystagmus. In A–D, the top trace is a time marker in secs; the second trace is the electronystagmogram with time constant 1.5 sec; the third trace shows the eye velocity of the slow phase. In C and D, the bottom trace is a photocell recording in which light on is indicated by upward deflection and light off by downward deflection. This is also indicated with black dots in A–D.

field potentials were recorded (Fig. 1B). This indicates that the CF pathway to the flocculus was interrupted.

The lesion of IO, however, was found not to be effective on VS of nystagmus in 6 of 12 cats in which the dorsal cap involving the caudal part was destroyed. This can be seen in Fig. 2. The slow phase velocity of caloric nystagmus toward the right and the left direction are reduced during the period when an animal was in the light before (Fig. 2A and B) and after (C and D) lesion of the dorsal cap of the left IO.

In 4 of 12 cats, the lesion was produced in the rostral part of IO, but VS of caloric nystagmus was not lost. In the remaining 2 animals, the lesion was found outside of IO. These 2 animals were discarded from the data.

These findings suggest that the CF pathway has no relevance to VS of caloric nystagmus and is in accord with the previous reports (Lisberger and Fuchs, 1974 and Ito and Miyashita, 1975).

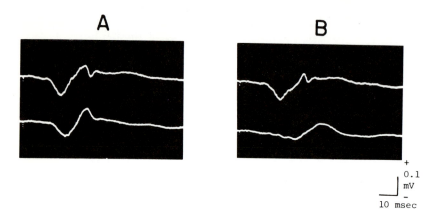

Fig. 3. Field potentials recorded in the flocculus following flash stimulation and averaged during 20 successive sweeps. A: the field potentials following flash stimulation to both eyes before (upper trace) and after (lower trace) the lesion of the left superior colliculus. B: the field potentials following flash stimulation to the right eye before (upper trace) and after (lower trace) the lesion. The early component is reduced after the lesion of the left superior colliculus. This reduction is prominent in the right eye stimulation.

VS After SC Lesion

The ventral part of the flocculus receives visual signals only through the CF pathway from the ipsilateral eye (Maekawa and Simpson, 1973), while the dorsal part receives those through both the MF pathway from both eyes and the CF pathway from the contralateral eye (Maekawa and Takeda, 1976). Furthermore, electrical stimulation of SC, even after destruction of the accessory optic tract (AOT), evokes field potentials resulting in MF activation in the dorsal part of the flocculus (Maekawa and Takeda, 1975). Thus, it is certain that SC projects to the flocculus via the MF pathway. But whether it sends visual signals responsible for modification of the vestibulo-ocular reflex still remains unsolved. By way of clarification experiments were carried out on 12 cats with electrolytic destruction of unilateral SC.

Fig. 3 shows the visually induced field potentials recorded from the flocculus. The early component was reduced after the lesion of SC (Fig. 3B). After the lesion of unilateral SC, VS of caloric nystagmus with the quick phase toward the contralateral side to the lesion was lost (Fig. 4D), while that towards the ipsilateral side to the lesion was preserved (Fig. 4C). As can be seen from Fig. 4C, the velocity of slow phase toward the right side was reduced by light

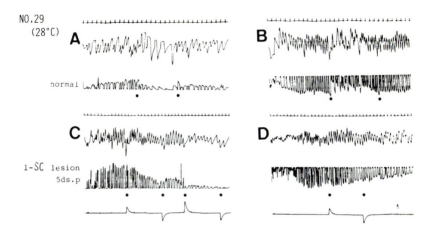

Fig. 4. Visual suppression of caloric nystagmus and effect of the lesion of the left superior colliculus. A and B: visual suppression of caloric nystagmus before the lesion of the superior colliculus. C and D: caloric nystagmus after the lesion of the left superior colliculus. Note that visual suppression of caloric nystagmus toward the right side is not reduced. The composition of the figure is the same as that of Fig. 2.

illumination and increased again after the light was turned off. On the contrary, the velocity of slow phase toward the left side was not reduced by light illumination as illustrated in Fig. 4D.

In 8 of 12 cats, VS of caloric nystagmus was abolished after lesion of the rostral part of SC. In 6 of these 8 animals, the extent of SC lesion was confirmed histologically to be large enough to cover the rostral half of SC and loss of VS of nystagmus persisted for more than 2 months after the lesion of SC. In the remaining 2 animals, the lesion was limited to a small area of SC and loss of VS of nystagmus was again observed. In another 4 animals, VS of nystagmus was preserved even after the lesion of SC, which was found to be very small.

Possible Pathway Relevant to VS

Loss of caloric nystagmus was observed after lesion of SC large enough to cover the rostral half, while it was not observed after IO lesion. These findings suggest that the MF pathway is relevant to VS of nystagmus, while CF pathway is not. This is supported by the findings of Lisberger and Fuchs (1975) and also Ghelarducci *et al.* (1975) that the complex spike activity of the floccular Purkinje cell is not related to immediate modification of vestibulo-ocular reflex by vision.

There is anatomical evidence that SC projects to the lateral reticular nucleus (LRN) (Kawamura *et al.,* 1975) and that LRN sends their fibers to the flocculus (Alley *et al.,* 1975). Hence, this pathway is the most likely candidate for VS of caloric nystagmus. Indeed, we recorded visually induced field potentials in LRN (unpublished). Recently, it has been reported that the nucleus of the basal optic root (nBOR) projects monosynaptically to the vestibulo-cerebellum (Brauth, 1977). Furthermore, the early component of the floccular fields potentials evoked by stimulation of the optic disc is reduced after the lesion of AOT (Maekawa and Takeda, 1975). Thus, AOT projections to the vestibulo-cerebellum should also be considered as the candidate for the pathway relevant to VS of caloric nystagmus.

The pathway responsible for VS of nystagmus could not be clearly established in this study. But it may be very probable that SC conveys at least a part of visual signals relevant to VS of nystagmus to the cerebellar flocculus.

References

Alley, K., Baker, G. and Simpson, J.I. (1975): Afferents to the vestibulo-cerebellum and the origin of the visual climbing fibers in the rabbit. *Brain Res.* **98**, 582-589.

Brauth, S.E. (1977): Direct accessory optic projections to the vestibulo-cerebellum: A possible channel for oculomotor control system. *Exp. Brain Res.* **28**, 73-84.

Brodal, A. (1940): Experimentelle Untersuchungen uber die olivo-cerebellare Lokalisation. *Z. ges. Neurol. Psychiat.* **169**, 1-153.

Ghelarducci, B., Ito, M. and Yagi, N. (1975): Impulse discharges from floccular Purkinje cells of alart rabbits during visual stimulation combined with horizontal head rotation. *Brain Res.* **87**, 66-72.

Ito, M. (1976): Cerebellar learning control of vestibulo-ocular mechanisms. *In* T. Desiraju (Ed.), Mechanisms in transmission of signals for conscious behaviour. Elsevier Scientific Publishing, Amsterdam/Oxford/New York, pp. 1-22.

Ito, M. and Miyashita, Y. (1975): The effects of chronic destruction of the inferior olive upon the visual modification of horizontal vestibulo-ocular reflex of rabbits. *Proc. Jap. Acad.* **51**, 716-720.

Kawamura, K., Brodal, A. and Hoodevik, G. (1975): The projection of the superior colliculus onto the reticular formation of the brain stem. An experimental anatomical study in the cat. *Exp. Brain Res.* **19**, 1-19.

Lisberger, S.G. and Fuchs, A.F. (1974): Response of flocculus Purkinje cells to adequate vestibular stimulation in the alart monkey: fixation vs. compensatory eye movements. *Brain Res.* **69**, 347-353.

Maekawa, K. and Simpson, J.I. (1973): Climbing fiber responses evoked in vestibulocerebellum of rabbit from visual system. *J. Neurophysiol.* **36**, 649-666.

Maekawa, K. and Takeda, T. (1975): Mossy fiber responses evoked in the cerebellar flocculus of rabbit by stimulation of the optic pathway. *Brain Res.* **98**, 590-595.

Maekawa, K. and Takeda, T. (1976): Electrophysiological identification of the climbing and mossy fiber pathway from the rabbit's retina to the contralateral cerebellar flocculus. *Brain Res.* **109**, 169-174.

Takemori, S. and Cohen, B. (1974): Loss of visual suppression of vestibular nystagmus after flocculus lesion. *Brain Res.* **72**, 213-224.

3. Adaptation in the caloric response

G.R. BARNES, A.J. BENSON

Royal Air Force, Institute of Aviation Medicine, Farnborough, Hants. U.K.

Introduction

Stimulation of the receptors of a semicircular canal by irrigation of the external canal with fluid at a temperature above or below that of the body is a familiar clinical test of vestibular function. Various measures of the evoked response are employed; for example, in Fitzgerald and Hallpike's (1942) version of the test, the duration of the response is determined by direct observation and is typically 100 sec, although when the evoked nystagmus is recorded by electro-oculography, in the absence of visual fixation, the average duration of the response is about 180 sec (Stahle, 1958). These figures are, however, substantially shorter than the persistence of the thermal stimulus which Cawthorne and Cobb (1954) have shown, by direct measurement, to be of the order of 10 min. Indirect evidence for the longevity of the basic stimulus has been obtained by Oosterveld and van der Laarse (1969) who showed that nystagmus could be evoked for up to 20 min after irrigation by repeated exposure to high levels of linear acceleration (2.5 *g*). More recently Hood (1973) reported the persistence of nystagmus for at least 10 min when the subject was moved from the prone to the supine position at regular intervals following irrigation.

These observations, as well as those of Jongkees (1960), Yuganov (1965) and Oman (1972) strongly suggest that the nystagmus evoked by a caloric stimulus is substantially modified by an adaptive process. A mathematical description of the adaptive processes observed in the response to angular acceleration has been devised by Young and Oman (1969) and Malcolm and Melvill Jones (1970), but there is no unambiguous evidence that the model is applicable to the caloric response; the studies of Oman (1972) were not conclusive and Hood (1973) presented only qualitative data. Accordingly, an experiment was carried out in order to obtain quantitative information which would allow the adequacy of contemporary models of both adaptation and the thermal stimulus to be assessed. The experimental situation was similar to that employed by Oman (1972) and Hood (1973) in that it involved a reorientation of the subject with respect to the gravity vector at regular intervals following irrigation.

Method

Experimental Conditions

The subject was seated within a framework attached to a turntable which could be rotated about an earth horizontal axis, the body being constrained to move in the sagittal plane. The head and body were firmly clamped to the framework. The experiment was conducted in a darkened room with the eyes closed; alertness was maintained by carrying out simple exercises in mental arithmetic. The subjects were eight healthy members of staff (2 female, 6 male), without neuro-otological defect or diseases of the middle or external ear. Some reported slight nausea during the test procedure, but none failed to complete the experiment.

Procedure

The caloric stimulus was an irrigation of the left ear with water at 44°C for 30 seconds. The stimulus was administered with the subject in a near-supine position with the coronal plane of the head at 60° to the vertical. In this '60° back' position the plane of the lateral canals was approximately vertical and thus the caloric stimulus was maximally enhanced by gravity. Each subject was exposed to two experimental conditions separated by a period of at least 24 hours. One condition was a control in which the subject remained in the 60° back position for a period of 10 minutes. In the other (referred to as the reorientation condition) irrigation was carried out in the 60° back position, but 60 seconds after the start of irrigation the subject was moved in the sagittal plane to a position 30° forward of the vertical (the positions are indicated at the foot of Fig. 2). In the 30° forward position the plane of the lateral canals was approximately horizontal and thus the effective stimulus to the cupula, attributable to the density gradient, was reduced to zero. The subject was moved thereafter at intervals of 1 minute between the 60° back and 30° forward positions for a period of 9 minutes. Half of the subjects experienced the control condition first and half the reorientation condition first in order to balance out the effects of habituation.

Instrumentation

Eye movements were transduced by conventional DC electro-oculography and recorded on an FM tape recorder. Records were analysed by measuring representative slow phase eye velocity at equal time intervals: these being every 5 seconds for the reorientation condition and every 10 seconds for the control condition. Each experimental run was preceded and followed by a calibration of the eye movements.

Results

Control Condition

Typically the response of the eyes to the caloric stimulus was a nystagmus, initially with a slow phase component to the right. The mean slow phase eye velocity (Fig. 1) rose to a maximum of approximately 25°/sec some 60 sec after the start of irrigation and thereafter decayed steadily to reach zero velocity on average after 220 sec. However, some 250–300 sec after the start of irrigation a reversal of nystagmus, with slow phase to the left, was observed in all subjects.

Reorientation Conditions

As was to be expected, during the first 60 sec from the start of the irrigation the nystagmus was not dissimilar to that observed in the

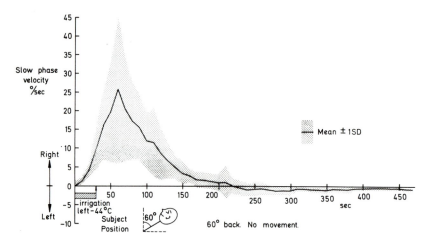

Fig. 1. The slow phase angular velocity of the eye (mean of 8 subjects) following irrigation of the left external ear with water at 44°C for 30 seconds. Subject maintained in 60° back position.

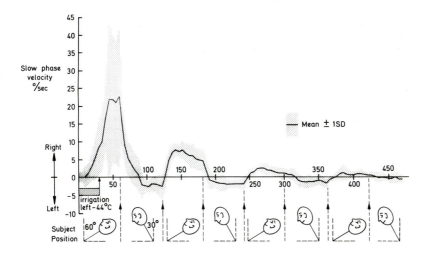

Fig. 2. The slow phase angular velocity of the eye (mean of 8 subjects) following irrigation of the left external ear with water at 44°C for 30 seconds. Subject moved in sagittal plane at regular 1 min intervals between initial 60° back position and 30° forward position, as indicated.

control condition. However, at the first movement to the 30° forward position, which occurred when the nystagmus response was maximal, there was a rapid decay of the slow phase velocity to the right with reversal to a slow phase left nystagmus some 20–25 sec after the reorientation (Fig. 2). Typically, the maximum velocity of this slow phase left nystagmus was 10–15% of the peak slow phase right response.

On return to the original (60° back) position after 120 sec, the slow phase right nystagmus returned within a few seconds to reach a velocity which was greater than that achieved in the comparable period of the control condition. This pattern of response was observed with subsequent changes in head position, though the intensity of the nystagmus progressively declined. It is noteworthy that a slow phase right nystagmus occurred on each occasion the subject was moved to the 60° back position and was detectable for up to 7 min after irrigation. In each 60 sec period there was a significant difference ($p < 0.05$ by Wilcoxon Test) in the mean slow phase velocity of the nystagmus recorded during the control and reorientation conditions, with the exception of the first 60 sec, when the experimental conditions were identical, and for the periods beginning at 300 sec and 420 sec, when the response in both conditions was characterised by a slow phase left nystagmus.

Discussion

The pattern of the nystagmus elicited in subjects whose orientation to gravity was changed at regular intervals following irrigation of one ear for 30 sec, have demonstrated that this thermal stimulus can be effective for at least 9 min. This conclusion is in agreement with the direct measurements of the temperature change within the membranous labyrinth made by Cawthorne and Cobb (1954) as well as the electro-nystagmographic studies of Hood (1973).

It is most probable that the relatively rapid decay of nystagmus which occurs when there is no alteration of head position or change in force environment following irrigation is due, primarily, to neural adaptation (Oman, 1972; Hood, 1973; Benson, 1974). The same process would also account for the reversal of nystagmus observed in the control condition of the present experiment as well as the augmented responses and nystagmus of opposite sign that occurred in the 60° back and 30° forward positions respectively.

Analysis of the oculomotor response to rotational stimuli allowed Young and Oman (1969) and Malcolm and Melvill Jones (1970) to develop a describing function of the adaptation process $A'(s)$ which was of the form:

$$A'(s) = \frac{T_A s}{1 + T_A s} \quad \dotsc\dotsc\dotsc\dotsc\dotsc\dotsc\dotsc\dotsc \quad (1)$$

Representative values for T_A, the time constant of adaptation, ranged between 80 and 120 sec.

In order to assess the applicability of this adaptation model to the caloric response it is necessary to have describing functions for the heating effect $(H(s))$ and for the dynamics of the semicircular canals $(C(s))$. The latter has been extensively studied (summarized by Barnes (1976)) and has been shown to be of the form:

$$C(s) = \frac{K T_B (1 + T_D s)}{(1 + T_B s)(1 + T_C s)} \quad \dotsc\dotsc\dotsc\dotsc\dotsc\dotsc\dotsc\dotsc \quad (2)$$

where $K \cong 0.7$

$T_C \cong 0.01$ sec and $T_D \cong 0.1$ sec so the contribution of these short time constant lag and lead terms may be ignored in the computation of the response to a slowly changing stimulus. The long time constant of the semicircular canals (T_B) is of the order of $15-20$ sec.

Thus, the response of a canal and the adaptation process may be combined and represented by a describing function of the form:

$$A(s) = \frac{KT_A \, T_B s}{(1+T_A s)(1+T_B s)} \quad \dots\dots\dots\dots\dots \quad (3)$$

The heating effect ($H(s)$) may be represented by:

$$H(s) = \frac{(1+T_E s)}{(1+T_F s)(1+T_G s)} \cdot \cos \psi \quad \dots\dots\dots\dots \quad (4)$$

where ψ is the angle made by the plane of the lateral canal with the gravitational vertical.

When $T_E = 67$ sec, $T_F = 230$ sec and $T_G = 44$ sec, the describing function was found to model the data of Cawthorne and Cobb (1954) much more closely than the simpler function proposed by Steer (1967) and subsequently used by Oman (1972).

As the data presented in Fig. 1 and 2 are the arithmetic mean of the responses of 8 subjects, each of whom was likely to have slightly different adaptation and canal dynamics, the adequacy of the model was assessed against the plot of nystagmus slow phase velocity of one subject (Figs. 3 and 4). Optimisation procedures gave values for T_A and T_C of 90 sec and 17 sec respectively, which are not dissimilar to the values obtained by others (vide supra) for modelling the responses to rotational stimuli.

It may be seen that the model effectively predicts the main features of the oculomotor response in both the control and reorientation conditions, both with regard to the timing of nystagmus reversals and the amplitude of the slow phase velocity. The fit is, of course, not perfect; in particular the model predicts a slightly more rapid decay and earlier reversal of nystagmus than was found experimentally following movement of the subject to the 30° forward position. This disparity may be caused by an alteration of the adaptive time constant with head position which is attributable to an interaction between canal and otolithic afferents (Benson, 1974). Nevertheless, the ability to model the nystagmus induced by a thermal stimulus, both when the effective stimulus to the cupula changed relatively slowly and when the stimulus was periodically removed, implies that the adaptation transfer function derived from studies of the system response to rotational stimuli is no less applicable to the less physiological, but clinically more useful, thermal

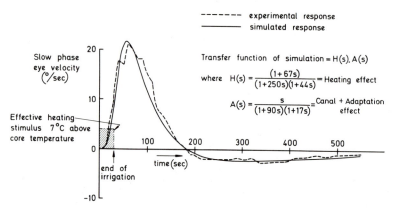

Fig. 3. A comparison of the experimentally determined slow phase eye velocity of one subject (S7), resulting from caloric irrigation, with that predicted by the mathematical model (transfer functions as indicated). Subject maintained with lateral body plane in 60° back position.

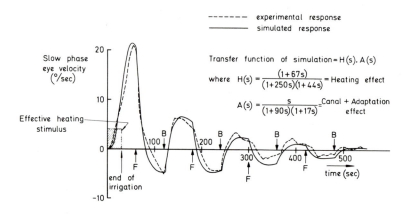

Fig. 4. A comparison of the experimentally determined slow phase eye velocity of one subject (S7), resulting from caloric irrigation, with that predicted by the mathematical model (transfer functions as indicated). Subject initially positioned with lateral body plane at 60° to the vertical and moved forward (F) through 90° and backward (B) to original position at 1 min intervals, as indicated.

stimulus. Our findings thus corroborate those of Oman (1972) who concluded that the process of adaptation is the same for both caloric and rotational responses. However, unlike Oman (1972), we do not find the need to propose the existence of a mechanism which inhibits secondary nystagmus when a unilateral stimulus is employed.

The locus of the adaptive process in the vestibulo-ocular pathway is a topic for speculation. Hood (1973) argues that it lies in the sensory cells of the crista, a view which receives some support from the electrophysiological studies of Goldberg and Fernandez (1971) who have shown that some, but not all, primary vestibular afferents in the squirrel monkey exhibit adaptation with an average adaptive time constant of 80 sec. This adaptation may be an essential feature of the stimulus response relationship of the sensory cells; alternatively, it may reflect a modification of their behaviour by efferent pathways (Schmidt, 1963). While accepting that adaptation does occur in the peripheral receptors, the presence of an adaptive coupling at a higher level within the afferent vestibular projection cannot be excluded. Indeed, the substantially shorter adaptive time constant for the sensations than for the nystagmus evoked by vestibular stimuli implies that some adaptive processing of vestibular information occurs within the central nervous system.

Conclusion

The present experiment confirms that the nystagmus elicited by a thermal stimulus, such as is commonly employed in clinical tests, is substantially modified by adaptive processes. Furthermore, an adequate stimulus to the ampullary receptors, which is assumed to be evoked by alterations in the thermal environment of the lateral canal, can be detected for at least 9 min in a normogravic force environment.

These findings have implications for the conduct and interpretation of the clinical caloric test. First, a period of 5 min between the administration of consecutive caloric stimuli, regarded by Hallpike *et al.* (1951) as the minimum interval to ensure negligible interaction, is probably insufficient. It is recommended that at least 10 min be allowed between irrigations, particularly when the response is recorded by electro-oculography and there is no suppression of low velocity eye movements by visual fixation, as in the Fitzgerald and Hallpike procedure. Second, it is important to recognise that the intensity and duration of the nystagmus evoked by a thermal stimulus represents not just the intrinsic response of the sensory epithelium whose sensitivity and adaptation dynamics may be modified by disease processes, but also the influence of neural components within the vestibulo-ocular pathway and of higher centres which can influence the adaptive mechanism.

References

Barnes, G.R. (1976): Vestibulo-ocular responses to head turning movements and their functional significance during visual target acquisition. Ph.D. Thesis University of Surrey, Guildford.

Benson, A.J. (1974): Modification of the response to angular accelerations by linear acceleration. In: Handbook of Sensory Physiology, 6, Part 2, 281-320. Ed. Kornhuber, H.H. Heidelberg: Springer-Verlag, Berlin.

Cawthorne, T. and Cobb, W.A. (1954): Temperature changes in the perilymph space in response to caloric stimulation in man. Acta Otolaryng. 44, 580-588.

Fitzgerald, G. and Hallpike, C.S. (1942): Studies of human vestibular function: Observations on the directional preponderance (Nystagmusbereitschaft) of caloric nystagmus resulting from central lesions. Brain. 65, 115-131.

Goldberg, J.M. and Fernandez, C. (1971): Physiology of peripheral neurons innervating semicircular canals of the Squirrel Monkey. 1. Resting discharge and response to constant acceleration. J. Neurophysiol. 39, 635-684.

Hallpike, C.S., Harrison, S.M. and Slater, E. (1951): Abnormalities of the caloric test results of certain varieties of mental disorder. Acta Oto-Laryng. 39, 151-159.

Hood, J.D. (1973): Persistence of response in the caloric test. Aerospace Med. 44, (4), 444-449.

Jongkees, L.B.W. (1960): On positional nystagmus. Acta Oto-Laryng. 159, 78-83.

Malcolm, R. and Melvill Jones, G. (1970): A quantitative study of vestibular adaptation in humans. Acta Oto-Laryng. 70, 126-135.

Oman, C.M. (1972): Dynamic response of the semicircular canal and lateral line organs. Ph.D. Thesis, Massachusetts Institute of Technology, Cambridge, Mass.

Oosterveld, E.J. and van der Laarse, W.D. (1969): Effect of gravity on vestibular nystagmus. Aerospace Med. 40, 382-385.

Schmidt, R.S. (1963): Frog labyrinthine efferent impulses. Acta Oto-Laryng. 56, 51-64.

Stahle, J. (1958): Electro-nystagmography in the caloric and rotary tests. Acta Oto-Laryng. Suppl. 137.

Steer, R.W. (1967): The influence of angular and linear acceleration and thermal stimulation on the human semicircular canal. Sc.D. Thesis. Massachusetts Institute of Technology (NVT-67-3).

Young, L.R. and Oman, C.M. (1969): Model for vestibular adaptation to horizontal rotation. Aerospace Med. 40, 1076-1080.

Yuganov, Ye.M. (1965): The problem of the functional characteristics and interaction of the otolith and cupular portions of the vestibular apparatus under conditions of altered gravity. In: Problemy Kosmicheskoy biology. Moscow: 'Nauka' Press, 4, 54-69. (English translation: Problems of Space Biology 4, Washington, D.C.: NASA, TT F-368, 48-63 (1966)).

4. The effect of mental activity on thermally induced nystagmus under changed test conditions

P. STRAUSS, A. MEYER ZUM GOTTESBERGE

E.N.T. Clinic, University of Düsseldorf, Moorenstr. 5, D–4000, Düsseldorf 1

Material and Methods

The right ear of 30 healthy subjects (15 males and 15 females), ranging in age between 20 and 30 years, was stimulated with water at 30°C. The nystagmic response was recorded electro-nystagmographically (AC-Amplifier). The water application was applied by filling the ear-canal for 20 or 30 seconds followed by a rinse of 30 sec. duration. The rinse was administered through a polyethylene-catheter attached to the head of the test subject. After each test each subject was given a 7 minute rest period. Two tests were carried out:

1. a change in the visual environment through changing the fixation and illumination, and
2. an increase in stimulus intensity through increasing the time period of filling and rinsing the ear-canal.

Each of the tests was carried out twice. In the first test the subject was in a relaxed state (dream) and in the second one the subject was asked to exercise an arithmetic task (continuous subtraction).

In the analysis of the nystagmus the following parameters were evaluated: total duration, total beat, total amplitude, maximum frequency within the culmination interval and the optimal reaction time; i.e. the time period from the end of the stimulation till the median of the culmination interval.

The maximum amplitude within the culmination interval corresponds, according to our own study (unpublished data), approximately to the maximum velocity of the slow phase; i.e. the angular velocity in regard to the distribution and the variation coefficient.

Results

Change in Visual Environment

Subjects tested in the dark room with their eyes open and performing an arithmetic exercise showed a statistically significant increase in regard to the stimulus response. For the statistical evaluation a twotailed STUDENT t-test was used; the error probability was always smaller than 5% and usually in the 1.0 to 0.1% range.

This enhancement has also been described by Collins (1962), Sokolovski (1965) and Henriksson (1975). The most significant increase of the response is found in the total amplitude, the increase is nearly the same with respect to maximal amplitude during the culmination interval (Fig.1).

Illuminating the eyes with Frenzel-glasses and performing an arithmetic exercise while eliminating fixation did not increase the amplitude any further (Fig. 2). Duration and frequency, however, were still further increased.

If additional to the illumination and arithmetic exercise the eyes fixed a point, the duration and frequency were no longer increased. The result is an inversion of the previously observed effect. Now, however, mental exercise decreases the intensity of the response in regard to the frequency and this decrease is statistically significant (Fig. 3).

Provided that illumination and fixation are varied, Fig. 4 indicates two probable reasons that might cause the change of parameter values during the switch from dreaming to mental exercise; thus in illuminating the eyes through Frenzel-glasses and eliminating fixation the amplitude is increased in relationship to the dark room, consequently a further increase through changing the dreaming state into a mentally more active state (calculating) is impossible. The absolute values are approximately $600°$ degree for the total amplitude and approximately $180°$ for the maximum amplitude. When the eyes, besides being illuminated, are additionally fixed on to a point almost all parameters decrease in intensity. Now the arithmetic exercise leads to a further decrease, most likely caused by fixation related inhibition in the brainstem.

Increase in Stimulus Intensity

When the thermal stimulus is increased the stimulus response increases almost all parameters. Again, a particularly strong increase can be observed in relationship to the amplitude. With increase in stimulus intensity the degree of a further increase due to a change from dreaming to calculating is lowered, especially in regard to the amplitude. The cause for this might be again the large absolute values of the amplitude that allow of little further increase.

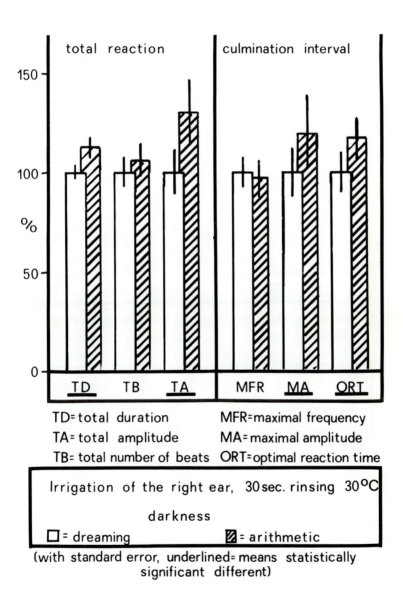

Fig. 1. Effect of mental activity

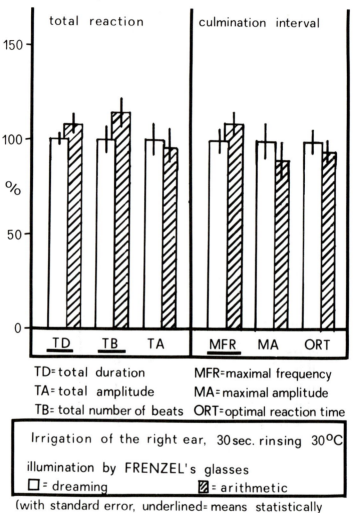

TD= total duration   MFR= maximal frequency
TA= total amplitude   MA= maximal amplitude
TB= total number of beats ORT= optimal reaction time

Irrigation of the right ear, 30 sec. rinsing 30°C

illumination by FRENZEL's glasses
□ = dreaming   ▨ = arithmetic

(with standard error, underlined= means statistically
significant different)

Fig. 2. Effect of illumination by Frenzel's glasses

Distribution of Parameters

The variance of a parameter is of interest to the clinician in order to discriminate between healthy and pathological results. We had hoped that the activation of the brainstem through mental exercising would reduce the variance. The arousal of the test subject through mental activity is, however, not constant, hence the variance is not reduced.

The variance is expressed as the standard deviation divided by the mean; i.e. through the variation coefficient. The comparison of variances was calculated according to a method by Schmitz (1976) using Pearson's correlation coefficient (Table 1). During the dark room tests as well as during illumination of the eyes with Frenzel-glasses the variance of the duration and amplitude is significantly

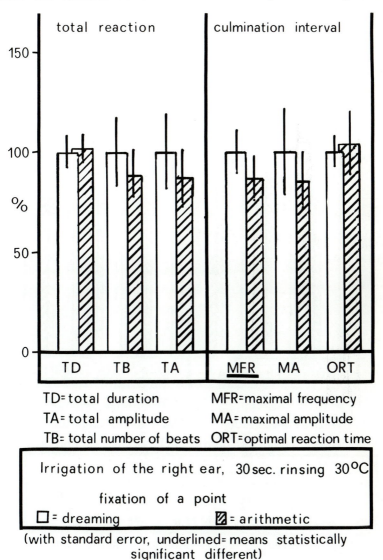

TD= total duration MFR=maximal frequency
TA= total amplitude MA= maximal amplitude
TB= total number of beats ORT= optimal reaction time

Irrigation of the right ear, 30 sec. rinsing 30°C

fixation of a point

□ = dreaming ▨ = arithmetic

(with standard error, underlined= means statistically significant different)

Fig. 3. Effect of fixation upon a point

increased by arithmetic exercise. This increase of the variance is most likely caused by an enhancement of the response by the change from dream to mental exercise. This assumption is supported by the observation that during fixation on a point the change from dreaming to mental exercising lowers the response intensity. During this time the variance is also significantly decreased.

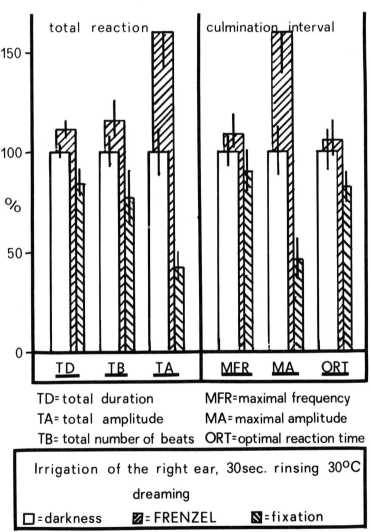

TD= total duration   MFR= maximal frequency
TA= total amplitude   MA= maximal amplitude
TB= total number of beats   ORT= optimal reaction time

Irrigation of the right ear, 30 sec. rinsing 30°C

dreaming

□ = darkness   ▨ = FRENZEL   ◩ = fixation

(with standard error, underlined= means statistically significant different)

Fig. 4. Relative effects of illumination and fixation

TABLE 1

Variation Coefficient (s/x) of some Parameters under Various Test Conditions
(thick lined: statistically significant difference)

	darkness		FRENZEL		fixation	
	dream	arith.	d.	a.	d.	a.
T D	0.12	0.18	0.16	0.24	0.31	0.27
T B	0.29	0.30	0.37	0.36	0.65	0.51
T A	0.42	0.47	0.43	0.58	0.75	0.63
MFR	0.29	0.36	0.35	0.30	0.43	0.49
MA	0.48	0.58	0.50	0.58	0.85	0.65
ORT	0.39	0.33	0.34	0.32	0.30	0.58

Conclusion

In comparing the variance of the duration with the variance of the amplitude one tends to accept the duration as the more exact measure, due to its much smaller distribution. The low distribution of the duration is caused, however, by the limiting increase of the duration in general. It follows therefore that differences in excitability will not be revealed by the duration alone.

The results of this study clearly indicate a preference for carrying out ENG investigations in a dark room. The patient should be relaxed (dreaming) and with his eyes open. An arithmetic exercise is only given when the response is so small that its evaluation would cause considerably difficulties.

References

Collins, W.E., Guedry, F.E. and Posner, J.B. (1962): Control of caloric nystagmus by manipulating arousal and visual fixation distance. *Ann. Otol.* 71, 187-202.

Henriksson, N.G. and Afzelius, L.E. (1975): Effect of eye-closure on vestibular nystagmus reflecting alertness and personality. Proc. Barany Society, Kyoto, 180-186.

Schmitz, H. (1976): Personal Communication.

Sokolovski, A. (1965): The influence of mental activity and visual fixation upon caloric-induced nystagmus in normal subjects. *Acta Otolaryngol.* 61, 209-220.

Optokinetic responses

1. Optokinograms in clinical documentation of vestibular disorders

J. STAHLE and K. MIZUKOSHI

Departments of Otorhinolaryngology, Akademiska sjukhuset, Uppsala, Sweden and Niigata University, School of Medicine, Niigata City, Japan

Introduction

Focal nervous system lesions can often be revealed through abnormal results of optokinetic and eye-tracking tests (Carmichael *et al.*, 1955, Enoksson, 1956, Kornhuber, 1966, Ino, 1970, Baloh *et al.*, 1977). Numerous variants of optokinetic (OK) tests have been described but neither the OK stimulus nor the interpretation of the responses has yet been fully standardized, for clinical use. The degree of acceleration and the constant velocity of the stripes, as well as the instructions given to the test subjects, strongly influence the optokinetic response (Honrubia *et al.*, 1968). Variations in any of these factors complicate comparison between different tests. Thus there would seem reason to assume that a standardized OK test would be appreciated, in view of the wide acceptance of the Fitzgerald and Hallpike caloric test.

The aim of this paper is to present an optokinetic test suitable for clinical use and a new way of documenting the optokinetic response.

Method

A slit-projector[1], giving an image pattern of black and white stripes on the inner surface of a cylindrical screen, was used. Only horizontal nystagmus was recorded[2].

*This work was supported by the Swedish Medical Research Council (Project B78-17X-3908-06A).

1. Slit-projector Type OK 1 b, ServoMed AB, PO Box 110, S-162 12 Stockholm-Vallingby, Sweden.
2. ELEMA Mingograph Model 34.

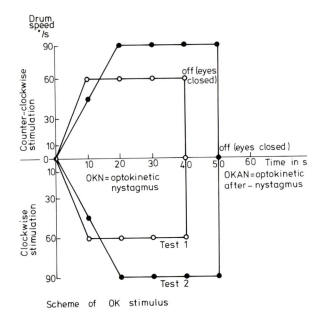

Scheme of OK stimulus

Fig. 1. The test subjects were exposed to two different stimuli, applied in both a clockwise and a counter-clockwise direction. In Test 1 the optokinetic stimulation starts with acceleration at $6°/sec^2$ for 10 sec, followed by rotation at a constant speed of $60°/sec$ for 30 sec. Test 2 comprises 20 sec of acceleration at $4.5°/sec^2$ up to a speed of $90°/sec$, followed by rotation at a constant speed for 30 sec.

The test subjects and patients were instructed not to follow the revolving stripes, but to keep their gaze straight ahead and count the stripes moving by. This method corresponds to the "stare" test (Honrubia *et al.*, 1968). After cessation of the OK stimulation, the subjects were told to close their eyes and the optokinetic after-nystagmus (OKAN) was recorded for about 100 sec.

Two different OK stimuli were used in the search for a suitable method (Fig. 1). Common to both of them is that they contain both acceleration and constant velocity. In the two stimuli the final velocities are $60°/sec$ and $90°/sec$ respectively. The choice of $60°/sec$ was based on reports that this is normally the upper limit for conformity between the speed of the stimulus and the eye-speed in the slow nystagmus phase (Jung, 1953, Honrubia *et al.*, 1968), and the choice of $90°/sec$ on the view that higher speeds increase the diagnostic possibilities (Enoksson, 1956, Kornhuber, 1966).

The reason that OKN was also recorded during the acceleration was an attempt to determine when the eyes would fail to keep up with the speed of the stimulus.

Assessment of the recordings

Comparison between maximum eye-speed in the slow phase, frequency and amplitude have shown that the first mentioned factor varies least in normal individuals (Mizukoshi *et al.*, 1977). This factor also revealed a greater number of abnormalities than the other two in a pilot study and has consequently been assumed to be the most suitable of the three for clinical evaluation of the OK response.

The Normal Values

1. The mean maximum eye-speeds in Test 1 (rotation speed of 60°/sec) are presented in Fig. 2. These values comprise the mean of the three to four fastest beats during a 10-sec period. Thus during acceleration the highest values were recorded at the end of the period. The mean slow-phase speeds of the eyes almost equalled the speeds of the optokinetic stimulus. Only in two individuals were

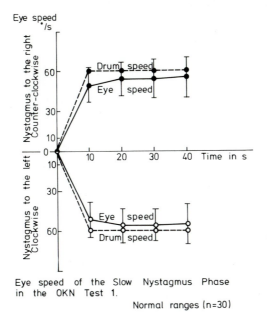

Fig. 2. Mean values and normal ranges (± 2 SD) for the maximum speed of the eyes in the slow nystagmus phase. The mean eye-speed (continuous line) almost equalled the drum speed (line of short dashes). Thirty normal subjects.

marked deviations between the eye-speed and drum-speed observed; in these cases the eyes were only able to follow the stimulus up to 40°/sec.

At a rotation speed of 90°/sec (Test 2) the mean maximum eye-speeds were somewhat higher (60-65°/sec during a 10-sec period) and the individual variations greater. Only in 4 of the 30 normal subjects were the eyes able to conform with the speed of the stimulus during the entire acceleration up to 90°/sec. We therefore decided to base our clinical test on a stimulus speed of 60°/sec (Test 1).

2. We have named the *upper limit for consistency* between the eye-speed in the slow nystagmus phase and the speed of the OK stimulus the "Optokinetic Fatigue Threshold (OFT)". We are not yet prepared to give an opinion on the diagnostic significance of large discrepancies of this threshold.

3. *The limits for normality.* The formula for caloric directional preponderance recommended by Jongkees and Philipszoon (1964) can also be applied to the OK response. On the basis of the results in our normal material it may be stated that the difference in maximum eye-speed with stimuli to the left and to the right should not exceed 10%. The disadvantage of this mode of evaluation is that it gives no information on abnormally weak reactions (diminution).

The Optokinogram

This is a new way of presenting the OK response. The results are plotted in a diagram, which illustrates the reaction simply and clearly. For clinical use we have also constructed a form (Fig. 3), which includes space for noting any optokinetic inversion and long-standing OKAN (> 30 sec). The normal range (2 SD) for maximum eye-speed is 40-67°/sec, which is enclosed in the hexagonal area on the optokinogram.

Clinical application of the new OK test

The test was applied in two groups of patients:
1. 68 patients with disorders of the inner ear and the peripheral neuron- including 43 patients with Meniere's disease and 2) 25 patients with vertigo or dysequilibrium caused by disorders of the central nervous system (CNS).

OK directional preponderance and unilateral or bilateral diminution was found in 37% of the Meniere patients and in 32% of the

OPTOKINOGRAM

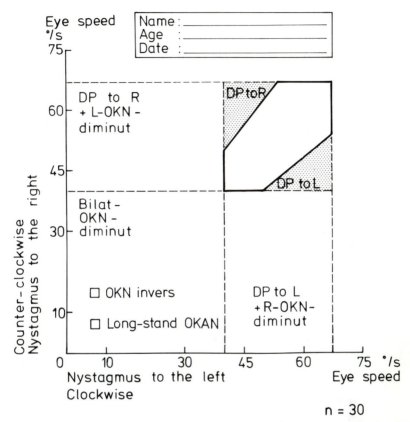

Fig. 3. Form for optokinogram, based on the maximum eye-speed in the slow nystagmus phase in Test 1. The normal range is 40-67°/sec. Values falling within the hexagonal area are classified as normal. The shaded areas indicate directional preponderance (DP) to the right alone and to the left alone. The other three areas include bilateral diminution of the OKN (lower left square) and unidirectional diminution combined with DP. R and L OKN diminution mean abnormal reduction of the right/left-beating optokinetic nystagmus, respectively.

other patients with different peripheral disorders. Optokinetic inversion did not occur and longstanding OKAN was only recorded in one case in this group. A total of 35% of the patients with peripheral disorders displayed an abnormal optokinogram. This was an unexpected result.

In patients with CNS disorders the number of pathological optokinograms was considerably higher, as expected (Fig. 4). A total of

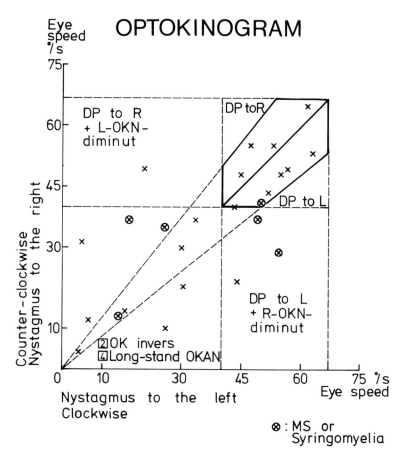

Fig. 4. OK test results from 25 patients with CNS disorders presented together as one optokinogram. Abnormal optokinetic responses were recorded in 17 patients. Optokinetic inversion was observed in two and longstanding OKAN in four patients.

71% of the patients in this group had a pathological optokinogram.

Comments

1. Our finding of numerous abnormal OK responses among patients with vertigo or dysequilibrium due to CNS disorders was to be expected and is in line with previous experience. It is worth pointing out, however, that directional preponderance alone was uncommon, whereas bilateral diminution of the OK response was found in one-third of the patients with CNS disorders.

2. Abnormal optokinograms in 35% of the patients with peripheral vestibular disorders is a remarkable finding. Our results contradict the experience of Baloh *et al.,* (1977) that "patients with chronic peripheral vestibular disorders usually have normal optokinetic nystagmus".

3. Some uncertainty prevails as to whether the optokinetic and vestibular systems are related, or whether they function independently of one another. Dix *et al.,* (1949) found normal OKN in cases with severe streptomycin intoxication in spite of abolition of both caloric and galvanic nystagmus. They therefore concluded that the brain stem mechanism of OKN was entirely separated from the vestibular nuclei. The observation of Baloh *et al.,* (1977) is well compatible with this view. On the other hand it has been found that experimental labyrinthine lesions can give rise to OKN abnormalities (Cohen *et al.,* 1973). The high frequency of pathological optokinogram in our Meniere patients indicates, in fact, that the optokinetic and vestibular reflex arcs are integrated. Recent findings of discrete ultrastructural hair-cell changes in patients with Meniere's disease support our theory that the abnormal responses emanate from the labyrinth (Rosenhall *et al.,* 1977).

References

Baloh, R.W., Honrubia, V. and Sills, A. (1977); *Ann. Otol. Rhinol. Lar.* **86**, 108-115.

Carmichael, E.A., Dix, M.R. and Hallpike, C.S. (1955): *J. Lar. Otol.* **64**, 269-276.

Cohen, B., Uemura, T. and Takemori, S. (1973): *Int. J. Equil. Res.* **3**, 88-93.

Dix, M.R., Hallpike, C.S. and Harrison, M.S. (1949): *Brain* **72**, 241-245.

Enoksoon, P. (1956): *Acta ophthal.* **34**, 163-184.

Honrubia, V., Downey, W.L., Mitchell, D.P. and Ward, P.H. (1968): *Acta. oto-lar.* **65**, 441-448.

Ino, H. (1970): *In:* "Vestibular Function on Earth and In Space" (ed. J. Stahle), pp. 209-214, Pergamon Press, Oxford, New York.

Jongkees, L.B.W., and Philipszoon, A.J. (1964): *Acta. oto-lary. Suppl.* **192**, 168-170.

Jung, R. (1953): *In:* "Handbuch der inneren Medizin" (ed. G.V. Bergman *et al.*) 4th edn. V/1 pp. 1325-1379, Springer, Berlin-Gottingen-Heidelberg.

Kornhuber, H.H. (1966): *In:* "Hals-Nasen-Ohrenheilkunde" (ed. J. Berendes *et al.*) III/3, pp. 2150-2351, Georg Thieme Verlag, Stuttgart.

Mizukoshi, K., Fabian, P. and Stahle, J. (1977): *Acta. oto-lar.* **84**, 155-165.

Rosenhall, U., Engstrom, B. and Stahle, J. (1977): *Acta. oto-lar.* **84**, Nov.-Dec.

2. Optokinetic nystagmus in normal human subjects

S. HOLM-JENSEN and E. PEITERSEN

University ENT-clinic, Copenhagen City Hospital, DK 1399, Copenhagen

Introduction

Since Robert Barany's classic works (Barany, 1920) on optokinetic nystagmus (OKN) in the 1920's, a vast literature on this subject has evolved, and the optokinetic responses are now investigated as a routine test in neuro-otological examinations. Despite this, few attempts have been made to standardize the test and pathological reactions are often identified by the investigator's clinical experience alone due to lack of exact criteria on pathology. The requirements of a standardised procedure must be, that the optokinetic responses in normal subjects are regular with the slightest possible variation of eye speed in the slow phase and the slightest possible variation of the frequency, thus creating optimal conditions.

The two stimulus variables of major significance in determining the regularity of the optokinetic responses are target speed and target frequency.

Material and Method

Changes in the optokinetic responses due to alterations of these two factors, were investigated in 6 normal humans with variation of the target speed from 5°/sec to 120°/sec and variation of frequency of the targets from 1/3 per sec to 24 per sec.

The optokinetic nystagmus was produced by a rotator which projected either 24, 36 or 72 lightslits on a semi-circular screen. The eye velocity of the slow phase was calculated according to Kestenbaum (1924), without regard to the duration of the fast phase. Eye speed was calculated on a 10 sec period of even response. If this could not be achieved, the results were rejected.

Eye deflections were recorded by an Elema Mingograph 34 AC-

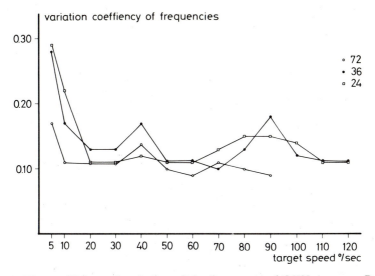

Fig. 1. The coefficient of variation of the frequency of OKN: − o − : Rotator with 72 lightslits (targets) per 360 degrees. − ● − : 36 targets per 360 degrees. − □ − : 24 targets per 360 degrees.

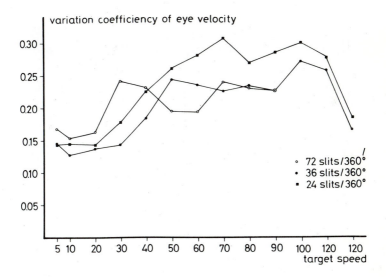

Fig. 2. The coefficient of variation of the slow phase velocity of the OKN. − o − : Rotator with 72 lightslits (targets) per 360 degrees. − ● − : 36 targets per 360 degrees. − □ − : 24 targets per 360 degrees.

amplifier with a time constant of 2.5 sec. Calibration of eye deflections was performed every 30 sec to allow for any changes in the corneo-retinal potential, as the nature of the test makes it impossible to secure total darkness.

Frequency

The coefficient of variation of the frequency of nystagmus was relatively constant except for the slowest target speeds, that is, slower than 20°/sec (Fig. 1). There were no significant differences in these measures between the tests carried out with the 3 rotators.

Eye speed of the slow phase

Two levels of the coefficient of variation were found (Fig. 2). One − low − for targets speeds slower than 30°/sec and one − high − for the faster speeds. The figure shows a rise of the coefficient of variation for the rotator with 72 slits, which began earlier than for

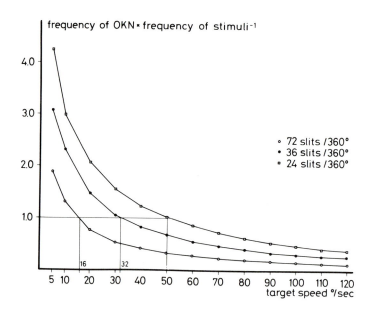

Fig. 3. The correlation between the frequency of the targets and the frequency of the OKN. − o − : 72 lightslits (targets) per 360 degrees. − ● − : 36 targets per 360 degrees. − □ − 24 targets per 360 degrees.

the other two rotators. The fall of the coefficient for the fast speeds is an artefact, due to rejection of an increasing number of tests as it was impossible to obtain the necessary periods of even responses. At the fastest target speed investigated (120°/sec) and at a target frequency of 24 Hz only 5 of 36 tests were accepted, as short periods of reaction was interrupted by irregular eye deflections with no sign of optokinetic response, thus making estimates of the true eye speed uncertain. This pheomenon makes the diagnostic value of the optokinetic fusion limit doubtful. (Blomberg, 1960).

Influence of target frequency on nystagmus frequency

It is often stated, that target frequency does not influence the frequency of optokinetic nystagmus (Honrubia *et al.*, 1967). This is only true for relatively fast target speeds. At slow speeds, target frequency may have a significant influence on response frequency. The correlation between the two factors, target frequency and frequency of the responses is shown in Fig. 3, where the quotient: frequency of optokinetic nystagmus divided by target or stimulus frequency, is drawn as a function of target speed. At slow speeds, the quotient is over 1. At target speeds of 50, 32 and 16°/sec respectively for the 3 rotators the quotient is 1 (synchronous reaction), and at faster target speeds the quotient is less than 1.

Primary and secondary beats

Working inside the upper limit for synchronous reaction, the optokinetic response in normal humans may be dominated by either primary beats, which are beats generated by transit of one target before the eyes, or by secondary beats unrelated to the targets (Fig. 4).

Responses, entirely built up of primary beats, as in the upper trace of Fig. 4, were rarely seen. If this type of reaction in fact dominated the response one might doubt the reflex nature of the optokinetic nystagmus. The majority of records showed primary as well as secondary beats, without the subject having knowledge of the secondary beats. In a few cases, the reaction consisted entirely of secondary beats without any evident correlation between the transit of the targets and the optokinetic eye movement; an example of this type of response is shown by the lower trace in Fig. 4. In a series of 75 persons, each tested 4 times, the last mentioned type of reaction was found 6 times in the 10 sec period. Reactions consisting only of primary beats were found 66 times.

PATTERNS OF OPTOKINETIC RESPONSE.

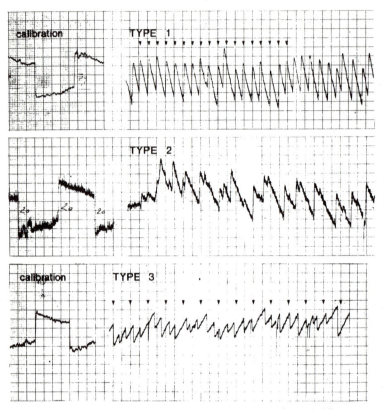

Fig. 4. Examples of OKN patterns. Upper record: each target (indicated by ▼) induces one nystagmic beat, (primary beats). Middle record: the OKN is composed of large primary beats and smaller secondary beats. Lower record: the nystagmic beats are unrelated in time to the targets (secondary beats).

The remaining 278 tests revealed primary and secondary beats in varying proportions. This finding implies that the frequency of the optokinetic nystagmus is of no special interest as a measure of normality.

Synchronous reaction

Synchronous optokinetic response may be defined as an optokinetic response either as one beat or as a sequence of beats following each transit of targets. Test conditions, securing synchronous reaction of the optokinetic response, make it possible, that the eye can follow the moving target, and that it can cope with the frequency of the targets. Target speeds and frequencies beyond the fields of synchronous reactions produce unnecessary variations in the eye speed of the normal response which might be interpreted as pathology. Consequently tests of optokinetic nystagmus ought to be carried out at one specific target speed and frequency. Working with a target speed of 20°/sec, or less, and a target frequency of 20 per sec, or less, secures enough room for the varying number of secondary beats that might occur to create a synchronous reaction within the maximum limit of response frequency of 3.2 – 3.4 Hz. Too slow a target speed and too low a target frequency (i.e. less than 10°/sec and 10 targets per sec) should be avoided, because the response though synchronous tends to be highly irregular due to drifting of the eyes from one target to another (Mioyshi, 1976). This phenomenon is responsible for the large coefficient variation found at the low stimulus speeds as is shown in Fig. 1.

Width of the targets

In another series of 10 normal humans the effect of the width of the targets on the regularity of the OKN was tested.

At 20°/sec and at 10°/sec, with a target frequency of 20 per second, the variance of amplitudes did not change with an alteration of the width of the targets from 1/2 degree to 5 degrees. At 30°/sec and a target frequency of 30 per second, the variance of the amplitudes were significantly larger and increased with a reduction in the width of the target. This indicated a greater difficulty in coping with the frequency of the targets at the higher target speed, where a synchronous reaction is unsecure.

Habituation of OKN

Test conditions securing a synchronous OKN (i.e. 20°/sec and a target frequency of 20 per sec) neutralise habituation of the optokinetic response (Miyoshi *et al.*, 1973). 10 normal humans took part in daily habituation trials of clockwise rotation, each of 30 sec duration for 10 consecutive days, with no trace of any alteration of eye speed or frequency of the OKN.

Interaction with vestibular nystagmus

Synchronous optokinetic nystagmus, secured by a strong stimulus, hardly interferes with nystagmus of vestibular origin (Fig. 5). In 10

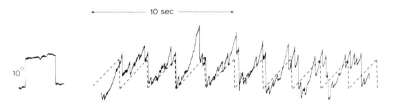

SIMULTANEOUS CALORIC- AND OPTOKINETIC NYSTAGMUS

IRRIGATION: LEFT EAR, 44°C. → NYSTAGMUS TO THE LEFT.

O.K. STIMULATION: CW ROTATION →   ″   ″   ″   ″
(5°/sec, 5 Hz.)

----- : THEORETIC SYNCHRONOUS OPTOKINETIC RESPONSE.

Fig. 5. Caloric nystagmus superimposed upon OKN of the same direction.

normal persons the right ear was irrigated with water at 44°C with the eyes closed. At the peak nystagmus the eyes were opened and an optokinetic stimulus of 5°/sec, 10°/sec and 20°/sec was presented either in the same or in the opposite direction to that of the caloric nystagmus.

At 20°/sec, no interference from the caloric nystagmus could be demonstrated, but in 6 cases an interference of the two types of nystagmus took place at lower target speeds. This was not a true interaction with summation of eye speeds, as previously has been claimed (Jones, 1966), but rather there was a superimposition of the vestibular nystagmus upon the recorded optokinetic nystagmus.

Conclusion

The purpose of this paper has been to emphasise the significance of the target speeds and target frequencies. Conditions evoking a synchronous optokinetic response will ensure:

1. an even optokinetic nystagmus of the alerted subject with

a) no habituation and
b) undetectable vestibular-optokinetic interference.

References

Barany, R., (1920): Zur Klinik und Theorie des eisenbahn Nystagmus. *Acta Otolaryng.* (Stockh.) **3**, 260-265.

Blomberg, L.H., (1960): The Optokinetic fusion limit. *Acta Otolaryng.* (Stockh.) **51**, 455-466.

Honrubia, V., Barbara, J.S. and Ward, P.H. (1967): Experimental studies on optokinetic nystagmus. I. Normal cats. *Acta Otolaryng.* (Stockh.) **64**, 388-402.

Jones, G.M. (1966): Interactions between optokinetic and vestibuloocular responses during head rotations in various planes. *Aerospace Med.* **37**, 172-177.

Kestenbaum, A. (1924): Frequenz und amplitude des Nystagmus. *Arch. f. ophthalm.* **114**, 550-582.

Miyoshi, T. (1976): The importance of the point of fixation in optokinetic nystagmus. *ORL* **38**, 148-156.

Miyoshi, T., Pfaltz, C.R. and Piffko, P. (1973): Effect of repetitive optokinetic stimulation upon optokinetic and vestibular responses. *Acta Otolaryng.* (Stockh.) **75**, 259-265.

3. The effect of optokinetic training on vestibular responses

C.R. PFALTZ and B. NOVAK

Department of O.R.L. (Head Prof. Dr. C.R. Pfaltz), University of BASEL, Switzerland

Introduction

In a previous study on vestibular habituation in man we investigated the influence of unidirectional optokinetic training (OKT) on vestibular responses, induced by repeated angular accelerations (Pfaltz and Kato, 1974). We were able to demonstrate a facilitating effect of OKT on vestibular habituation; however, the response decline was bidirectional and not unidirectional, as observed by Young and Henn (1974). These authors were able to show a selective unidirectional habituation of vestibular nystagmus by visual stimulation, i.e. a transfer of habituation across sensory modalities.

In order to find an explanation of our conflicting results we have reinvestigated the problem of whether or not a unidirectional visual stimulus would modify the response to a subsequent vestibular stimulus strictly in one direction.

Methods and experimental procedure

20 test subjects ranging in age from 18 − 45 years, participated in the experiment. They were divided into 4 groups (5 persons per group) and subjected to the experimental procedure shown in Fig. 1.

Results

We have made an attempt to reinvestigate the effect of repeated uni- and bidirectional optokinetic training (OKT) on the vestibular responses induced by positive and negative angular acceleration. In order to assess the difference between the vestibular responses

This Research Project was sponsored by the Schweiz. Nationalfonds zur Forderung der wissenschaftlichen Forschung.

EXPERIMENTAL PROCEDURE

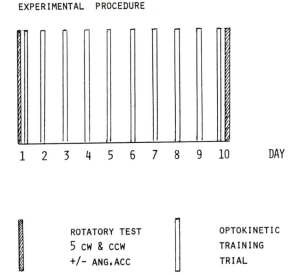

1	2	3	4	5	6	7	8	9	10	DAY

ROTATORY TEST
5 CW & CCW
+/- ANG.ACC

OPTOKINETIC
TRAINING
TRIAL

Fig. 1. Experimental procedure.

before and after OKT we have analyzed the results by the parameter of the *average slow phase velocity of vestibular nystagmus,* recorded during the *culmination period* of perstimulatory nystagmus (i.e. 5 s before and after the end of positive and negative angular acceleration). The results are exhibited in Table 1.

TABLE 1

Average slow-phase velocity ω of vestibular nystagmus to the right (index R) and to the left (index L) during the culmination period in the rotatory tests before (index B) and after (index A) OKT.

Rotat. Test	ω RB (Deg. Sec.$^{-1}$)	ω RA (Deg. Sec.$^{-1}$)	ω LB (Deg. Sec,$^{-1}$)	LA (Deg. Sec.$^{-1}$)
Group A	14,0	14,3	17,1	5,7
Group B	15,9	42,8	12,5	13,9
Group C	6,3	14,5	5,8	13,5
Group D	7,4	7,9	6,5	5,8

Group A showed a *unidirectional response decline* of vestibular nystagmus beating in the opposite direction to the foveal OKN induced during unidirectional OKT.

Group B showed a *unidirectional response enhancement* of vestibular nystagmus, beating in the same direction as the foveo-peripheral OKN, induced during unidirectional OKT.

Group C showed a *bidirectional response enhancement* of vestibular responses, following bidirectional foveo-peripheral OKT.

In control group D responses to both sides were unchanged.

Discussion

In the present study we were able to show that vestibular responses can be modified unidirectionally by repeated optokinetic stimuli. This observation is in agreement with the findings of Young & Henn (1974) but contradicts our own results published previously (Pfaltz and Kato, 1974). This disagreement is most probably due to a different experimental procedure: in our first experimental series repeated bidirectional rotatory stimulation was carried out after unidirectional OKT, thus inducing a bidirectional vestibular response decline. This phenomenon was more marked after OKT indicating a facilitation of vestibular habituation by repeated O.K. stimulation, i.e. transfer of habituation. However, our present findings disagree with some observations made by Young and Henn (1974), because we have not only observed a unidirectional response decline but also a unidirectional enhancement of vestibular responses. The former was induced by foveal OKT, the latter by foveo-peripheral OKT.

How can we explain this unexpected response enhancement? OKN consists of two separate and distinct mechanisms: foveal and peripheral nystagmus. Attempts to distinguish between these two forms have been made by many investigators (Miyoshi, 1975; Robinson, 1975; Miyoshi and Pfaltz, 1973, a, b, 1974; Miyoshi *et al.,* 1973). Foveal OKN is induced by one single object moving within the visual field which, according to Robinson (1975), does not test the OK-system but the pursuit system. Foveo-peripheral nystagmus is induced by the movement of the entire visual field. It is the result of stimulation of the OK-system, which is subcortical and operates on visual signals from the entire retina, not just the fovea. This system has developed as a companion of the vestibular system. The two are intimately coupled to each other and serve the same purpose; namely to determine the angular speed of self-rotation in a stationary visual environment. Thus the real purpose of the OK system is not to track a moving visual environment while the observer is stationary. Its purpose is to use vision to help the vestibular system to assess self-rotation within the environment and generate appropriate eye movements (Robinson, 1975).

As shown in previous experiments (Miyoshi, *et al.,* 1973) OK-training results in a definite response increase which we interpreted as the result of a positive learning process which probably allows the visual system to improve its ability to pick up the periodicity of simple motion patterns. This response enhancement obviously subserves the improvement of the *gain of the vestibulo-ocular reflex,* i.e. the ratio of eye to head movement. The vestibulo-ocular reflex developed in evolution to allow animals and men to keep a stable image on the retina. Head movements in one direction are countered by eye movements in the opposite direction, so that objects in the visual fields remain clear (Barr, Schultheis and Robinson, 1976). The ratio between *slow-phase eye velocity* and *head velocity* is called the *gain of the vestibulo-ocular reflex.* As may be seen from table II foveal OKT does not change the gain of the vestibulo-ocular reflex whereas unidirectional foveo-peripheral OKT induces a corresponding unidirectional gain increase. These

TABLE II

Influence of OKT on the gain of the vestibulo-ocular reflex.

Group	Nystagmus → Right		Nystagmus → Left	
	Gain before	After OKT.	Gain before	After OKT.
A unidirectional CCW Fov.OKT.	0.14	0.14	0.17	0.06
B unidirectional CCW Fov.per.OKT.	0.16	0.43	0.12	0.14
C bidirectional Fov.per.OKT.	0.06	0.15	0.06	0.14
D control No OKT.	Vest. resp. 1 0.08	Vest. resp. 2 0.08	Vest. resp. 1 0.06	Vest. resp. 2 0.06

findings are in agreement with the statement of Robinson (1975), according to whom the optokinetic system is a subcortical system which has to be separated from the smooth pursuit system. From the work of Young and Henn (1975) we know that one of the basic functions of the vestibular system is to convey information about self-motion. Receptors for such information mainly are the eyes and the labyrinths. At some level information from these two systems has to converge. Experimental evidence shows that such convergence has already taken place at the level of second order vestibular neurons. There are probably 2 systems projecting from the visual to the vestibular system: one which determines frequency and amplitude of OKN — another which can modify the activity of second order units. Dichgans *et al.,* (1973) and Henn *et al.,* (1974) demonstrated that the activity of neurons in the vestibular nuclei responding to rotation is *enhanced* when OK stimuli are given which produce OKN in the same direction as nystagmus induced by rotatory stimuli. These experimental findings may help to explain our observation that unidirectional foveo-peripheral OKT leads to a corresponding unidirectional enhancement of vestibular responses.

The next question which arises is the following: is response enhancement a phenomenon which is compatible with habituation? Collins (1974) emphasises a modified view of habituation, because repeated stimulation does not induce merely a simple "dropping out of responses" (i.e. response decline). Instead there is a gradual inhibition of the original response as the opposing reaction becomes more fully developed. These opposing reactions appear most clearly under two non exclusive conditions.

1. When there is an element of conflict between vestibular and visual signals.

2. Where the organism is attempting to adapt to an unusual vestibular environment.

Considering these reflections we may assume that both foveal and foveo-peripheral OKT modify the initial vestibular response. *Repeated foveal stimuli* induce a *unidirectional response decline,* corresponding with the vestibular nystagmus beating in the opposite direction to the OK-nystagmus elicited during OK-Training.

Repeated foveo-peripheral stimuli, however, induce a *unidirectional enhancement* of vestibular responses, corresponding in direction with the OKN elicited during OKT.

Both phenomena seem to subserve an improvement of the gain of the vestibulo-ocular reflex in one direction. This is reflected by a marked shift of directional preponderance which corresponds with the direction of the OKN elicited repeatedly during OKT. These mechanisms help the vestibular system to improve the assessment of self-rotation within the environment in order to impede visual-vestibular conflicts.

References

Barr, C.S., Schultheis, L.W. and Robinson, D.A. (1976): Voluntary, non-visual control of the human vestibulo-ocular reflex. *Acta Otolaryngol.* **81**, 365-375.
Coats, A. (1966): Directional preonderance and spontaneous nystagmus. *Ann. Otol.* **75**, 1135.

Cohen, B. (1975): Discussion of "signals processed in vestibulo-ocular reflex", Proceedings of the Barany Society. *International J. of Equilibrium Research,* Suppl. **139**, Kyoto.

Collins, W.E. (1974): Habituation of vestibular responses with and without visual stimulation. *In:* "Handbook of Sensory Physiology," Vol. VI/I, pp. 369-388. (Ed. Kornhuber, H.H.), Springer Verlag, Berlin.

Dichgans, J., Schmidt, C.L. and Graf, W. (1973): Visual input improves the speedometer function of the vestibular nuclei in the goldfish. *Exp. Brain Res.* **18**, 319-322.

Henn, V. Young, L.R. and Finley, C. (1974): Vestibular nucleus units in alert monkeys are also influenced by moving visual fields. *Brain Research.* **71**, 144-179.

Jongkees, L.B.W. (1973): The caloric test and its value in evaluation of the patient with vertigo. *In:* "Otolaryngologic Clinics of North America, " Vol. **6**, pp. 73-93. Publisher Philadelphia-London-Toronto.

Miyoshi, T. and Pfaltz, C.R. (1973a): Upon the Correlation between the Optokinetic Stimulus and the Induced Optokinetic Nystagmus: I. Influence of O.K. Targets. *ORL* **35**, 52-64.

Miyoshi, T. and Pfaltz C.R. (1973): II The Influence of the Visual Fields upon the Optokinetic Response. *ORL* **35**, 350-362.

Miyoshi, T. and Pfaltz C.R. (1974): III The Influence of Repetitive Narrow and Wide-Angle Stimuli upon OKN and Vestibulospinal Function. *ORL* **36**, 65-75.

Miyoshi, T., Pfaltz, C.R. and Piffko, P. (1973): Effect of repetitive optokinetic stimulation upon optokinetic and vestibular responses. *Acta. Otolaryng.* **75**, 259-265.

Miyoshi, T. (1975): Foveal and peripheral nystagmus; Proceedings of the Barany Society. *Intern. J. of Equilibrium Research,* Suppl. pp. 171-174,

Pfaltz, C.R. (1974): Quantitative Parameters in Nystagmography: II Nystagmus amplitude. *ORL* **36**, 46-52.

Pfaltz, C.R. (1977): Vestibular Habituation and Central Compensation. *Adv. Oto-Rhino-Laryng.* **22**, 136-142.

Pfaltz, C.R. and Kato, I. (1974): Vestibular Habituation − Interaction of visual and vestibular stimuli. *Arch. Otolaryngol.* **100**, 444-448.

Robinson, D.A. (1975): How signals are processed in the vestibulo-ocular reflex: Proceedings of the Barany Society. *Intern. J. of Equilibrium Research.* Suppl. pp. 130-141.

Young, L.R. and Henn, V.S. (1974): Selective Habituation of vestibular nystagmus by visual stimulation. *Acta. Otolaryng.* **77**, 159-166.

Young, L.R. and Henn, V.S. (1975): Effects of moving visual fields and body rotation on sensation, nystagmus and vestibular nucleus activity: Proceedings of the Barany Society. *Intern. J. of Equilibrium Research.* Suppl. pp.106-111.

4. Foveal and peripheral vision in optokinetic nystagmus

T. MIYOSHI, M. SHIRATO, S. HIWATASHI

Fukui Red Cross Hospital, Japan

Introduction

It is a well known fact that not only the fovea but also the peripheral retina play an important role in the formation of optokinetic nystagmus (De Kleyn, 1920; Ohm, 1922; Ter Braak, 1936; Hood, 1967; Miyoshi, and Pfaltz, 1973). For the sake of clarification of the roles played by various portions of the retina, a variety of methods have been devised to separate foveal vision from peripheral vision (Ter Braak, 1936; Aso, 1956; Hood, 1967; Asano 1969; Miyoshi and Pfaltz, 1973). None of them, however, was successful in complete isolation. Recently, the authors succeeded in perfect separation and reported it at the Fifth Extraordinary Meeting of Barany Society under the title of "Foveal and peripheral nystagmus" (Miyoshi, 1975). This report, however, was merely a qualitative one. The authors investigated this matter in detail by employing the reported method in combination with the overlapping method.

Test Procedure

In the present series of experiments, the authors examined six persons with normal vestibular and visual function. The apparatus consisted of a projection type optokinetic simulator, a masking or erasing device, a photosensor and a DC electronystagmograph (ENG) (Fig. 1). The projector projects vertical stripes. An opaque area on the erasing device blocks the projection on the way to the screen. The mask is driven in the same direction and with the same angular excursion as the eye movement by the output of the DC nystagmograph. Thus a certain portion of the visual field, within which an optokinetic stimulus is presented, is constantly blocked

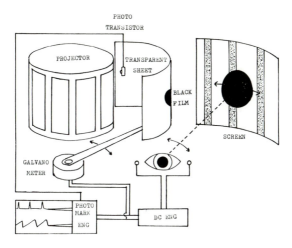

Fig. 1. *Diagram of apparatus.* An opaque area on a transparent sheet blocks projection of the optokinetic stimulus on its way to the screen. The transparent sheet is moved by a galvanometer which is driven by the output of a DC Electronystagmograph (ENG). Thus the shadow cast by the opacity moves on the screen in the same direction and through the same angle as the eye ball, and erases a certain portion of the stimulus field. A photo-transistor in front of the projector detects the stripes and its output is recorded with the ENG.

by the shadow of an appropriate mask.

A photo-transistor is set up just in front of the projector so that the passing of each stripe can be marked on the electro-nystagmogram. With this mark and (the ENG) calibration, the displacement of the stripe can be easily drawn on the nystagmogram. The crossing point of the base line and a vertical line which is drawn from the photo-mark indicates the moment when the stripe passes through the mid-line of the visual field. The angle of inclination of the trace of the stripe can be readily calculated from the eye displacement calibration and paper speed of the nystagmograph. This method of indicating stripe displacement on the nystagmogram is named the "overlapping method" by the authors and allows the relationship between the movement of the eye and of the target to be displayed on the nystagmogram. In the method, DC recording of the eye movement is essential. Double paste type zinc-zinc sulphate electrodes were used for this purpose.

Stimulation of the central visual field was achieved by fitting a black sheet having a round window of 20° in visual angle on the erasing device. On the other hand, stimulation of the peripheral

OKN

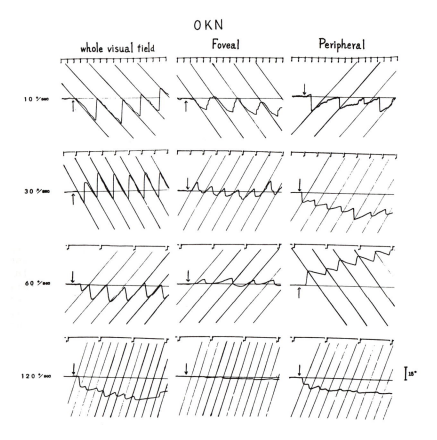

Fig. 2. *Nystagmus at the start of rotation.* Straight lines show the displacement of stripes. Arrows indicate the start of rotation.

visual field was obtained by fitting a black disc of 60° in visual angle on the erasing device. The stripes which were projected on the screen each had a visual angle of 3° and were separated by 30°. The projector used in the present test was able to start rapidly to achieve a given speed of rotation and also to reverse its direction of rotation with equal rapidity. In the present trial, it was rotated at uniform speeds of 10°, 30°, 60° and 120°/sec; the effect of instant reversals in the direction of rotation was also examined. The responses obtained with occlusion of the peripheral or foveal fields were also compared with the optokinetic nystagmus induced by stimulation of the whole visual field.

Results

A. Eye movements at the start of rotation (Fig. 2 and Table 1-A)

1. Nystagmus induced by whole visual field optokinetic stimulation. In the slow speed range of stimulation, about half the records of nystagmus began with a slow component. As the speed of stimulation increased the initial response was more commonly a saccade.
2. *Nystagmus induced by foveal stimulation.* At each speed of rotation nystagmus beginning with a slow component was much more frequent than that which begain with a fast component. When the projector was rotated at a speed of 120°/sec, the induced nystagmus was so minute that fast and slow phases could not be differentiated.
3. *Nystagmus induced by peripheral stimulation.* Most of the records showed a nystagmus which began with a fast component irrespective of stimulus velocity. At 60°/sec and 120°/sec nystagmus always began with a fast component.

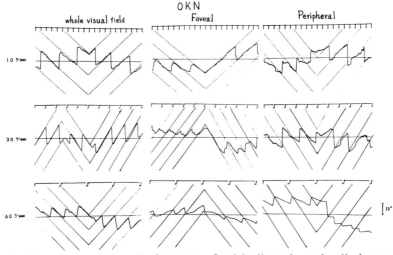

Fig. 3. *Nystagmus at reversal of rotation.* Straight lines show the displacement of stripes. Intersections of lines indicate the moments of reversal.

B. Eye movements at the reversal of rotation (Fig. 3 and Table 1-B)

1. *Whole visual field stimulation.* At stimulus velocities of 10 and 30°/sec, more than two-thirds of the nystagmus records showed reversal of the slow components on reversal of the stimulus, though at the higher speed of 60°/sec reversal was more commonly achieved by means of a fast component.

TABLE I – A: AT START

Eye movements during optokinetic stimulation

	10°/sec		30°/sec		60°/sec		120°/sec	
	Slow Phase	Fast Phase	Slow Phase	Fast Phase	Slow Phase	Fast Phase	Slow Phase	Fast Phase
OKN (whole visual field)	46%	54%	38%	62%	15%	85%	13%	87%
Foveal OKN	64%	36%	65%	35%	68%	32%	(—)	
Peripheral OKN	22%	78%	16%	84%	0%	100%	0%	100%

TABLE B: AT REVERSAL

	10°/sec		30°/sec		60°/sec	
	Slow Phase	Fast Phase	Slow Phase	Fast Phase	Slow Phase	Fast Phase
OKN (whole visual field)	72%	28%	58%	42%	21%	79%
Foveal OKN	94%	6%	76%	24%	87%	13%
Peripheral OKN	5%	95%	13%	87%	7%	93%

2. *Foveal stimulation.* A majority of the responses were characterised by a reversal of the slow component irrespective of the speed of stimulation.

3. *Peripheral stimulation.* In contrast to the nystagmus elicited by the foveal stimulus, reversal of the peripheral visual field stimulus commonly produced a fast component eye movement.

C. Eye Deviation (Figs. 2 and 3)

1. *Whole visual field stimulation.* In most tests the mean eye deviation was in the direction of the fast component.

2. *Foveal stimulation.* In this condition the mean eye deviation was always in the direction of the slow component.

3. *Peripheral stimulation.* In the absence of a foveal stimulus the mean eye deviation was always in the direction of the fast component.

D. Eye velocity of slow component (Figs. 2 and 3)

With the foveal stimulus the eye velocity of the slow phase of nystagmus, at low stimulus speeds, was equal to the speed of the target, such that the eye accurately followed the target. At the higher speeds the eye velocity fell below that of the target speed. With peripheral vision, slow phase eye velocity was often slower than the speed of the target even in the slow speed range.

E. Waveform of nystagmus (Fig. 2)

When the stimulus was confined to the fovea, the fast component was often fragmented into several steps, especially at low stimulus velocities. Furthermore, there was, typically, a lack of constancy of slow phase velocity during each nystagmic beat with a reduction in eye speed over the latter half of each movement. In contrast to the foveal stimulus, the nystagmus induced by a peripheral stimulus was not apparently distorted.

Discussion and conclusion

The role played by the fovea and the peripheral retina in the generation of optokinetic nystagmus has yet to be clarified. Ter Braak (1936) stated that there were two kinds of optokinetic nystagmus, subcortical and cerebral nystagmus. He stated, furthermore, that the slow phases of both kinds of nystagmus were fixating movements and that the rapid phases were only rhythmical interruptions attributable to a central rhythm. He said that the slow component of the cerebral nystagmus brought the target to the fovea and retained it there. Many investigators have agreed with him, but no proof of foveal retention has been obtained. The eye-mark camera or overlapping method revealed the true nature of foveal vision (Nakano, 1977; Miyoshi and Pfaltz, 1973; Miyoshi, 1976). Combination of "the separation of visual field" and the "overlapping method" revealed the properties of .nystagmus induced by foveal vision and by peripheral vision.

The nystagmus induced by foveal stimuli begins with a slow component, whereas the nystagmus evoked by a peripheral field stimulus begins with a fast component. In the slow speed range of stimulation, foveal vision is primarily responsible for fixation, therefore, the nystagmus induced by a stimulus to the whole visual field typically begins with a slow component. However, the importance of foveal mechanisms wanes as the stimulating velocity is increased when nystagmus, characteristically, begins with a fast component rather than a slow tracking eye movement. The obtuseness of the beginning of the slow component of nystagmus, observed when the optokinetic stimulis is confined to the foveal area, indicates the inability of the foveal mechanism to achieve quickly accurate foveal fixation of the target. In contrast, the sharpness of the beginning of the slow component with a peripheral stimulus shows the ability of peripheral vision to give support to foveal 'catch'.

These findings are in accord with the report of Watanabe (1960). He stated that the discharge from the area close to the fovea was increased by foveo-fugal stimulation and, conversely, that the discharge from the peripheral retina was increased by foveo-petal stimulation. With a peripheral optokinetic stimulus the eyes are attracted by the stimulation of the peripheral retina and deviate in the direction of the fast component. Because of the lack of this peripheral stimulation, the eyes deviate in the direction of the slow component in foveal nystagmus. These facts coincide well with the clinical studies of Nakano (1977). He examined the optokinetic nystagmus of a patient with central scotoma and another patient with tunnel vision and found that the eye deviation exhibited by the former patient tended to be in the direction of the fast component and by the latter to be in the direction of the slow component.

The comparison of the nystagmus induced by whole visual field stimulation, by foveal stimulation and by peripheral stimulation, reveals that the coordination between foveal and peripheral visual mechanisms in optokinetic nystagmus is not additional but multi-plicative.

References

Aso, T. (1956): Analytic observation on the labyrinthine nystagmus by electro-nystagmography. *Acta Medica et Biologica* **2**, 93-112.

Asano, N. (1969): Upon the macular vision and peripheral vision in the opto-kinetic nystagmus. *Vestibular Research* **24**, 120-121 (in Japanese).

Braak, J.W.G. Ter. (1936): Untersuchungen uber optokinetischen Nystagmus. *Arch. Neerl. Physiol.* **21**, 309-376.

Hood, J.D. (1967): Observation upon the neurological mechanism of opto-kinetic nystagmus with especial reference to the contribution of peripheral vision. *Acta otolaryngol.* (Stockh.) **63**, 208-215.

De Kleyn, A. (1920): Uber die Unabhangigkeit des Dunkelnystagmus der Hunde vom Labyrinth. *Arch. Ophthal.* (Berlin) **101**, 228-234.

Nakano, K. (1977): Visual fixation patterns in optokinetic nystagmus. *Pract. Otol.* Kyoto, **70**, 147-179.

Miyoshi, T., Pfaltz, C.R. (1973): Studies of the correlation between optokinetic stimulation and induced nystagmus. II. *ORL* **35**, 350-362.

Miyoshi, T. (1975): Foveal and peripheral nystagmus. *Proceedings fifth extra-ordinary meeting of the Barany Society.* 171-174.

Miyoshi, T. (1976): The importance of the point of fixation in optokinetic nystagmus. *ORL* **38**, 148-156.

Ohm, J. (1922): Die klinische Bedeutung des optischen Drehnystagmus. *Klin. Mbl. Augenheilk.* **68**, 323-330.

Watanabe, A. (1960): Some observations on the neuronal mechanism of opto-kinetic nystagmus. *Jap. Jour. Otol.* Tokyo. **63**, 1163-1180. (In Japanese).

Head Movement Perception

1. Disorders of head movement

M. GRESTY and M. HALMAGYI

Medical Research Council, Hearing and Balance Unit, Institute of Neurology, National Hospital, Queen Square, London WC1N 3BG, England

Objective observations have been made of head movement and posture in patients suffering a variety of nervous diseases producing symptoms of disordered movement control, postural instability and tremor. Choreiform movements and torticollis have, for the present, been excluded.

The recording technique employed was that of Gresty *et al* (1976) which made use of a Schottky barrier photodetector to transduce the movement of a small lamp mounted firmly on the patient's occiput by means of a head band. The patient was seated in an armchair which restricted torso movement and was presented with the task of executing rapid step-like head movements on command. The displacements subtended angles up to a maximum of approximately 60 - 70°, and could be in the horizontal or vertical plane. Observations were also made of tremor, instability of maintained posture and the ability to regain postural equilibrium following a sudden push by a lever placed under the patient's chin. The experiments were conducted in the presence and absence of vision.

The data was analysed using techniques of systems analysis in an exploratory attempt to provide a unified explanation of the apparent diversity of head movement disorders.

Voluntary head movement approximates to the response of a critically damped second order system in which duration of voluntary head movement is approximately constant irrespective of amplitude (Gresty, 1974) implying that head movement is associated with a particular frequency which is the natural resonant frequency of the head-neck system. For normal subjects this is an average of 2Hz. The patients examined executed head movements with durations ranging between 350 and 600 msec. which corresponds to a frequency range of 1.66 - 2.85 Hz. and is within the normal range.

In certain nervous diseases an oscillation of the head may be seen when the patient tries to turn his head quickly sideways or tries to perform a locomotor activity which gives rise to jarring movements of the spine such as walking down stairs. The appearance is that the head wobbles to and fro. Such movements were studied in one patient with spino-cerebellar degeneration and a second with ophthalmoplegia and cerebellar degeneration, who failed to maintain a steady head position after movement. They instead suffered damped oscillations at 2 Hz and 2.2 Hz respectively (Fig. 1). Similar oscillations at the natural frequency of the head

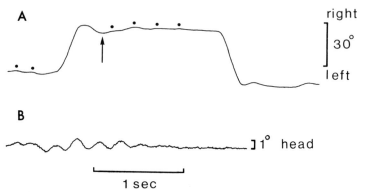

Fig. 1. A. Stepwise, voluntary displacement of the head in the horizontal plane (yaw) made by a patient with a diagnosis of cerebellar disease as part of an ophthalmoplegia plus syndrome. Following the movement the head makes a damped oscillation, indicated by the arrow, with a frequency of approximately 2 Hz. Superimposed upon the movement and posture is a tremor, of which successive cycles are indicated by black dots, at a frequency of approximately 4 Hz. B. An amplified recording of the head tremor taken during the same recording session when the tremor was of largest amplitude.

neck system were found in patients with multiple sclerosis and defective labyrinths as a result of recent streptomycin intoxication. It was apparent that in these patients, head movement approximated the response of a second order system which was underdamped and hence oscillated for a short time following abrupt disturbances. The cause of oscillations of this nature may be attributed to a reduction in the viscosity of the musculature in the head neck system which arises from inappropriate muscle tension.

There is evidence that the labyrinths are of prime importance to the maintenance of the appropriate visco-elastic properties of the head neck system and of postural equilibrium. In a patient with oscillopsia who had total bilateral loss of labyrinthine function following a recent course of streptomycin, an abrupt disturbance to the chin in the vertical plane produced damped oscillatory head movements at a frequency of 1.8 Hz, a duration of 1 - 2 sec and peak amplitude of 10°. In the same situation a normal subject would suffer 3° of movement for only a quarter of a second. The patient's response was independent of vision. In contrast, a patient with multiple sclerosis having a head titulation at 2 Hz which was triggered by body movement, and oscillopsia arising from lesions of the central pathways for the vestibulo-ocular reflex, could control her head oscillations much better in the presence of vision. These comparative observations suggest that visual control of head posture is less effective if there is loss of signals from the vestibular end organ and hence in the vestibulo-spinal pathways.

Head tremor at the frequencies indicated was measured in patients with the following symptoms or diagnoses (in all cases the tremor was approximately sinusoidal):

Suspected cerebellar degeneration (3 - 4 Hz horizontal)

Cerebellar degeneration as part of an ophthalmoplegia plus syndrome (4.25 Hz horizontal)

Cerebellar disease (5 - 5.6 Hz horizontal)

Startle myoclonus (3 - 4 Hz horizontal)

Roussy Levy Syndrome (4 - 4.6 Hz horizontal and vertical)

Vertebro-basilar stroke (2.5 - 5.4 Hz oblique)

"Torticollis" and nodding (4 Hz horizontal)

Neck dystonia and head tremor (5.5 - 6 Hz horizontal)

It is evident that most of the tremors occurred within a quite narrow frequency band of 3 - 5 Hz. In the apparent exceptions, e.g. vertebro-basilar insufficiency, the oblique tremor appeared to result from the beating of two fundamental frequencies of approximately 3.5 and 4.5 Hz which were executed in the vertical and horizontal planes. In each patient the frequency of individual tremor was approximately double the estimated natural frequency of the patient's head neck systems and is thus the second harmonic (Fig. 1).

Barnes and Rance (1975) (and personally communicated) have demonstrated in normal subjects that when the body is passively oscillated the head shows oscillations at a fundamental resonant frequency which is usually between 1.4 and 2 Hz with an additional resonance close to the second harmonic which results from the geometry of the head neck articulation. The experimental evidence together with the data from patients, allow a hypothesis to be formulated that voluntary head movement approximates to the response of a critically damped second order system. Certain disease states can render the damping ratio less than unity, in which case damped oscillations of the head may be seen during voluntary or passive movements. In addition, by virtue of its geometry, the system possesses a higher frequency resonance which is evident upon forced oscillations but which is suppressed or "turned out" during everyday locomotion. It is possible that the neural circuit responsible for suppressing the resonance, when disordered, produces head tremor at the same frequency as the resonance. The variations in tremor frequencies may reflect the individual differences in mass and musculature of the patient's heads and necks.

In this analysis the observed disorders of head movement are simply related to the fundamental dynamics of the head neck system. The causes of disordered head movements are twofold. A disease of the central nervous system may produce titubation of the head by altering the visco-elastic properties of the neck muscu-lature or by producing oscillations in a neural circuit which is specifically tuned to counter-effect natural resonances.

References

Barnes, G.R. and Rance, B.H. (1974): Transmission of Angular Acceleration to the Head in the seated human subject. *Aerospace Medicine* **45**, 411-416.

Gresty, M.A. (1974): Co-ordination of head and eye movements to fixate continuous and intermittent targets. *Vision Research* **14**, 395-403.

Gresty, M., Leech, J., Sanders, M. and Eggars, H. (1976): A study of head and eye movement in Spasmus Nutans. *British Journal of Ophthalmology* **60**, 652-654.

2. Representation of movement direction and plane by vestibular and cervical afferents to the posterior cerebellum in the pigeon*

D.W.F. SCHWARZ, R.D. TOMLINSON, A.C. MILNE

Department of Otolaryngology, University of Toronto

Although no knowledge is available concerning functional operations of the cerebellar cortex it is generally agreed that it subserves motor control. The clearest probable indication of the kind of control provided is given by saccadic eye movements for which the cerebellar cortex adjusts muscular force to account for conditions not primarily entering the saccadic program itself, such as visco-elastic properties of orbital tissues (Ritchie, 1976). To perform this adjustment appropriate parameters about the executed movements must enter the 'neuronal machine' (Eccles, Ito and Szentagothai, 1967). E.g. the cerebellar portion adjusting saccades is informed by eye muscle stretch receptors about the plane and direction of movement (Schwarz and Tomlinson, 1977; Tomlinson *et al* this volume). If plane and direction are critical parameters for cerebellar operations a study of semi-circular canal input seems particularly promising, since all the afferent fibers in one canal nerve provide information about direction of angular movement in a specified plane.

The first goal in our study of cerebellar utilization of canal information was to determine how the representation of the six canals in the vestibulocerebellum is organized, more specifically if the geometrical arrangement of cortical elements is somehow matched by a microgeometry of this plane and direction specific input. Although our anatomical studies on this question are not yet completed, our physiological data, based on stimulation of individual canal nerves and microelectrode recording in the pigeon's vestibulocerebellum, disappointingly support earlier reports suggesting a wide overlap of canal afferents (Carpenter, *et al* 1972; Wilson,

*Supported by M.R.C. of Canada

et al 1974).

It seemed particularly discouraging that our data supported the earlier report by Wilson, *et al* (1974) that lateral canal input occupies by far the greatest volume of the bird's vestibulocerebellum. This seems odd for an animal having to move in all three dimensions of space. The birds flight behaviour can, on the other hand, also be cited to require a particularly efficient control machinery for adjustment of head and body in the normal horizontal plane thus accounting for the great volume of vestibulocerebellar tissue dedicated to horizontal canals.

If our assumption is correct that movement adjustment by the cerebellum requires organisation of neural activity in terms of plane and direction, the circuitry controlling position of head and body should receive afferent input from movement and position receptors in the labyrinth and neck with matching plane and direction characteristics.

In order to examine if this is true it was first necessary to see where canal- and neck proprioceptors converge in the cerebellum. We investigated this question by recording responses of single units in the posterior cerebellum of pigeons to electrical stimulation of the vestibular nerve and to stretch of neck muscles (musculi digaster, splenius and complexus cervicis on either side). The birds were anaesthetized with Ketamine (0.3 mg/kg) and halothane-$N_2 O$, the halothane being discontinued before recording. Unitary recordings were obtained with glass microelectrodes from lobules VI to X (Larsell, 1967), the location of recorded units being histologically verified. The vestibular nerve was stimulated via two fine silver wires implanted on the nerve leaving the horizontal canal crista (0.1 ms duration pulses, maximal current 0.3 mA). Neck muscles were stretched by attaching their severed tendons to a vibrator driven by a function generator delivering variable ramp stretches of maximally 2mm amplitude and 40 cm/sec velocity. Neuronal responses to a number of identical stimuli (usually 64 or 128) were summated by computer to provide average responses in form of peristimulus time histograms.

The responses of a neuron in the Purkinje cell layer of lobule IXA (including IXa and b of Larsell, 1967) are shown in Fig. 1. The top trace shows a single response to a double pulse stimulus of the contralateral vestibular nerve as it is seen on the oscilloscope screen. A window discriminator selected the two large spikes which were counted by the computer producing the histogram in the second trace from 128 such stimuli. An excitation starting after 17 msec is evident. The excitation in response to ipsilateral vestibular nerve

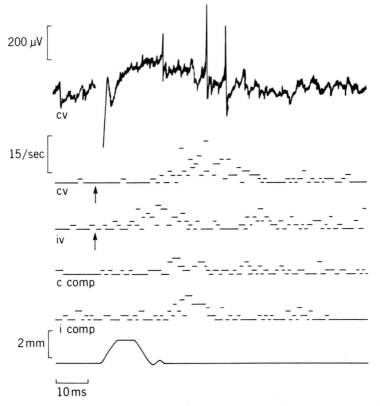

Fig. 1. Response of a neuron in lobule IXA of the pigeon's uvula. Stimuli corresponding to the responses shown are indicated below each trace: cv = contralateral vestibular nerve; iv = ipsilateral vestibular nerve; c comp. = contralateral complexus cervicis; i comp. = ipsilateral complexus cervicis. The time scale applies to all six traces and the amplitude calibration bar to all four histograms. Cf. text.

stimulation seen in the third trace has a shorter latency of 11 msec. Ipsilateral vestibular nerve stimulation typically causes shorter latency responses. The fourth and fifth traces show histograms in response to stretch of the contra- and ipsilateral complexus cervicis muscles with the stimulus being represented by the bottom trace which is the output of a length detector coupled to the stretch stimulator.

Neurones exhibiting this kind of convergence between neck proprioceptive and vestibular afferents were found in lobules VII, VIII, IX and X. Note that only lobules X and the ventral portion of IX receive direct vestibular fibers (Whitlock, 1952; Schwarz and Schwarz, in preparation). It is interesting that only very few of these 135 convergent cells (5%) were located in the nodules (lob. X). The majority of them were found in the uvula (68%), particularly its portion IXc and d. That does not, however, imply that the vestibular input to these elements is less direct than the neck input; the opposite seems true: the latency distribution for vestibular responses had its mode between 2 and 4 msec, whereas the mode for neck input was found between 16 and 32 msec (means between 8 and 16 msec, and 16 and 32 msec respectively).

It can be concluded that movement and position of head and neck are integrated in large areas of the posterior cerebellum with the uvula more and the nodulus less involved than other lobules. Therefore we searched for directional specificity mediated by semicircular canal- and neck proprioceptors throughout the posterior lobe, with most of our microelectrode tracks terminating in the uvula. In these experiments the pigeons were placed on a servo-controlled rotation table with the axis of rotation passing through the center of the head and the plane of the lateral canals adjusted to be parallel with the plane of rotation.

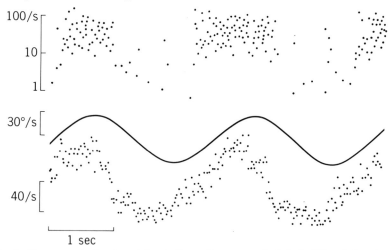

Fig. 2. Response to horizontal rotation of a neuron in lobule IXc of the pigeons uvula. Top: Instantaneous frequency plot for a single response (note logarithmic scale of y-axis). Middle: head velocity. Bottom: average of 16 responses. Time scale applies to all traces.

Stimuli were sinusoidal rotations at 0.25 Hz or 0.5 Hz with maximal angular velocities of 60°/sec. Only units responding to these stimuli were selected for further study. An example is shown in Fig. 2. The sine wave of the middle trace represents head velocity (output of a tachometer coupled to the rotation chair axis), the top plot illustrates an individual response of this unit in the form of a diagram of instantaneous frequency versus time and the bottom plot shows the average of 16 such responses as a computer generated histogram. Although this unit clearly shows a strong response to lateral canal stimulation it is not permissable to conclude that it is only or even mainly caused by horizontal canal activity on the basis of this histogram. Early during this study we decided upon the following criteria for identification of lateral canal activity:

1. the unit should not respond to lateral tilting movements of the head about the roll axis;

2. the phase angle between stimulus in the horizontal plane and response should indicate a reasonable correlation between unitary activity and head velocity;

3. when the pigeon's head was tilted about the roll axis the amplitude of the neurons response to horizontal rotation should drop according to a cosine function.

To our surprise we recorded no unit which satisfied the latter criterion. Fig. 3 illustrates a characteristic deviation from the expected behaviour of canal afferents: there is a strong response encoding head velocity to the contralateral side when the head is kept horizontal. However, with ipsilateral tilt of 30° the response almost disappears in the background noise, and with a 30° contralateral tilt no response is seen. According to the cosine function 87% of the maximal response should still be present with a 30° tilt. It may be objected that a cosine function cannot be applied to the neuronal response in Fig. 3 since only part of a sine wave is displayed as response. Most of our units responded in form of such sine wave segments. The amplitude of the complete sinewave obtainable by regression from a plot such as shown in Fig. 3 can be calculated using the following relationship

$$r = \frac{y}{1 - \cos x,}$$

where r is the peak amplitude, y the observed amplitude and x half of the response duration. When the calculated complete amplitudes were used to compare responses, amplitude reduction caused by lateral tilt was always far greater than predicted: mean values for 88 responses were, reduction to 65% with a 10° tilt, 46% for 20°, and 33% for 30°; that is to say, responses at 10° tilt behaved according to the cosine function, as if the head was tilted by 47°, as if it was tilted 63° for 20°, and 72° for 30° (Fig. 4). Thus the plane of

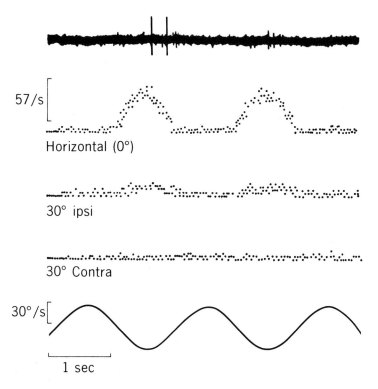

Fig. 3. Response of a neuron in lobule IXb to horizontal rotation with the head kept horizontally and tilted by 30° to either side. Top: Specimen recording. 1st histogram lateral canals in the horizontal plane; 2nd histogram lateral canal plane tilted 30° ipsilaterally; 3rd plot 30° tilt contralaterally. Bottom: head velocity. Time calibration applies to all traces.

rotation is specified far more precisely by semicircular canal afferent information available to the cerebellum than predicted according to the classical torsion pendulum model. It is uncertain at the present time if this high degree of plane specificity is available in the primary vestibular afferents, or if contrast enhancing circuitry within the brain is responsible.

Since cerebellar units exhibit greater plane specificity than prescribed by the cosine function, our third, less rigorous criterion for horizontal canal responses was that the maximal amplitude was indeed obtained in the horizontal plane. Of 96 horizontal canal cells, 41 received neck afferent input as well. This was examined by manually moving the body, which was embedded in a plaster cast, with respect to the immobile head about three mechanically predetermined axes of yaw, roll and pitch. Movements were registered

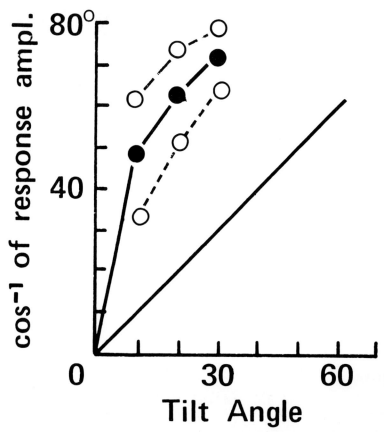

Fig. 4. Plane specificity mediated by horizontal canal input for neuronal responses in the posterior cerebellum of the pigeon. Y axis gives the arc cos value for the response amplitude normalized according to the maximal amplitude (in the horizontal plane) being equal to 1.X axis: angle of tilt out of the horizontal canal plane. Solid line connects mean values, broken lines standard deviations. The more vertical these lines are, the greater is the plane specificity of the response population. Plane specificity predicted by cosine function is given by the straight line. No plane specificity would correspond to a horizontal line.

electronically as voltage shifts across a potentiometer coupled to the axis. All of the 41 neurons exhibiting convergence between neck and horizontal canal inputs responded to neck movement about the yaw axis with only 3 responding also to roll movements starting from normal head and body positions. All these responses were directionally specific, neck bending towards ipsilateral being excitatory and towards contralateral inhibitory or vice versa. The directional specificity encoded in neck responses did however, not match that displayed in the horizontal canal responses in a systematic fashion: about as many activations with neck movements in yaw towards ipsilateral converged with canal activation due to ipsilateral head rotation as did those with head rotation towards the contralateral side. That is to say, the chances that information from neck is cancelled by the labyrinth due to subtraction when the pigeon moves its head towards one side are about as great as those of the generation of a stronger signal due to summation of both inputs.

It is noteworthy that these convergence patterns represent only a carefully selected group of neurons. Many other response patterns were seen which are not easily interpreted. It is sufficient to mention that vestibular neurons responding to tilt about the roll axis always responded to neck rotation about roll or pitch axes, provided neck input was present at all.

A brief theoretical assumption can be formulated as a conclusion to the data presented here and earlier (Thomlinson, *et al* this vol.): cerebellar elements must be organised according to the plane and direction of the movement they control. Further details on this organisation must be disclosed before cerebellar operations can be understood.

References

Carpenter, M.B., Stein, B.M., and Peter, P. (1972): Primary vestibulocerebellar fibers in the monkey: Distribution of fibers arising from distinctive cell groups of the vestibular ganglia. *Am. J. Anat.* **135**, 221-250.

Eccles, J.C., Ito, M., and Szentagothai, J. (1967): The cerebellum as a neuronal machine. Springer, Berlin/Heidelberg/New York.

Larsell, O. (1967): The comparative anatomy and histology of the cerebellum from myxinoids through birds. (Ed. J. Jansen). *The University of Minnesota Press,* Minneapolis.

Ritchie, L. (1976): Effects of cerebellar lesion on saccadic eye movements. *J. Neurophysiol.* **36**, 1246-1256.

Schwarz, D.W.F. and Tomlinson, R.D. (1977): Neuronal responses to eye muscle stretch in cerebellar lobule VI of the cat. *Exp. Brain Res.* **27**, 101-111.

Whitlock, D.G. (1952): A neurohistological and neurophysiological study of afferent fiber tracts and receptive areas of the avian cerebellum. *J. Comp. Neur.* **97**, 567-635.

Wilson, V.J., Anderson, J.A. and Felix, D. (1974): Unit and field potential activity in the pigeon vestibulocerebellum by stimulation of individual semicircular canals. *Exp. Brain Res.* **19**, 142-157.

3. A comparison of nystagmus and turning sensations generated by active and passive turning*

*F.E. GUEDRY, Jr., **C.E. MORTENSEN, †J.B. NELSON, ††M.J. CORREIA

*Naval Aerospace Medical Research Laboratory, Pensacola, Florida, **Emory University, Atlanta, Georgia, †Louisiana State University, Baton Rouge, Louisiana, †† University of Texas Medical School, Galveston, Texas

Introduction

It is well known that deceleration from prolonged whole-body rotation in one direction produces a false sensation of rotating in the opposite direction. Recently we have found that this perceptual after-effect is not always in the opposite direction when the whole-body rotation is actively generated. This paper reviews part of a preceding study and also describes results of further observations in which nystagmus was recorded in active and passive modes of vestibular stimulation.

Methods

Subjects in both studies experienced two types of rotation: active and passive. For active turning, subjects were instructed to turn smoothly with head level at moderate speed within the confines of a 50cm diameter circle outlined on the floor. After brief practice, subjects completed two active trials, one clockwise (CW) and one counterclockwise (CCW), of eight turns, separated by 3 minutes' rest.

In the first study (Correia et al 1977) only part of which is described herein, passive rotation was accomplished with subjects standing upright, but firmly secured to the rotating structure by straps and pads at the head, trunk and legs. Body weight was supported primarily by the feet and legs. In the second study, a Stille-Werner chair was used to produce passive rotation. Subjects were

*Opinions or conclusions contained in this paper are those of the authors and do not necessarily reflect the view or endorsement of the Navy Department.

Table I

Percentage of Reports of ASI, SI, or No Clear

Sensation Following Active and Passive Rotation

	ASI	SI	O or D*	
STUDY I (N = 40)	73	15	12	} Active Rotation
STUDY II (N = 26)	50	25	25	
STUDY I (N = 40)	12	85	3	} Passive Rotation
STUDY II (N = 26)	4	96	0	

- - - - - - - - - -

*O signifies no turning sensation and D signifies dizziness without a

clear turning sensation.

seated, secured by a lap belt, with the head supported at the center of rotation by an occipital headrest.

Average angular velocities of the active CW and CCW trials were calculated and duplicated in passive CW and CCW rotation trials, each also of eight complete turns. In all trials, vision was excluded by face masks. Horizontal nystagmus was recorded by electro-nystagmography in the second study.

Results

Perceptual Effects

Table 1 summarizes results on postrotatory sensations of turning. In the passive trials, sensations of turning in a direction opposite to that of the stimulus rotation, referred to as the somatogyral illusion (SI), occurred in 85% of the trials in the first study, and in 96% of the trials in the second study. The relatively low 85% reporting of the traditional SI in the first study may be due to the standing posture during passive trials.

In the active trials, reports of postrotatory sensations were predominantly of turning in the same direction as the preceding direction of physical rotation, a perceptual effect referred to herein as the antisomatogyral illusion (ASI). The predominance of ASI over

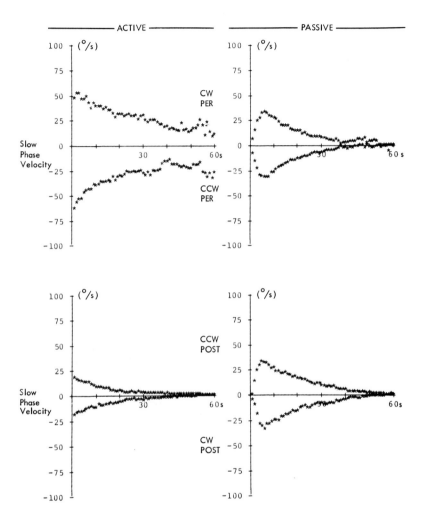

Fig. 1. Comparison of mean per- and postrotatory nystagmus slow phase velocity in the active and passive rotation trials. Due to different active-turning rates, duration of turn varied between subjects; for this reason, N decreases beyond 30 seconds.

SI reports in active trials, though clearly present in both studies, was greater in the first than in the second.

Nystagmus

Fig. 1 shows mean nystagmus slow-phase velocity during and after

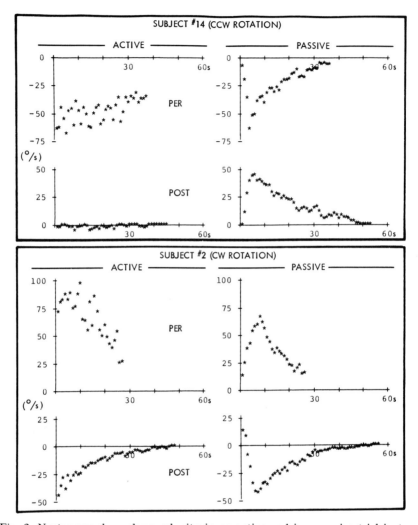

Fig. 2. Nystagmus slow phase velocity in an active and in a passive trial in two subjects who represent extremes of individual differences in postrotatory suppression of nystagmus following active turning. Both of these subjects experienced the ASI.

active and passive turning trials for the 26 Ss of the second study. In the active trials, per-rotatory nystagmus was elevated, whereas postrotatory nystagmus was suppressed relative to passive stimulation responses. In only one S was nystagmus direction following active turning reversed relative to a 'normal' response, and in this S the reversed response was weak. Thus, postrotatory nystagmus, though usually suppressed in active trials, did not match the direction of the ASI. Pronounced individual differences in per-rotatory augmentation and postrotatory suppression of nystagmus were not clearly indicative of whether the ASI or the SI was reported. Most Ss with strong suppression of postrotatory nystagmus following active turning reported either the ASI or no clear turning sensation (S   14 in Figure 2). However, of Ss with little or only moderate suppression, a number reported the ASI (S   2 in Figure 2), but some reported the SI.

Torsional movements of the head and body

The head, in Study 1 (Nelson 1976), and torso, in Study II, were observed for torsional deceleratory reflexes (Roberts, 1967) in the active trials. Reflexes were not apparent in 38% of the observations. When detected, 64% were in the classical direction, but 36% were in opposite direction. Such inconsistency is to be expected (cf; Peitersen, 1974) when voluntary and reflex control are in opposition. It is noteworthy that the ASI was predominantly present irrespective of the overt manifestation of these reflexes.

Discussion

Because our active-turn results are contrary to expectations, analysis of cupula-endolymph responses in our active-turn condition in relation to theoretical cupular dynamics seems appropriate. During prolonged active rotation, cupular deflection would decay toward the null position with superimposed cyclic variation related to perturbations in head velocity relative to the average active-turn head velocity; and because of the time-dependent decay, deceleration would produce a cupular overshoot (solid χ-line, Figure 3) that is ordinarily associated with a sense of turning and nystagmus fast phase opposite in direction to the preceding rotation.

The nature of sensorimotor input-output conflict in our active-turning condition can be appreciated by comparing a typical, active turn through a short arc (e.g., 180°) (dotted ω-curve in Figure 3) with our prolonged active-turn condition. Short turns are accomplished precisely without perceptual or equilibratory aftereffects, yet the peak velocity in a 180° turn is typically at least as great as the peak velocities attained during our prolonged active turns. Therefore, the angular momentum of the body, and hence the muscular torque required to stop the body, would be the same or nearly the same. However, the vestibular information is grossly

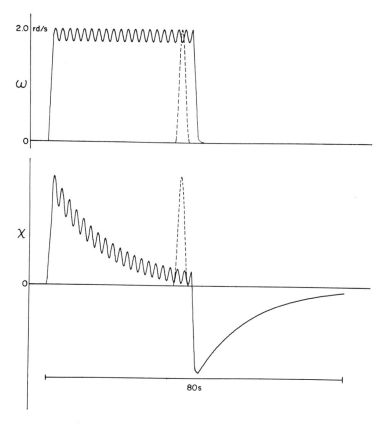

Fig. 3. Angular velocity (ω) and cupula deflection (χ) during and after a prolonged (solid lines) and short (dotted lines) active turn. Peak angular momentum
of body, and hence required stopping torques, for a short turn would equal
that for a prolonged turn. Vestibular information would be accurate during
and after a short turn but would lead to 1) underestimation of required stopping
torque for the prolonged turn and 2) conflictual vestibulospinal after-effects.

different. In the short turn, the vestibular information (dotted χ-
curve in Figure 3) is accurate during and after the turn. If the
vestibular information is instrumental in preprogramming (cf. Melvill
Jones and Watt, 1971) the torque required to stop the body, the
stop would be accomplished with precision. On the other hand, in
the prolonged active-turn condition, vestibular information (solid
χ-curve in Figure 3) would lead to preprogramming of far less
muscular stopping torque than is required to stop the body. Moreover, when the cupular overshoot occurs, the classical deceleratory
reflexes (Roberts, 1967) elicited would tend to twist the body still

further in the same direction as the twist produced by partially un-compensated angular momentum.

An interpretation by Melvill Jones of recent findings on motor control suggests speculations concerning the ASI. Studies by Towe and his associates (cf. Evarts *et al.,* 1971) indicate that the cortico-spinal pyramidal tract not only generates motoneurone activity to drive skeletal muscles, but also sends collateral branches which influence sensory activity in dorsal column nuclei; i.e., pyramidal tract output can enhance its own afferent input. Similarly, central coactivation of alpha and gamma motoneurones may result in nulling out of sensory discharge changes from muscle spindles, that would otherwise be elicited by mechanical changes in the main muscle, when movement proceeds as "anticipated by the controlling higher center" (Matthews, 1972, p. 573). Thus, "If all went ac-cording to plan, then the CNS would not be bothered with un-necessary sensory information. By contrast, if the 'intended' (sic) response was not achieved, then needed sensory information would indeed reach the CNS which, in turn, would presumably modify the next motor command" (Melvill Jones, 1974, p. 848). After prolonged turning, the stopping torque and corollary "feedforward" signals would be low if their preprogramming were influenced by the vestibular input when the subject was told to stop (note difference between solid and dashed χ-curves in Figure 3). The resulting mismatch between feedforward and feedback signals may enhance afferent input to the sensorimotor cortex and bring about re-evaluation in that part of the nervous system where adjustment is required (MacKay, 1962, 1966). Domination of the perceptual experience by the spinal feedback to the sensorimotor cortex would serve to readjust motor control to overcome both the under-estimated inertial torque and the counterproductive vestibulospinal effects produced by cupular overshoot.

In the passive condition, the rotary structure and restraint system acted on the body as a whole and controlled its state of motion. Voluntary muscular torques would have been ineffectual in changing the state of motion of the body and were not required to overcome the inertial torque of the body during deceleration or to counteract conflictual deceleratory vestibulospinal reflexes. Presumably without the necessary conditions for a feedforward/feedback mismatch to enhance the spinovestibular feedback to the sensorimotor cortex (Bizzi and Evarts, P. 41, 1971; Adkins *et al.,* 1966), the perceptual experience is dominated by more direct vestibular cortical projection (Fredrickson *et al.,* 1966).

The nystagmus data suggest that proprioceptive feedback associated with active turning and stopping can augment per-rotatory vestibular nystagmus and suppress postrotatory vestibular nystagmus. This conclusion should be regarded tentatively, however, because of potential stimulus artifacts such as axis wobble during active turning that might induce 'barbecue' nystagmus (Stockwell *et al.,* 1972) or head tilt following rotation that could suppress postrotatory nystagmus (cf. Benson, 1974). These potential artifacts can only be properly evaluated by more careful measurement, but our current opinion is that they were insufficient to be of critical importance. Moreover, there is no evidence of which we are aware that such artifacts could produce the ASI (or a reversed nystagmus in the one individual who exhibited this effect). The lack of correlation between compensatory reflexes and concomitant sensations suggests predominance of subcortical control over vestibulo-ocular and vestibulospinal reflexes and that any cortical servo-assistance (cf. Matthews, 1972) in this control, though perhaps reflected in a reversed sensation e.g., ASI, must join with subcortical mechanisms to yield reflexes relatively appropriate to the situation, e.g., per-rotatory augmentation and postrotatory suppression of nystagmus. With habituation, it is likely that reflexes would improve in adequacy and automaticity while false sensations would disappear.

Finally, we suggest that the present results have practical implications for predicting sensations and reflex action to be expected during active control of motion during vestibular pathology or during normal vestibular responses to bizaare stimulation encountered in ice-skating, aviation, et cetera.

References

Adkins, R.D., Morse, R.W., and Towe, A.L. (1966): Control of somatosensory input by cerebal cortex. *Sc.'ence,* **153**, 1020-1022.

Benson, A.J. (1974): Modification of the response to angular accelerations by linear accelerations. *In:* Handbook of Sensory Physiology, V1/2 (H.H. Kornhuber, Ed.) Berlin/Heidelberg/New York: Springer-Verlag. Pp 281-320.

Bizzi, Emilio, and Evarts, E.V. (1971): Translational mechanisms between input and output. *Neurosciences Res. Prog. Bull;.* **9**, (1) : 31-59.

Correia, M.J., Nelson, J.B., and Guedry, F.E. (1977): The antisomatogyral illusion. In press, *Aviat. Space Environ. Med.*

Evarts, E.V., Bizzi, Emilio, Burke, R.E., DeLong, Mahlon and Thach, W.T., Jr. (1971): Central Control of Movement. *Neurosciences Res. Prog. Bull.,* **9** (1).

Fredrickson, J.M., Figge, U., Scheid, P. and Kornhuber, H.H. (1966): Vestibular nerve projection to the cerebral cortex of the Rhesus monkey. *Exp. Brain Res.,* **2**, 318-327.

MacKay, D.M. (1962); Theoretical models of space perception. *In:* Aspects of the Theory of Artificial Intelligence (C.A. Muses, Ed.) New York: Plenum

Press. Pp 83-104.

MacKay, D.M. (1966): Cerebral organization and the conscious control of action. *In:* Brain and Conscious Experience (J.C. Eccles, Ed.) New York: Springer-Verlag. Pp 422-445.

Matthews, P.B.C. (1972): Mammalian Muscle Receptors and Their Central Actions. London: Edward Arnold Ltd.

Melvill Jones, G. (1974): Adaptive neurobiology in spaceflight. *In:* The Proceedings of the Skylab Life Sciences Symposium, JSC09275, TMX-58154.

Melvill Jones, G., and Watt, D.G.D. (1971): Observations on the control of stepping and hopping movements in man. *J. Physiol.,* **219**, 709-727.

Nelson, Julie B. (1976): Comparison of subjective responses following active vs. passive turning. Master's Thesis, Louisiana State University, Baton Rouge, Louisiana.

Peitersen, E. (1974): Measurement of vestibulo-spinal responses in man. *In:* Handbook of Sensory Physiology, V1/2 (H.H. Kornhuber, Ed.) Berlin/Heidelberg/New York: Springer-Verlag. Pp267-280.

Roberts, T.D.M. (1967): Neurophysiology of Postural Mechanisms. New York: Plenum Press.

Stockwell, C.W., Guedry, F.E., Turnipseed, G.T., and Graybiel, A. (1972): The nystagmus response during rotation about a tilted axis. *Minerva Otohinolaryng.,* **22**, 229-235.

4. Hysteresis in orientation to the vertical (the effect of time of preceding tilt on the subjective vertical)

S. LECHNER—STEINLEITNER and H. SCHÖNE

Max-Planck-Institut für Verhaltensphysiologie, Seewiesen

Introduction

For many decades the perception of the vertical has been a topic of psychological as well as of physiological investigations (review see Guedry, 1974). The phenomena of deviation of the perceived vertical from the true vertical were described quite early (Aubert, 1861, Müller, 1916). They have been named as Aubert- and Müller-phenomena after the authors. It has been shown that several input systems are involved in perception of the vertical. The labyrinths, in particular the statolith organs, as well as the somesthetic receptor systems, play a role.

The subjective vertical is a function of body tilt and of duration of tilt (Schöne and Udo de Haes, 1969, Lechner-Steinleitner, 1977). It is furthermore a function of the preceding tilt. This has the consequence that differences in the subjective vertical appear when the position is reached from different turning directions. In other words, we find a hysteresis of the subjective vertical (Schöne and Lechner-Steinleitner, 1977). Effects of the preceding tilt have been reported also for the postural vertical (Clark and Graybiel, 1964) and for the visually adjusted vertical (Day and Wade, 1966, Wade, 1968, 1970), both with respect to tilt into the normal upright body position.

The hysteresis effect may be demonstrated by a series of illustrative sketches (Fig. 1). The upper line of heads refers to changes of position in counterclockwise direction, the lower to a clockwise sequence. Each vertical pair of figures refers to the same body position. The arrows in front of the heads indicate the subjective vertical. A comparison of the upper and lower setting in each pair reveals a difference in subjective vertical. It is larger at larger angles

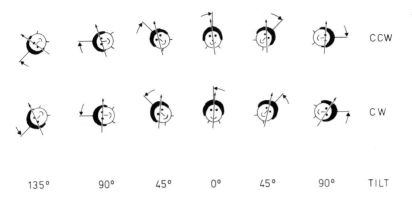

Fig. 1. Subjective vertical (straight arrow) at different tilt postions of body. Tilt reached in clockwise (lower) or counterclockwise sequence (upper) respectively.

of body tilt. But even in the upright postion (0°) there is a significant hysteresis effect. The subjective vertical deviates from the true vertical either to the right or to the left if there was a pretilt to the right or to the left respectively. In parenthesis it might be noted that this effect in the upright position cannot be classified in terms of the Aubert and Müller notations because the definition of these terms presupposes a tilt position of the body. In order to find out more about the mechanisms involved we had a closer look at the effect of the time relations of the pretilt events.

Method

For measuring the perceived or subjective vertical (SV) the method of adjusting a luminous line to the vertical was used. The angle ß between this setting and the body axis was recorded and used as a measure for the SV. In a setup which has been described in a previous paper (Lechner-Steinleitner, 1977), the subjects could be turned into different positions of side tilt. They were kept in this pre-tilt position for a period of one or 8 minutes respectively, after which they were moved into the end position. There they adjusted the SV 6 times during two minutes.

Three end positions were investigated, 0° (i.e. normal upright standing), 60° tilt to the right and 120° tilt to the right. The pretilt positions were at the left and at the right side of each end-tilt. Thus for the 120° -end position, the pre-tilts were 90° and 150°, for the 60° -end position 30° and 90°. For the 0° -end position there were four pre-tilt postions, 30° to the left and to the right and 60° to the left and to the right.

Results

Figure 2 summarizes the results of measuring the SV at the three end positions of body tilt, 0°, 60° and 120°. The triangles (upper

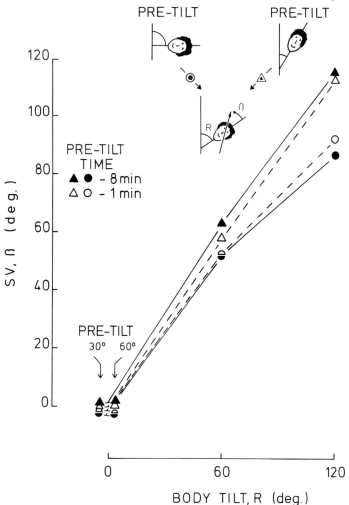

Fig. 2. Subjective vertical (ß) as a function of body tilt (end-tilt). End-tilt attained after pre-tilt conditions as indicated in Fig. 3; sketches refer to 60° of end-tilt. Each point represents the mean of the respective time curve of Fig. 3.

curves) indicate the settings after the pre-tilt angle left of end-tilt angle, whereas the circles (lower curves) refer to the records after pre-tilt angles to the right of end-tilt. At 60° end position, for instance, the triangles indicate SV values after 30° of pre-tilt, the circles, values obtained after 90° of pre-tilt.

Obviously the differences between triangles and circles, that is the effect of pre-tilt, increases from 0° to 120° end position. Also with respect to pre-tilt time there is a clear effect: 8 min. of pre-tilt (filled symbols) has a larger effect than 1 min. pre-tilt (open symbols).

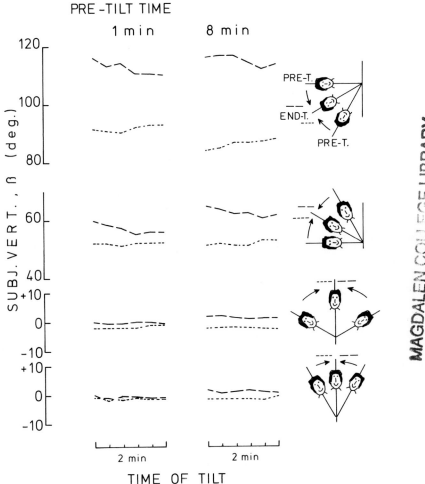

Fig. 3. Subjective vertical (ß) as a function of time in end-tilt position. End-tilt taken after pre-tilt conditions as indicated. Average of data of several Ss (number of Ss cf. Tab. 1).

Thus the hysteresis effect is more pronounced when the subject is maintained for longer time in the pre-tilt position. The details of the settings are elaborated further in the next figure (3) which shows the single settings during the two minutes of recording in end position. The four lowermost pairs of curves refer to 0° -end position. After 8 minutes of pre-tilt, as seen on the right side, the curves of both pre-tilt positions, 30° and 60°, differ. In the 1 min. pre-tilt experiments, left side, only the curves of 60° pre-tilt run separately, the curves of 30° pre-tilt, however, merge into each other. A statistical evaluation of the data is offered in table 1.

TABLE 1

t-Test evaluation (significance level) of differences in SV as recorded at an end-tilt position which has been reached after pre-tilt to the left (a) or the right (b) of the end-tilt. Based on SV means of the 2-min. measurements (Fig. 3).

End-Tilt (deg.)	Pre-Tilts (deg.)	Number of Ss	Sign. Level of ß-Diff. a-b after Pre-tilt time of		Sign. Level of ß-Diff. 1-8 min.
			1 min.	8 min.	
1	2	3	4	5	6
0	a) 30 left b) 30 right	4	-	0,5%	a) 5% b) -
0	a) 60 left b) 60 right	6	5%	1%	a) 2,5% b) -
60	a) 30 right b) 90 right	6	0,5%	0,5%	a) 0,5% b) -
120	a) 90 right b) 150 right	5	5%	5%	a) - b) 1%

Discussion

The findings indicate that the time which has been spent in the pre-tilt position magnifies the hysteresis effect of SV. As far as the 0° -end position is concerned, it is the more distant pre-tilt of 60° which is more effective than the closer pre-tilt of 30°.

We attribute these results to the influence of the somesthetic input. Former investigations have shown that the SV changes with time of tilt (Schöne and Udo de Haes, 1969, Lechner-Steinleitner, 1977). This temporal change of SV has been related to adaptational processes in the somesthetic system. In our experiments such adaptation occurs in the pre-tilt position. When the subject is moved into the end position the somatoreceptors are already pre-adapted to some extent. This has the consequence that the positional information stemming from the somatoreceptive system differs as a function of pre-tilt position. This results in different settings of subjective vertical and thus in hysteresis.

It is an open question if also the labyrinthine input is involved in this phenomenon.

References

Aubert, H., 1861: Eine scheinbare bedeutende Drehung von Objekten bei Neigung des Kopfes nach rechts oder links. *Virchows Arch.* **20**, 381-393.

Clark, B. and Graybiel, A., 1964: Perception of the postural vertical following prolonged bodily tilt in normals and subjects with labyrinthine defects. *Acta Otolaryng.* (Stockholm) **58**, 143-148.

Day, R.H. and Wade, N.J., 1966: Visual spatial aftereffect from prolonged head tilt. *Science* **154**, 1201-1202.

Guedry, F.E., 1974: Psychophysics of vestibular sensation. *In:* Handbook of Sensory Physiology, vol. V1/2 3-154. Springer Berlin, New York.

Lechner-Steinleitner, S., 1977: Interaction of labyrinthine and somatoreceptor inputs as determinants of the subjective vertical. *Psychol. Res.* **40**. In Press.

Muller, G.E., 1916: Uber das Aubert'sche Phanomen. *Z. Sinnesphysiol.* **49**, 109-244.

Schone, H. und Lechner-Steinleitner, S., 1977: The effect of preceding tilt on the perceived vertical. *Acta Otolaryng.* **85**, 68-73.

Schone, H. and Udo de Haes, H.A., 1971: Space orientation in humans with special reference to the interaction of vestibular, somaesthetic and visual inputs. *Biokybernetik III, Materialien* **2**. *Internat. Sympos. Biokybernetik, VEB Fischer Jena,* 172-191.

Wade, N.J., 1968: Visual orientation during and after lateral head, body and trunk tilt. *Percept. Psychophysics* **3**, 215-219.

Wade, N.J., 1970: Effect of prolonged tilt on visual orientation. *Quart. J. Exp. Psychol.* **22**, 425-439.

Postural Control

1. Head movement while "marching in place".

M. KITAHARA and H. MATSUBARA

Department of Otolaryngology, Faculty of Medicine, Kyoto University, Japan

Introduction

In observations of the righting reflex of the human body, equilibrium in movements back and forth or to the right and left of the body are usually seen as being asymmetrical. A one-leg test has thus been employed using the above mentioned principle. However, in this test, an unstable posture makes for variations in normal persons so that the test itself has no practical value.

"Marching in place" consists of alternate, continuous repetition of standing on the right foot and then the left foot and the equilibrium in the one leg standing appears to be more stable than that in the one-leg test.

Using two averagers, we analyzed head movement while marching in place and the clinical value of this approach is discussed.

Method

The subjects were instructed to march fifty paces in place and head movements were measured using an unbonded strain-gauge-type linear accelerometer. The results were averaged respectively as the subject stood on each alternate foot. Figure 1 shows a block diagram of this study. For registering acceleration of head movement from side to side, the accelerometer is attached in such a way that the direction of sensitivity is parallel to the frontal plane of the head. The output from the accelerometer is connected to two electric averagers. One averager is actuated by a trigger mechanism which is released as one foot is lifted. The trigger mechanism of the other averager is released when the other foot is lifted. Marching in place is carried out in the same way as in Fukuda's stepping test.

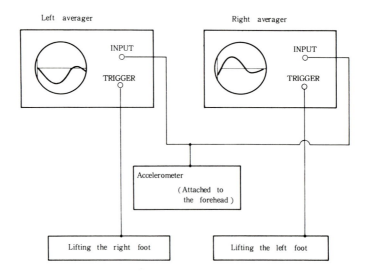

Fig. 1. Block diagram of the averaged acceleration registrograms.

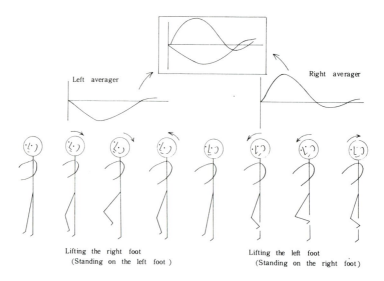

Fig. 2. The first two steps in marching in place.

Figure 2 shows the first two steps. The head movement while standing on the left foot is registered on the oscillograph of the left averager for 400 msec by lifting the right foot from the iron plate. Next, the head movement while standing on the right foot is registered on the oscillograph of the right averager for 400 msec by lifting the left foot. This marching is continued for 50 steps. Thus the acceleration registrograms during 25 left foot standings are averaged on the right averager and vice versa. Both averaged registrograms are photographed on a polaroid film. The same procedure is carried out with eyes closed and the averaged acceleration registrograms are compared with those taken with eyes open.

Results

(1) Results of Normal Subjects. Twenty normal healthy adults were tested. The acceleration registrograms during fifty paces of marching in place with eyes open were compared with those with eyes closed.

Figure 3 shows the averaged acceleration registrograms of a normal healthy man, 28 years of age. Head movements while standing on one foot were recorded for 400 msec after the foot lifting. Two gradations on the oscillograph are calibrated to indicate 0.25g.

In both figures, the averaged registrograms above the base line indicate the head movement while standing on the right foot and the registrograms below the base line indicate the head movement while standing on the left foot. Since the zero-line indicates the upright head position, the upper and lower registrograms from the base line indicate respectively, the inclinations of the head to the right and left.

As an index of the deviation of the head while marching in place, the ratio of the maximum deviation is defined as follows. The ratio of the maximum deviation is the percentage of the difference of the maximum deviations when standing on the right foot and standing on the left foot divided by the distance between the maximum deviations when standing on each foot. In cases when the direction of the deviations when standing on each foot are the same side, the sum of the maximum deviations is used instead of the difference.

In this study, the difference of the ratio of the maximum deviation between eyes closed and eyes open was noted.

Summarizing the results in twenty normal healthy adults;
1. Averaged registrograms taken with the subject standing on each foot show a repetitive, individual idiosyncrosy. The amplitudes of the registrograms are greater in males than in females.

eyes open   eyes closed

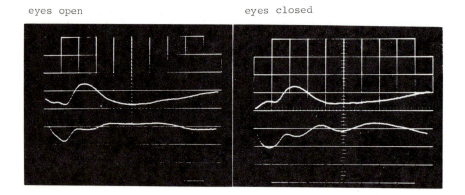

Fig.3. The averaged acceleration registrograms of a normal healthy man, 28 years of age. Comparing the marching with eyes open and eyes closed, the difference of the ratios is 7.9% to the left.

2. Comparing the marching with eyes closed and open, the ratio of the maximum deviation increases with eyes closed. The difference of the ratios of the maximum deviation between eyes closed and eyes open is from 1.3% to 12.5%. According to statistical analysis, 95% of the normal population falls below 9.4%. Therefore, the value of 9.4% is defined as the upper limit of normal range.

(2) Results of Pathological Cases. (Case 1) S.T. male, 40 years old.
A postoperative patient who underwent translabyrinthine removal of acoustic naurinoma on the right side. He was tested 4 months after surgery. Then he was able to walk without disturbance, although he did sometimes feel unstable.

Neuro-Otological findings; Otoscopic findings were negative. He was deaf in the right ear. The Romberg test was within normal limits, the Mann's test with eyes closed revealed a falling tendency to the right, the one-leg test with eyes closed revealed a falling tendency to the back and to the left. In the stepping test with eyes closed, when 50 steps were completed, the angle of rotation was 0°, the angle of displacement 0° and the distance of displacement forward 0.5m. Neither spontaneous nor positional eye nystagmus were observed. There was no response to caloric stimulation in the right ear.

eyes open   eyes closed

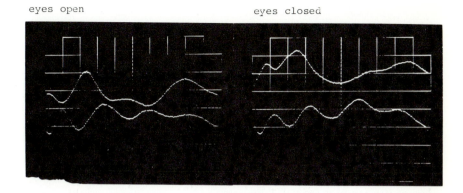

Fig. 4. The averaged acceleration registrograms of a man with translabyrinthine removal of acoustic neurinoma on the right side. Comparing the marching with eyes open and eyes closed, the ratio of the maximum deviation increases to the right side with eyes closed. The difference of the ratios of the maximum deviation is 23.3% to the right.

Results of the averaged acceleration registrograms; (Figure 4). The difference of the ratios of the maximum deviation between eyes closed and eyes open was 23.3% to the right. In this case, the Mann's test and the one-leg test revealed a falling tendency on opposide sides while the stepping test showed no deviation. That is, these former tests showed no definite direction of deviation.

In 22 patients with labyrinthine dysfunction, the following was revealed; Averaged registrograms taken with the subject standing on each foot show repetitive, individual indiosyncrosies and the deviation of averaged registrograms while standing with eyes closed, on the foot the same side as the dysfunctional labyrinth is greater than on the opposite foot. This was observed even in cases with indefinite findings in static or kinetic functional tests.

Discussion

In observation of the righting reflex, especially that involving the labyrinth, the main objective is to watch for an ataxia usually seen as being asymmetrical to the front, back, right and left of the body. Thus the tests regarding the labyrinthine reflex are usually performed in a static condition, although the Romberg test tends to be too stable and the one-leg test tends to be too unstable and has little clinical value. However, the one leg standing while walking or marching in place is more stable and patients usually feel dizzy or ataxic in kinetic conditions.

While stepping or walking, the head inclines a little to the right side when the right foot is set down and the left foot lifted. The tonic labyrinthine and neck reflexes induced by the inclination increase the extensor tone of the two limbs on the right side and contractive tone of the two limbs on the left side and with such reflexes, walking becomes smooth. The same effect occurs during the right foot lifting. In cases where a one side labyrinthine function is hypoactive, ataxia and deviation of the body occur. In order to compensate for the ataxia and deviation, it is considered that inclination of the head to the labyrinthine hypoactive side is increased when the foot on the same side is put down, i.e. decrease of the righting reflex of the head. In our study, head movements while marching in place were recorded by an accelerometer which was attached to the subject's forehead. This method clearly indicates the relation between the direction of gravity and head position. In normal cases, the deviation of the averaged registrograms above or below the base line show right or left inclination of the head during right or left foot standing. In cases of labyrinthine dysfunction, the definite increase of deviation of the averaged registrograms to the dysfunctional side during the one foot standing on the same side, without significant ataxia or deviation of the body, can be regarded as support for the above mentioned hypothesis.

The results of averaged registrograms can be summarised as follows:
1. Averaged registrograms taken with the subject standing on each foot show a repetitive, individual idiosyncrosy. Amplitudes of the registrograms are larger in males than in females.
2. Comparing the marching with eyes closed and open, the ratio of the maximum deviation of the averaged registrograms while standing on the left and then the right foot is similar in normal persons.
3. In the case of labyrinthine dysfunction, deviation of the averaged registrograms while standing with eyes closed on the foot the same side as the dysfunctional labyrinth, is greater than standing on the opposite foot. This is observed even in cases with indefinite findings in static or kinetic functional test.

Based on the above mentioned results, the averaged registrograms are considered to be an excellent parameter of the labyrinthine righting reflex.

References

Fukuda, T. The stepping test; Two phases of the labyrinthine reflex. *Acta otolaryngol.* **50**, 95-108, 1958.

Kitahara, M. Acceleration registrography; a new method of examinations concerned with the labyrinthine righting reflex. *Ann Otol.* **74**, 203-214, 1965.

2. Galvanic body-sway test for the differential diagnosis of vertigo.

S. HONJO, T. SEKITANI, M. TANAKA, K. SHIMAMOTO

Department of Otolaryngology, Yamaguchi University Medical School, Ube city, Japan.

Introduction

The galvanic test, as generally accepted, is used to differentiate disease of the labyrinth from the affections of the vestibular nerve (retrolabyrinthine lesions). The test is therefore indicated in a case in which, for example, the labyrinthine excitability under caloric and rotatory stimulation is absent, so that it becomes important to know whether or not the galvanic reaction can be elicited. A positive response indicates a labyrinthine disease; a negative reaction points to the possibility of retrolabyrinthine lesion.

As one of the routine tests in otoneurological examination, we have developed and have been using a so-called "computer Galvano-ARG Test" for detecting galvanic body-sway, qualitatively and quantitatively. A weak electric current stimulation, i.e. 0.6 mA and 2-6 volts, did not produce any noticeable complaint, such as local pain or discomfort.

The paper briefly presents the method of the computer Galvano-ARG Test and the findings in representative cases with various causes, i.e. Meniere's disease, vestibular neuronitis, acoustic neuroma, cerebellopontine angle tumor and congenital deafmute; and evaluates the results obtained from the 128 patients who were examined at the Otoneurological clinic of Yamaguchi University Hospital.

Methods and Materials

Recording of small Body-sway induced by weak electrical stimulation was done by acceleration registrography, abbreviated A.R.G.

It will be explained briefly as follows (Fig. 1): movements of the head and body are picked up with two accelerometers. These two accelerometers were fixed on the top of a light helmet which was fastened tightly to the head of the subject.

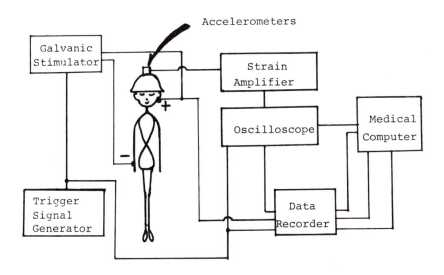

Fig. 1. Block diagram of "Computer Galvano-ARG Test", showing instrumentation and subject's posture.

In this way, it is possible to record the subject's body sway in two dimensions, lateral and anteroposterior planes, simultaneously.

The two accelerometers were connected with two dynamic strainmeters yielding the output of these accelerometers as electric potential. This electric potential was proportional to the range of head-body movement.

The output from the strainmeters was observed with an oscilloscope and simultaneously recorded on magnetic recording tape with a data-recorder.

In order to process and analyse (average summation), a medical data processing computer was used.

The program of the computer was set to calculate the average of each component of the head movement.

The first channel of the oscilloscope was used for lateral movement, the second for sagittal plane and the third for the stimulation marker (duration of stimulation).

Trigger mode was set on EXT., and was prepared to begin work at the trigger signal recorded on the magnetic tape of the data-recorder.

In this procedure, average data were obtained from eight sweeps.

Electrodes: The stimulating electrode was made of silver plate, 2x3cm.

Saturated salt solution was used. Electrodes were fixed with a rubber band at the postauricular skin on each side. One electrode was placed on the forearm as the indifferent electrode.

With this arrangement, skin resistance between the stimulating and indifferent electrodes was usually between 3000 and 5000 ohms. (Constant current stimulation was used).

Galvanic stimulator: As a galvanic stimulator, an electronic constant-current stimulator was used. Another electronic stimulator was used for the trigger signal generator at interval of 10 seconds, triggering the galvanic stimulator and Oscilloscope action.

The electric current yielded by the stimulator was recorded on the data-recorder as well as the output signal of the head-body sway response.

Test Procedure: Galvanic stimulation was delivered by anodal unipolar and double electrode technique.

In this study we used a stimulus of 0.6mA for 10 seconds with an interval of 15 sec.

All responses were obtained while the subject was standing with his feet parallel and touching; and his eyes closed. One series of eight stimulations, took about 3 min. so that a rest of at least five min. was given for each subject after every examination.

In the body sway recording, upward wave deflection of the oscilloscope trace corresponds to a sway of the body to the right side in the lateral plane.

Upward deflection in the second channel the anteroposterior plane, corresponds to a sway backward.

Results

The normal galvanic body-sway responses. It is a well-known fact, that body-sway occurs toward the stimulated side when anodal galvanic current is applied. When the anodal galvanic is off, the body sways away from the stimulated side.

Galvanic body-sway responses occurred in all of our normal subjects stimulated by the anodal electrode on one ear.

For example, when the right ear is stimulated, the body sways to the right side and when the left ear is stimulated the body sways to the left side in the lateral plane.

As far as body-sway induced by galvanic stimulation is concerned, it seems to be important to analyze the response wave at both onset and cutoff of the stimulus.

In other words, the following 4 divisions are analyzed, i) latent period after onset (0.1-0.8sec) (mean value: 0.36±0.1); ii) deviation (swayed) period (Maximum deviation. 1.0-3.0sec) (1.75±0.75); iii) latent period after cutoff. (0.4-1.0sec; 1.60±0.47) and iv) sway-back period (0.7-2.7sec; 1.60±0.47).

Eight traces of the original waves of body-sway elicited by unipolar anodal stimulation on the one side in the same normal subject were recorded on the magnetic tape of the data-recorder. The averaged wave from eight waves was obtained by means of a medical data-processing computer.

Clinical case presentation: The test was applied to 128 cases at the Otoneurological Clinic.

5 representative cases follow.

(Case 1): Meniere's disease.

A 35 years old woman with left sided Meniere's disease, who had bad recurrent attacks of vertigo with hearing loss and tinnitus on the left side, for the last 5 years. She had occasional unsteadiness of gait.

Otoneurological study showed right-beating spontaneous nystagmus and direction-fixed positional nystagmus. Caloric test showed no response on the left side. The right ear showed a normal response.

In this case, the computer Galvano-ARG Test showed normal galvanic body-sway responses on both sides. Furthermore, double electrode stimulation elicited no body-sway.

(Case 2): Vestibular neuronitis.

Sudden onset of vertigo occurred following "catching common colds". Hearing tests revealed hearing acuity within the normal range.

There was right-beating spontaneous and direction-fixed positional nystagmus.

Caloric tests revealed no response on the left side.

Computer Galvano-ARG Test with unipolar anodal stimulation on the affected (left) side showed that the duration of the body-sway (deviation) extended more than the normal range.

Stimulation on the non-affected side showed a normal response.

It seems to be important to note that anodal double galvanic stimulation elicited body-sway to the opposite side (right side).

This body-sway, beyond any doubt, is due to the response of the non-affected healthy side.

(Case 3): A 49-years-old woman with acoustic tumor.
   No body-sway response was detected on the affected side, at all.

*(Case 4): Cerebellopontine angle tumor (due to acoustic neuroma)
(Fig. 2).*

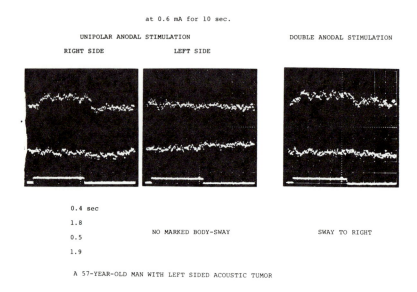

Fig. 2. "Body-sway response wave", average of 8 traces of A.R.G. recording of Galvanic body-sway by data-processing computer (case with left sided acoustic tumor).

A 57 years-old man, who had had persistent dull headache and tinnitus (on the left side) for the last 2 years. Recently, he began to have some unsteadiness of gait. The audiogram revealed total hearing loss on the left side. Caloric tests showed no response. Computer Galvano-ARG Test revealed no response wave on the left side.

(Case 5): Congenital deafmute.
   She showed disturbed balance with closed eyes, on Mann's posture standing test and goniometer test. There was no spontaneous or positional nystagmus on examination. No caloric response was present even with ice-water stimulation on either side. Unipolar anodal stimulation on each side did not yield any body-sway

response. Double galvanic stimulation did not yield any body-sway (deviation) at all.

In conclusion, as already mentioned, a computer Galvano-ARG Test for otoneurological examination has been devised, especially for differentiating labyrinthine lesions from retrolabyrinthine lesions.

The cases examined and diagnosed by various tests have been divided into two groups in a wide clinical sense, i.e. vertigo of labyrinthine-origin and retrolabyrinthine lesions.

As shown in Table 1, these labyrinthine-origin vertigo and diseased ear cases showed a low percentage of abnormal pathologic galvanic body-sway responses.

TABLE 1
Labyrinthine Lesion (82 cases)

	Normal	Abnormal
Canal Paresis	34	2
Dead Labyrinth	7	2
Sudden Deafness	8	2
B.P.P.V.	3	0
O.M.C. with Fistular Labyrinthitis	13	2
Others	8	1
	73	9
	89%	11%

By contrast, the group with retro-labyrinthine lesion disease (Table 2) show a high percentage of the abnormal body-sway resonses in surgically confirmed cases with acoustic tumor and cerebellopontine angle tumor. Even the vestibular neuronitis cases show a high percentage of abnormal pattern in the computer Galvano-ARG Test.

Above all, the computer Galvano-ARG Test is useful for different-ial diagnosis of vertigo of labyrinthine and retrolabyrinthine origin.

TABLE 2
Retro-Labyrinthine Lesion (46 cases)

	Normal	Abnormal
Vestibular Neuronitis	3	9
Acoustic Tumor	1	5
Cerebellopontine Angle Tumor	0	4
Cerebellar Ataxia	0	2
Head Trauma	5	2
Cerebral Arteriosclerosis1	7	3
Others	1	4
	17	29
	37%	63%

References

Cervantes, J.J. : Goniometry during test for Romberg's sign and in galvanic testing of vestibular apparatus. *Pro. Oto-Rhino-Laryngol.* **14**, 124, 1952.

Coats, A.C.: Galvanic Body-sway in normals and patients with 8th nerve lesions. *Adv. Oto-Rhino-Laryng.,* **19**, 318, 1973.

Dohlmann, G.: Some practical and theoretical points of galvanic stimulation of the labyrinth. *Proc. Roy. Soc. Med.,* **28**, 1371, 1935.

Hongo, S., Tanaka, M. and Sekitani, T.: Body-Sway induced by Galvanic stimulation. *Agressologie (Paris)* **17**, **A**, 77, 1975.

Kunke, E.: Ueber die durch den galvanischen strom bewirken Korperschwankungen. *Pfluger Arch. Ges. Physiol.,* **252**, 599, 1950.

Neumann, H.: Galvanischen nystagmus. *Monatschr. Ohrenth.,* **41**, 280, 1907.

Sekitani, T. and Tanaka, M.: Test for Galvanic Vestibular Responses – survey through our experimental and clinical investigation for last 20 years – *Bull. Yamaguchi Med. Sch.* **22**, 439, 1975.

Tanaka, M.: Investigation of galvanic test. *Bull. Yamaguchi Med.Sch.* **21**, 61, 1974.

Tanaka, M., Sekitani, T. and Honjo, S.: Clinical Significance of Galvanic Body-Sway. *Bull. Yamaguchi Med. Sch.* **22**, 495, 1975.

3.   Orthostatic postural activity disorders recorded by statokinesimeter in post-concussional syndrome following head injuries. Oculomotor aspect.

J.B. BARON, N. USHIO, M.J. TANGAPREGASSOM

Serv. Neuroophthal, CPSA 1, Rue Cabanis, Paris XIV, France

The purpose of this paper is to emphasize the relationship between the oculomotor system and the tonic orthostatic postural activity and especially the influence of their disorders, after head injuries, on body balance.

In France during the First World War many papers had been written on the topic of the post-concussional syndrome. Mainly two directions are found in the description of these disorders.

Mairet and Pieron (1915) described a permanent postural trouble in relationship with a permanent vertigo-like sensation.

Pierre-Marie (1916) described a transitory one with a temporary false sensation of dizziness appearing during head-rotation or position changing.

Our purpose is to study this syndrome, and its aetiology in regard to traffic injuries or work accidents, and to summarize a part of our work and of the team of our fellow-workers who are studying this problem from different points of view.

Amphoux (1975) considering the biomechanical data following head injuries demonstrates that the maximum effect of energy of a direct blow is found in the region of the brainstem. While according to Vedrenne and Chodkiewicz (1975), the midbrain is specially involved in head injury indicating the importance of a unilateral lesion in the same part of the nervous system.

In 1905 Thiele demonstrated in rats the relationship existing between the tonic postural activity, locomotor behaviour and brain-stem reticular formation. The unilateral electrical stimulation of the latter structure inducing an incurvation of the spinal column homolateral to the stimulation and circling motions of the animal in the same direction; unilateral lesions of the midbrain at the level of the

III nucleus provoking stable and heterolateral reactions. There is a disequilibrium between the tonus primarily of the paravertebral muscles, and secondarily of the abductor, adductor, flexor and extensor muscles of the limbs between the left and right sides. In 1975, Yamamoto and Yamada, Tangapregassom, Lantin *et al.,* (1975) stereotaxically reproduced this phenomenon. It seems that the muscle tonus in equilibrium depends in part on the midbrain structures and especially that the oculomotor nuclei play a predominant part in the mechanisms for regulating the tonic activity of the neck and paravertebral muscles between right and left sides.

Our findings, (1975), have shown a disturbance of function of the oculomotor muscles in the ocular sphere homolaterally to electrical stimulation, and controlaterally to destruction, characterized by a ptosis, an exophthalmos and an exophoria, this means an elongation of the adductor eye muscles and a contraction of the abductor; we use the term of exophoria in the sense of its Greek etymology: deviation of the eyeball without specifying its aetiology or its ophthalmological implications. These disturbances have been previously described by Baron in 1953 in fishes and mice. A tonic change in the balance between the abductor and adductor oculomotor muscles of both eyes provokes, when the deviation of the eyeball is less than 4°, a scoliotic attitude and a peculiar locomotor behaviour, characterized by circling motion, due to an effective change in the length of the spindles in the muscles supplied by the third nerve exciting reflexly a contraction of the neck muscles and of the paravertebral muscles contralaterally.

The oculomotor structures seem to have a special effect on steady body equilibrium and on the tonus of the axial muscles. The III, IV and VI nuclei are formed by a mixed-cell population: large cells having a motor activity and small neurons having a sensory function. Palkovits and Jacobowitz (1974), demonstrated their cholinergic property.

The continuity of the oculomotor nuclei with the mesencephalic reticular formation leads us to consider the underlying reasons for disturbances of motor skill following alterations of structures other than the "specific" ones involved in the control of equilibrium e.g. VIIIth nerve, cerebellum, basal ganglia.

In this context it is possible to study the changes of biogenic amines or their precursors, as it has been shown by Friedman and Everett (1964) inducing, homolaterally to the disturbance, a drop in acetylcholine, Michaelis, Arango and Gerard (1949), modifying the level of DOPA, Ungerstedt and Butcher *et al.,* (1969), Cools and Van Rossum (1970), Barbeau (1962), Costall, Naylor and Olley

(1972) and changes in the levels of both neurotransmitters. Corroborating partially such an hypothesis, Lantin, Tangapregassom *et al.*, (1975) and Poletto, Lantin *et al.*, (1925), working on centrally lesioned rats and mice, have observed stable variations of DOPA in the telecephalon and diencephalon.

Clinical features

The tonic orthostatic postural activity is a functional entity. This function is an archaic one and specifically human, characterized by the positioning and maintenance of the centre of gravity of the body over the base. In standing, the body is never still, it sways continuously, following peculiar and complex rhythms, the amplitude and frequency of which reflect the functioning of the different sensori-motor systems which control and maintain the body gravity center over the base. This motion can be recorded by a statokinesimeter, and the amplitudes and frequencies of the sway measured.

These systems are generally supposed to be related to the extrapyramidal idiokinetic system more than to the pyramidal holokinetic one, and from our point of view there appears to be a close relationship with the reticular formation and with the output from the oculomotor nuclei.

The functioning of tonic postural activity can be examined under different conditions:

a) standing:

With a statokinesimeter, spontaneous displacements of the body gravity center are recorded, the patient standing in a dark room, looking straight ahead at a vertical bar situated in the sagittal median plane of the base, the head being successively free, fixated or rotated, and the eyeballs straight ahead or deviated homolaterally or controlaterally to the head position. The associated displacements of the body axis to galvanic labyrinthine stimulation are also recorded.

b) standing up dynamically:

The differences of tension existing between the muscles of the right and left, superior and inferior limbs can be revealed in repeated movements. This is the aim of Fukuda (1957), in the "marking time" test on the inferior limbs, reported by Ushio, Matsuura *et al.*, (1975) and of Gagey, Baron and Ushio (1974) in the key test on the upper limbs.

Associated with neurological tests a classical ophthalmological examination should be performed paying particular attention to the functioning of the oculomotor system:

a) standing up:

This examination must be done both with the head free and after fixation by a neck collar to correct any deviant attitude of the head. This inspection allows us to discover a small unilateral paralysis affecting especially some motor units of the III or IV nucleus, provoking displacements of one eye of a few degrees (less than 4°). This paralysis can be disclosed by a convergence manoeuvre, on the side of the paralysis there is an hypoconvergence, Baron, Filliozat and Soulairac (1965). This phenomenon is different from the phoria of fusion perturbations as described by Vidal (1968). A compression of the eyeballs is also performed and the diameter of the pupil is measured.

b) sitting down:

The deviation of the eyeballs to the right or the left side provokes a difference of tonus between the flexor-extensor, abductor-adductor muscle system of the inferior right and left limbs, Baron (1959), and this postural reaction is disturbed after head injury, Gagey, Baron *et al.,* (1973, 1975).

Some other examinations must be associated:
— O.R.L. to test the vestibular apparatus.
— rheoencephalographic, Rouquet, Babic *et al.,* (1975), Boismare, Boquet and Courtin (1975), reporting simultaneously an aspect of the right and left deep brain vascularisation.
— radiographic to examine the functioning of atlas-axis articulation by tomography and the neck vertebrae, Gentaz, Goumot *et al.,* (1975) also the entire vertebral column, with and without correction of the oculomotor paralysis.
— psychiatric, personality and performance tests, Filliozat, Goumot *et al.,* (1975), Boquet-Masiee (1975), reporting the psychiatric aspect are also applied.

Results

All these examinations have been performed on 150 patients most of them suffering from pseudo vertigo but working again after head injuries. These traumata have produced in most of them a coma of more than half an hour. They may be recent, less than one month, or long standing, more than two years. From these results it can be assumed that 3 types of postural tonic activity troubles can be isolated in our population, Baron, Goumot *et al.*, (1975).

75% show a spontaneous twofold increase of amplitude of the body oscillations. This phenomenon is reproduced with electrical vestibular stimulation and motion of the eyeballs. Statically and dynamically these perturbations are always associated with partial unilateral paralysis of the III or the IV nerves indicating an alteration in the midbrain. When the compression of the eyeballs decreases the amplitude of the statokinesigram it may be inferred that an orthopaedic therapy by prismatic lenses will ameliorate the condition. The O.R.L., rheographic and psychiatric examination are then normal.

10% show an induced increase of the amplitude of the body oscillations when the head and the neck are rotated to one side, the rheographic examination is disturbed after the same manoeuvre in the same way. Simultaneously all the other examinations are normal. It can be assumed that a unilateral mechanical or reflex disturbance of the deep vascular system of the brain is induced by the rotation of the head similar to a Vertebro-Basilar Insufficiency syndrome, Boquet, Boismare *et al.*, (1975).

15% of the population show an anarchic and gigantic perturbation of the motion more than ten times the normal amplitude. All the psychiatric tests are disturbed. The O.R.L. the rheographic, radiographic examinations are very difficult to carry out, Soulairac, Noto *et al.*, (1977).

Therapy

From all these results some therapy can be suggested depending on the aetiology of the disturbance of tonic body activity.

In case of brainstem lesions, a therapy changing the level of the neurotransmitter amine concentration, precursor of adrenaline or acetylcholine, associated with energy increasing drugs such as Vitamin B. can be utilized or an orthopaedic therapy using prismatic lenses. This latter therapy, using an optomotor reflex which relieves the oculomotor tonic imbalance, corrects the conflict existing between afferences from the II, III, IV, VI, VIII, XI nerves and tonic postural orthostatic reactions responsible for standing. The functioning of the formation seems to become more normal. The pharmacological therapy has a similar effect. These results can be used either as a therapy or as a test of drug efficiency.

In cases of Vertebro-Basilar Insufficiency syndrome, a therapy with D.H.E. alone or in association with Raubasine or Vitamin C can be used.

In cases of psychiatric syndrome a psychoanalytic, psychomotoric, psychosociologic therapy can be prescribed.

As a result of 10 years of investigation it can be said that the post-concussional syndrome is not a subjective one and the pseudo vertigo which is associated with it can be ameliorated by suitable therapy when the differential diagnosis is made.

References

Amphoux, M., Sevin, A., (1975): Traumatismes cérébraux et focalisations céré-brales. *Agressologie* **16A**, 47-53.

Barbeau, A., (1962): The pathogenesis of Parkinson's disease; a new hypothesis. *Can. Med. Assn.* J. **87**, 802-807.

Baron, J.B., (1955): Muscles moteurs oculaires, attitudes et comportement moteur chez les vertébrés. *Thèse Doctorat Es-sciences,* Paris.

Baron, J.B., (1959): Données récentes sur l'équilibration et le vertige. *Psychol. Franç.* **4**, 3 : 205-211.

Baron, J.B., Filliozat, R., Soulairac, A., (1965): Séquelles tardives des trauma-tismes crâniens. *8è Congrés Int. Neurol. Vienne. Excerpta Med. Found. Amsterdam.* **1** V : 143-147.

Baron, J.B., Goumot, H., Gagey, P.M., Filliozat, R., Gentaz, R., Koitcheva, V., Rouquet, Y., Fouque, A., Bessineton, J.C., Pacifici, M., Ushio, N., (1975): Perturbations de l'activité tonique posturale d'origine oculomotirce due à un traumatisme crânien. Aspect neuro-ophtalmologique et pharmacolo-gique. *Agressologie* **16** D : 53-64.

Boismare, F., Boquet, J., Courtin, J., (1975): Aspects rhéographiques et phar-macologiques du syndrome subjectif chez le traumatisé crânio-cervical. *Agressologie* **16** D : 23-26.

Boquet-Masiee, F., (1975): Examen psychométrique de sujets atteints de syndrome post-commotionnel. *Agressologie* **16** D : 71-76.

Cools, A.R., Van Rossum, M.J., (1970): Caudal dopamine and stereotype behaviour of cats. *Arch. Int. Pharmacology* **187**, 163-173.

Costall, B., Naylor, R.J., Olley J.E., (1972): Catalepsy and circling behaviour after intracerebral injections of neuroleptic, cholinergic and anti-cholinergic agents into the caudateputamen, globus pallidus and substantia nigra of rat brain. *Neuropharmacology* **11**, 645-663.

Filliozat, R., Goumot, H., Gagey, P.M., Gentaz, R., Rouquet, Y., Baron J.B., (1975): Projet expérimental d'évaluation du syndrome dit subjectif des traumatises crâniens. *Agressologie* **16** A : 25-30.

Friedman, A.H., Everett, G.M., (1964): Pharmacological aspects of parkin-sonism. *In:* "Advances in Pharmacology" 83-127, V.3. Academic Press, N.Y. and London.

Fukuda, T., (1957): Réflexes statokinétiques dans l'équilibre et le mouvement. **1** *V 83-85.* Ed. Igaku Shoin. Tokyo.

Gagey, P.M., Baron, J.B., Amphoux, M., Blaizot, M., Gentaz, R., Goumot, H., (1975): Perturbations de l'activité tonique posturale des membres inférieurs en cathédrostatisme au cours des mouvements oculaires horizontaux soutenus, recontrés dans certains syndromes post-commotionnels d'origine tronculaire. *Agressologie.* **16** D : 77-82.

Gagey, P.M., Baron, J.B., Lespargot, J., Poli, J.P. (1973): Variations de l'activité tonique posturale et activité des muscles oculocéphalogyres en cathédrostatisme. *Agressologie.* **14** B : 97-96.

Gagey, P.M., Baron, J.B., Ushio, N. (1974): Activité tonique posturale et activité gestuelle. Le test de la clé. *Agressologie.* **6** (15), **5** : 353-358.

Gentaz, R., Gagey, P.M., Goumot, H., Rouquet, Y., Baron, J.B. (1975): La radiographie du rachis cervical au cours du syndrome post-commotionel. *Agressologie.* **16** A : 33-46.

Lantin, N., Tangapregassom, A.M., Tangapregassom, M.J., Ficek, W., Baron, J.B. (1975): Lésions stéréotaxiques tronculaires du rat provoquant des troubles toniques posturaux. III — Aspect biochimique. *Agressologie.* **16** A : 73-80.

Mairet, A., Pieron, H. (1915): Le syndrome commotionnel au point de vue du mécanisme pathogénique et de l'évolution. *Bull. Acad. Méd. in Rev. Neurol.* 1916, 4-5.

Marie, P. (1916): Les troubles subjectifs consécutifs aux blessures du crâne. *Rev. Neurol.* **2**, 616.

Michaelis, M., Arango, N.I., Gerard, R.W. (1949): Inhibition of brain dehydrogenases by "anticholinesterases". *Amer. J. Physiol.* **157**, 463-467.

Palkovits, M., Jacobowitz, D.M. (1974): Topographic atlas of catecholamine and acetylcholinesterase containing neurons in the rat brain. *Journal Comp. Neurol. I,* **157**, 29-41.

Poletto, J., Lantin, N., Tangapregassom, M.J., Ficek, W., Vedrenne, C., Baron, J.B. (1975): Troubles posturaux à la suite de traumatismes crâniens expérimentaux chez la souris. Aspects comportementaux et biochimiques. *Agressologie.* **16** A : 81-86.

Rouquet, Y., Babic, R., Marstal, N., Goumot, H., Gagey, P.M., Gentaz, R., Baron, J.B. (1975): Syndrome post-commotionnel. Aspects rhéographique et statokinésimétrique. *Agressologie.* **16** D : 15-22.

Boquet, J., Boismare, F., Courtin, P., Boquet-Masiee, F., Montier, J. (1975): Etude clinique des troubles de l'équilibre postural chez 40 sujets traumatisés cervicaux ou cranio-cervicaux présentant un syndrome subjectif. *Agressologie.* **16** D : 65-70.

Soulairac, A., Rouquet, Y., Noto, R., Baron, J.B., Babic, R. (1977): Etude des corrélations entre les réponses circulatoires cérébrales et les régulations posturales chez le sujet normal et déficitaire sénile. *Agressologie.* **18** A : 57-

Tangapregassom, M.J., Tangapregassom, A.M., Lantin, N., Ficek, W., Baron, J.B. (1975): Lésions stéréotaxiques tronculaires du rat progoquant des troubles toniques posturaux. I — Aspects comportementaux. *Agressologie.* **16** A : 55-62.

Tangapregassom, A.M., Tangapregassom, M.J., Lantin, N., Ficek, W., Baron, J.B. (1975): Lésions stéréotaxiques tronculaires du rat provoquant des troubles toniques posturaux. II — Aspects neuro-histologiques. *Agressologie.* **16** A : 63-72.

Thiele, F. (1905): On the efferent relationship of the optic thalamus and Dieter's nucleus to the spinal cord, with special reference to the cerebellar influx theory (Hughling's) and the genesis of decerebrate rigidity (Sherrington). *Proc. Roy. Soc. London. S.B.* **76**, 360.

Ungerstedt, U., Butcher, L.L., Anden, N.E., Fuxe, K. (1969): Direct chemical stimulation of dopaminergic mechanisms in the neostriatum of the rat. *Brain Res.* **14**, 461-471.

Ushio, N., Matsuura, K., Hinoki, M., Baron, J.B., Gagey, P.M. (1975): Deux phases de réflexe dans l'équilibre progoquées par les propriocepteurs des muscles oculaires. Analyse à l'aide du test de piétinement de Fukuda et du test de réflexe orthostatique. *Agressologie.* **16** D : 39-52.

Vedrenne, C., Chodkiewicz, J.P., (1975): Les lésions du tronc cérébral chez les traumatisés crâniens (étude anatomique). *Agressologie.* **16** D : 1-8.

Vidal, M. (1968): Perturbations non paralytiques de l'équilibre oculomoteur et traumatisme crânien. *Thèse Faculté de Médecine, Toulouse.*

Yamamoto, H., Yamada, K. (1976); Equilibrial approach to scoliotic posture. *Agressologie.* **17** D : 61-65.

4. Postural control of center-of-force trajectories in patients with peripheral, eighth nerve, and posterior fossa lesions.

F. OWEN BLACK, C. WALL III, D. P. O'LEARY

Raymond E. Jordan Clinical Vestibular Systems Laboratory, Division of Vestibular Disorders, Department of Otolaryngology, University of Pittsburgh School of Medicine and the Eye and Ear Hospital of Pittsburgh.

Introduction

Center-of-force trajectory characteristics from humans attempting to maintain standard and tandem Romberg positions have been recorded and computer analyzed immediately off-line (Black, O'Leary and Wall, 1977). This vestibulo-spinal stability test (VESST) technique has proven to be a useful research and clinical tool (Black, 1977) with a resolution sufficient to record visually undetectable postural center-of-force shifts secondary to Galvanic vestibular stimuli (Black *et al.*, 1977-2) induced by electrical implant stimulation of the vestibular system. This report will summarize a portion of the preliminary findings from a group of carefully documented patients with sensory and neural equilibrium control system disorders.

Methods

A. Patient groups

Fourteen patients who satisfied the American Academy of Ophthalmology and Otolaryngology criteria (Alford, 1972) for unilateral Meniere's disease were selected as subjects afflicted with a peripheral (intra-labyrinthine) vestibular lesion. Six subjects with surgically confirmed acoustic neuromas limited to the internal auditory canal

This project supported by grants from the Martha Edwards Lazear Foundation, George H. and Margaret McClintic Love Foundation, Richard King Mellon Foundation, The Deafness Research Foundation and the United States Department of Health, Education and Welfare, Public Health Service, National Institutes of Health #NS13286.

(and without brain stem compression) were chosen to represent an anatomical "first-order" vestibular afferent nerve lesion group. Another six subjects with surgically confirmed unilateral lesions of a cerebellar hemisphere were chosen to represent an abnormal "central" neuromuscular control system group. Postural center-of-force characteristics of these patients were compared with the performance of 76 age-matched normal subjects. The details of the test apparatus and methods have been previously published (Black *et al.*, 1977; Black, 1977).

B. Summary of Test Procedure

Instructions given to the subject were identical to those used to obtain an unrecorded Romberg test in the clinic, as follows: After removing shoes, the subject was instructed to stand with knees locked on the force platform in the standard (feet together) or tandem (heel-to-toe, dominant foot behind) foot positions, with eyes open or closed. Four maneuvers were recorded: (1) feet together, eyes open; (2) feet together, eyes closed; (3) feet heel-to-toe, eyes open; and (4) feet heel-to-toe, eyes closed. During each maneuver the subject was asked to perform the Jendrissik maneuver by hooking his hands by the fingers and laterally extending his arms in tension in order to reduce articulated pelvic, upper torso and head sway.

Each subject was tested using two 15-second trials per maneuver. Continuous display of center-of-force determinations throughout the testing procedure on the computer display enabled the technician to properly position the subject before recording each trial.

C. Data Analysis

The following data analyses were performed:
1. x-y plot of center-of-force.
2. Polar coordinates of center-of-force, i.e. length (r) and rotation angle (θ) of the radial vector plotted versus time.
3. Position and velocity of center-of-force plotted separately versus time.
4. Phase plane plots, i.e., velocity versus displacement. The phase plane plots diagramatically display stability characteristics of the subject's center-of-force in the x and y planes separately.
5. Power spectral density (PSD). The power spectrum of the x, y, and r center-of-force fluctuations were estimated using the fast Fourier transform. An estimate of the energy expended for

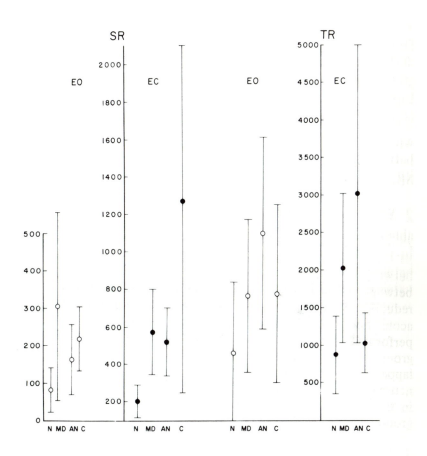

Fig. 1. Results of integrated power spectra plotted as means and standard deviations. Ordinate indicates power spectra integral in arbitrary units. SR: Standard Romberg; TR: Tandem Romberg; EO: Eyes open; EC: Eyes closed; N: Normal; MD: Meniere's disease; AN: Acoustic Neuroma; C = Central (posterior fossa) lesion. Comment in Text.

postural control was obtained by integrating the PSD plot.

The VESST results most easily related intuitively to clinically observed Romberg abnormalities appears to be the integral of the power spectral density plots and the ratio of the integrals between the various test conditions. In this report, data are summarized for only the polar vector (r) fluctuations.

Results

A Integrated Power Spectra

1. Standard Romberg (SR) Position, Eyes Open (EO). The integrated power spectra for the SR, EO trials (means and standard deviations) of both the Meniere's disease and acoustic neuroma group overlapped with the normal ranges group with a much greater variation recorded from the Meniere's disease group (Fig. 1). There was a minimal overlap of the posterior fossa (central) lesion group with the normal range, however, there were no significant differences between energy expended by the entire abnormal group for the SR, EO series.

2. SR, Eyes Closed (EC). Upon visual deprivation both normal and abnormal groups significantly increased energy expenditure relative to values determined with eyes open. There was much less overlap between normal and abnormal ranges and relatively less overlap between the "central" and "peripheral" lesion group (note scale reduction in Fig. 1). Performance of the Meniere's disorders and acoustic neuroma groups were virtually identical but both groups performed well outside normal ranges. The posterior fossa lesion group performed with a markedly increased variation which overlapped in the lower ranges with Meniere's disorder and acoustic neuroma groups. For the SR position, the greatest variation occurred in the Meniere's disease group with EO, and in the posterior fossa group with EC.

3. Tandem Romberg (TR), Eyes Open (EO). Energy expenditure during the more unstable TR, EO maneuvers corresponded in magnitude with the SR, EC trials, but with greater variance in the TR position. There was also considerable overlap in the performance of all groups, normal and abnormal, in the more unstable TR, EO series.

4. Tandem Romberg (TR), Eyes Closed (EC). Integrated power

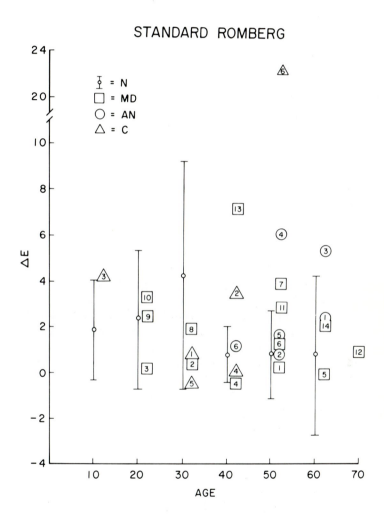

Fig. 2a. Standard Romberg Δ E abnormal group results plotted individually (symbols) to the immediate right of corresponding age matched normal subjects.

spectra means and standard deviations overlap considerably between normal and posterior fossa lesion groups but to a lesser extent with the Meniere's disease and acoustic neuroma groups. (Note second scale change in Fig. 1). Except for the central lesion group, the relative increase in energy expenditure from EO to EC test conditions was approximately the same for both SR and TR maneuvers.

B. Ratio Calculations

1. Relative Energy Expenditure with and without Visual Deprivation (Δ E). Integrated power spectral plots may be considered estimates of energy expenditure. Systematic changes in the integrated power spectra from maneuver to maneuver and trial to trial may be summarized by computing the difference between the eyes closed and eyes open trials as a ratio to the eyes open trial as follows:

$$\Delta \ E = \frac{\hat{E} \ closed - \hat{E} \ open}{\hat{E} \ open}$$

where: $\Delta \ E$ = relative energy change between trials
$\hat{E}$ = power spectrum integral

In the standard Romberg position, most of the acoustic neuroma and the posterior fossa lesion subjects fell outside normal $\Delta \ E$ ranges. Five well compensated or quiescent Meniere's disease patients fell within normal $\Delta \ E$ limited (Fig. 2a). Results for those subjects who could perform an eyes closed tandem Romberg series are plotted in Figure 2b. All of the six posterior fossa lesion patients fell at or below normal ranges. Responses from most of the remaining patient groups who could perform the maneuver were widely distributed relative to normal with four "inactive" Meniere's disorder patients recording within normal limits.

2. Differential Energy Expenditure of Normal and Abnormal Subjects. Ratios of the power spectral integrals (PSI) for the EO to EC are plotted (lower curves) in Fig. 3 as a function of subject group. There are no significant differences between the groups. The upper plot demonstrates the $\Delta \ E$ ratio for SR/TR maneuvers as a function of patient group.

Discussion

Power spectral density (PSD) analysis has been applied by several

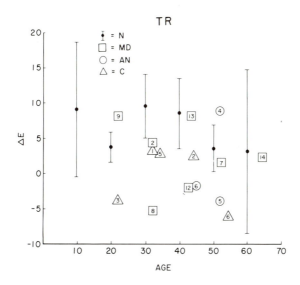

Fig. 2b. Tandem Romberg individual Δ E results. Only 15 of the 26 abnormal subjects could perform the TR maneuver. See text for discussion.

researchers to center-of-mass recordings in x and y planes in normal subjects (Bensel and Dzendolet, 1968; Scott and Dzendolet, 1972; and Leroux *et al.,* 1973). The highest PSD values plotted in the three studies varied between 0.0 and 0.4 Hz (Bensel and Dzendolet, 1968), 0.3 and 2 Hz (Scott and Dzendolet, 1972) and 0.0 to 0.2 Hz (Leroux *et al.,* 1973). Although close agreement was obtained for the frequency bandwidths among these laboratories, the PSD roll-offs ranged from -3 to -12 dB/octave among the three groups. Accordingly the results were interpreted as characterizations of first through fourth order control systems. Some variation was, in part, due to differences in the recording equipment and techniques, sampling methods, length of trials, and intersubject variability. Another reason for the difference in roll-offs reported may be secondary to the assumption that single plane (x or y) PSD estimates accurately reflect energy expenditure. In our opinion, polar co-ordinate fluctuations of the center-of-mass vector more accurately reflect a subject's energy expenditure, particularly if both normal and abnormal data are to be compared. (Unpublished observations). The data presented here represent the first step toward an attempt to determine which force vectors (r, x & y) are significantly altered

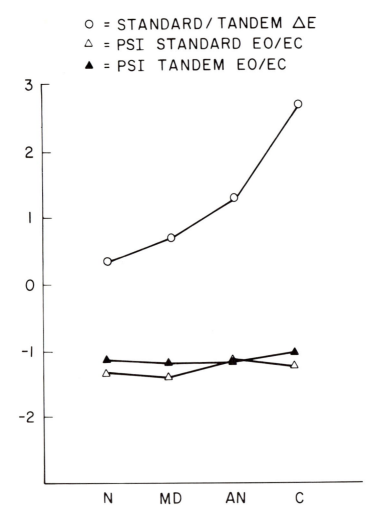

Fig. 3. Lower two curves are ratios of EO and EC power spectra for both SR and TR plotted as a function of patient classification. Upper curve reflects the ratio of SR to TR Δ E values.

by various types of equilibrium disturbances.

Particularly for normal subjects and the relatively stable postural maneuvers recorded from abnormal subjects, power spectral estimates were relatively band-limited compared to the more wide spectral bands recorded during relatively unstable maneuvers from both groups. These relationships will require continued study of a larger patient population before more exclusive quantitative characteristics of normal and abnormal postural control characteristics can be described. However Δ E data (Fig. 3) suggests that the *difference* between EO and EC trials PSI's may be a relatively sensitive indicator or predictor of equilibrium control system abnormalities.

Conclusions

Systematic, and apparently characteristic shifts in the energy expenditure required to maintain the Romberg positions occur in both normal and abnormal human subjects. Preliminary data from human upright postural center-of-force measures suggests several potentially fruitful approaches to the study of human vestibulo-spinal and musculo-skeletal control systems in normal and abnormal subjects. Careful analysis of the stability characteristics as reflected in center-of-force recordings appears to hold considerable promise for both clinical and research studies.

Acknowledgment

The excellent technical assistance of Mr. Frank Wimberly and Mrs. Betty Feltyberger is gratefully acknowledged.

References

Alford, B.R., (Chairman), (1972): Committee on Hearing and Equilibrium. Report of Subcommittee on Equilibrium and its Measurement. Meniere's Disease: Criteria for diagnosis and evaluation of therapy for reporting. *Trans. Am. Acad. Ophth. & Otol.* **76**, 1462-1464.
Bensel, C.K. and Dzendolet, E. (1968): Power spectral density analysis of the standing sway of males. *Percept. and Psychophy.* **4**, 285-288.
Black, F.O., O'Leary, D.P., Wall, C. III and Furman, J. (1977): The vestibulo-spinal stability test (VESST): Normal limits. *Trans. Am. Acad. Ophth. & Otol.* **84**, ORL 549-560.
Black, F.O. (1977): Present vestibular status of subjects implanted with auditory prostheses. *Ann. Otol. Rhinol. and Laryngol.* **86**, Suppl. 38 : 49-56.
Black, F.O., Wall, C. III, O'Leary, D.P., Bilger, R.C. and Wolf, R.V. (1977): Galvanic disruption of vestibulospinal postural control by cochlear implant

devices. Presented to American Neurotology Society, Boston, May, 1977. Submitted.

Leroux, J., Baron, J.B., Bizzo, G., Bessineton, J.C., Gueguen, R., Noto, R. and Pacifici, M. (1973): Etude spectrale des deplacements spontanes anter-posterieurs et lateraux du centre de gravite de l'home en orthostatisme. *Agressologie.* **14** C : 57-63.

Scott, D.E. and Dzendolet, E., (1972): Quantification of sway in standing humans. *Agressologie.* **13** B : 35-40.

Delayed Vertigo

1.   Delayed vertigo

T. KAMEI

Department of Otolaryngology, Gunma University Medical School, Maebashi, Japan

Introduction

Unilateral total deafness, indistinct in both etiology and time of onset, occurs in 0.1% of the school age population (Everberg, 1960). The afflicted children do not complain of any symptoms except for unilateral hearing loss (Everberg, 1960; Nandate, 1963). Nandate (1963) suggested calling this deafness, "juvenile unilateral total deafness of unknown etiology".

The aim of this report is to introduce a new clinical aspect of this deafness. Clinical experience has indicated that recurrent true vertigo develops preferentially in various adult stages of such juvenile unilateral total deafness during or after puberty. An illustrative case is presented in detail together with pertinent clinical statistics on this delayed onset vertigo.

An illustrative case

This was a 26-year-old male, first seen in June 1971 at the age of 20 years. His chief complaint was recurrent vertigo. His initial attack of vertigo occurred at age 16. The third attack occurred 3 days prior to his first visit. All attacks were described as being of violent rotatory vertigo continuing for 2 to 3 h, and accompanied by nausea and vomiting. However, cochlear symptoms did not occur concomitantly.

The patient's anamnesis revealed that he first became aware of total deafness of the left ear, without tinnitus, at the age of 5 when he found that he was unable to hear on the telephone with his left ear. At 8 he underwent audiometry by a specialist and was diagnosed definitively. However, history of a causal disease was lacking.

Examination at age 20 revealed normal tympanic membranes, normal hearing in the right ear and total deafness in the left ear

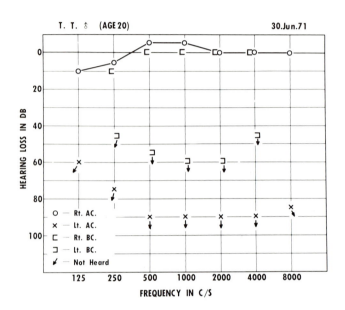

Fig. 1. Audiogram.

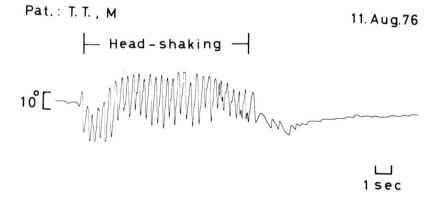

Fig. 2. Head-shaking nystagmus directed to the right (bitemporal electro-nystagmogram).

(Fig. 1). The left ear exhibited a slightly depressed response in the caloric test (stimulation with cold and warm water), while the right ear reacted normally. No abnormalities were observed with neurological tests, X-rays of the temporal bones, or electroencephalography. The Wassermann reaction was negative.

His course was followed subsequently to our initial examination. The patient complained of vertigo attacks, unaccompanied by cochlear symptoms, about 1 or 2 times per year. Spontaneous nystagmus or head-shaking nystagmus directed to the right (Fig. 2) was occasionally observed under Frenzel's glasses or by electronystagmography. Vestibular ataxia was not evident between attacks. Commencing in August 1976, the incidence of vertigo attacks increased. Since medicinal therapy lost almost all of its effectiveness, on January 14, 1977, at the age of 26, the patient was hospitalised; the afflicted ear causing vertigo was postulated to be the left one, and chorda tympanectomy was performed. No clear-cut attacks have occurred since then.

Statistical observations

During the period from April 1962 to March 1976, 89 patients with juvenile unilateral total deafness of unknown etiology were seen at the Gunma University Hospital. All patients conformed to the following four conditions: 1. Unilateral total deafness of unclear etiology and in which the onset of deafness could not be established to be other than very early in infancy; 2. Normal hearing in the other ear or, if deafness were present there also, normal hearing might be inferred to have existed in infancy; 3. Normal tympanic membranes; 4. Absence of central nervous symptoms.

Of these 89 cases of juvenile unilateral total deafness, recurrent vertigo was the chief complain of 27, or 30.3%. The age of onset ranged from 9 to 60 years. However, the majority of patients (70%) had their onset from 16 to 30 years (Table 1).

TABLE I

Age of onset of recurrent vertigo

Age	No. of cases (%)
9-15	3 (11.1%)
16-30	19 (70.4%)
31-45	4 (14.8%)
46-60	1 (3.7%)
Total	27

Although the frequency of vertigo attacks was variable, vertigo was rotatory without exception, and attacks were accompanied by nausea and vomiting. The duration of attacks was from 10 min to 24 h in 23 cases, from 1 day to 7 days in 2 cases, and of indefinite duration in 2 cases.

Vertigo attacks were actually observed in 7 patients. The type of spontaneous nystagmus during attacks was, without exception, horizontal nystagmus with rotatory components. However, there was no consistent relationship between the direction of nystagmus and the side of total deafness. Vestibular symptoms were normally not present between attacks.

Among these 27 patients with recurrent vertigo, fluctuating sensory-neural auditory disturbances were evident in the non-deaf side in 3 patients. Recruitment was present in all of them, and they were diagnosed as having Meniere's disease, transforming the ear with favorable hearing into a diseased one. In contrast, vertigo attacks in the other 24 patients were never accompanied by cochlear symptoms. However, 3 of these 24 patients exhibited mild sensory-neural deafness, not showing any fluctuation, in the side with favorable hearing. Recruitment was present in 2 of them. The onset of deafness in the originally non-deaf ear in all 6 out of the 27 patients reported here was during or after puberty.

Comment

The nature of vertigo attacks in all of the recurrent vertigo patients in this study could not be distinguished from that of Meniere's disease. This fact leads one to believe that the recurrent vertigo in these patients was labyrinthine in origin. However, except for the 3 patients diagnosed as having Meniere's disease and in which the ear with favorable hearing was the morbid one, the diseased ear responsible for vertigo could not be determined in any of the remaining 24 patients. The main reason for this was, of course, because cochlear symptoms did not accompany vertigo attacks in these patients. Another important reason was, however, the fact that caloric tests did not aid in determining the afflicted side for the following reason. Caloric tests were successful in establishing the presence of reduced response in the totally deaf side in 10 of these patients. However, it is a well-known fact that canal paresis of the totally deaf ear is frequently observed in cases of juvenile unilateral total deafness of unknown etiology (Tarkkanen and Aho, 1966). This indicates that, in patients in this study with vertigo and canal paresis of the totally deaf side, the side suffering complete hearing loss is not necessarily the morbid side causing vertigo.

Cases of vertigo similar to the recurrent vertigo in the present study have been reported recently by Nadol, Weiss and Parker (1975) and Wolfson and Leiberman (1975). The former report dealt with 12 cases of unilateral, sudden and profound sensori-neural hearing loss due to various causes. After a latency, true episodic vertigo developed in these cases. The latter report reviewed 5 cases of unilateral, severe hearing loss considered to be due to viral laby-rinthitis. It was reported that, after a period of several years, re-current episodic symptoms of Meniere's disease occurred in each case, showing no fluctuations in hearing acuity. Wolfson and Leiber-man took the view that vertigo was not accompanied by cochlear symptoms because the hearing ability of the morbid ear responsible for vertigo had already been lost in their cases.

Schuknecht (1976) offered an explanation for the pathogenesis of this vertigo: i.e. his concept of the delayed hydrops syndrome. He claimed that, regardless of the specific cause, this state may occur if the following two conditions are met: 1. the presence of a labyrinthine insult of sufficient magnitude to cause total deafness but preservation of vestibular function; and 2. the occurrence of delayed atrophy or fibrous obliteration of the endolymphatic resorptive system.

Schuknecht's concept of this delayed hydrops syndrome provides a possible explanation for the mechanism of onset in the 24 patients in this study with recurrent vertigo who had no fluctuations in cochlear symptoms.

However, we must not lose sight of the fact that, in 3 of these patients, hearing loss without any fluctuation was present in the ear with favorable hearing, and that the onset of this phenomenon was delayed, as in vertigo. Adequate consideration must also be given to the fact that there were 3 cases of Meniere's disease in the present study in which the ear with favorable hearing was the morbid one. This latter finding demonstrates that the favorable-hearing ear may be the morbid ear in certain cases of delayed onset vertigo with juvenile unilateral total deafness of unknown etiology.

References

Everberg, G., (1906): Unilateral anacusis. *Acta oto-laryng.* Suppl. **158**, 366-374.

Nadol, J.B., Jr., Weiss, A.D. and Parker, S.W. (1975): Vertigo of delayed onset after sudden deafness. *Ann. Otol.* **84**, 841-846.

Nandate, J. (1963): Juvenile unilateral total deafness of unknown etiology. *Jap. Jour. Otol.* Tokyo **66**, 281-287. (In Japanese).

Schuknecht, H.F. (1976): Pathophysiology of endolymphatic hydrops. *Arch.*

Oto-Rhino-Laryng. **212**, 253-262.

Tarkkanen, J. and Aho, J. (1966): Unilateral deafness in children. *Acta oto-laryng.* **61**, 270-278.

Wolfson, R.J. and Leiberman, A. (1975): Unilateral deafness with subsequent vertigo. *Laryngoscope* **85**, 1762-1766.

SUBJECT INDEX